Retinal Diseases: A Case-Based Approach

Retinal Diseases: A Case-Based Approach

Editor: Judi Graham

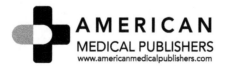

AMERICAN
MEDICAL PUBLISHERS
www.americanmedicalpublishers.com

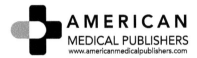

AMERICAN
MEDICAL PUBLISHERS
www.americanmedicalpublishers.com

Cataloging-in-Publication Data

Retinal diseases : a case-based approach / edited by Judi Graham.
    p. cm.
Includes bibliographical references and index.
ISBN 978-1-63927-797-1
1. Retina--Diseases. 2. Retina--Diseases--Case studies.
3. Eye--Diseases. 4. Ophthalmology. I. Graham, Judi.
RE551 .R48 2023
617.735--dc23

American Medical Publishers,
41 Flatbush Avenue,
1st Floor, New York,
NY 11217, USA

ISBN 978-1-63927-797-1 (Hardback)

Contents

Permissions

List of Contributors

Index

Preface

The retina is the light-sensitive innermost layer of tissue in the eyes of vertebrates and certain molluscs. Retinal diseases are the medical conditions affecting any part of the retina. There are many different retinal diseases and the majority of them cause visual symptoms. These may include a muted color vision, noticing flashes of light, straight lines that appear wavy, difficulty seeing in low light, etc. Some retinal conditions are more common as people develop diabetes or get older. Risk factors for these diseases can be genetic or hereditary, like retinitis pigmentosa. Fundus autofluorescence (FAF), MRI and CT, indocyanine green angiography, Amsler grid test, fluorescein angiography, ultrasound and other tests can be used to identify the location and severity of retinal diseases. The use of dietary supplements, intravitreal medicine like corticosteroid or anti-VEGF agents, and vitreoretinal surgery are some of the main modes of treatment for these diseases. This book contains some path-breaking studies on retinal diseases. It is appropriate for students seeking detailed information on these diseases as well as for experts.

This book is the end result of constructive efforts and intensive research done by experts in this field. The aim of this book is to enlighten the readers with recent information in this area of research. The information provided in this profound book would serve as a valuable reference to students and researchers in this field.

At the end, I would like to thank all the authors for devoting their precious time and providing their valuable contribution to this book. I would also like to express my gratitude to my fellow colleagues who encouraged me throughout the process.

Editor

Neuroprotective Strategies for Retinal Ganglion Cell Degeneration: Current Status and Challenges Ahead

Raquel Boia [1,2], Noelia Ruzafa [3], Inês Dinis Aires [1,2], Xandra Pereiro [3],
António Francisco Ambrósio [1,2,4], Elena Vecino [3] and Ana Raquel Santiago [1,2,4,*]

1   Coimbra Institute for Clinical and Biomedical Research (iCBR), Faculty of Medicine, University of Coimbra,
    3000-548 Coimbra, Portugal; raquelfboia@gmail.com (R.B.); inesaires9@gmail.com (I.D.A.);
    afambrosio@fmed.uc.pt (A.F.A.)
2   Center for Innovative Biomedicine and Biotechnology (CIBB), University of Coimbra,
    3000-548 Coimbra, Portugal
3   Department of Cell Biology and Histology, University of the Basque Country UPV/EHU,
    48940 Leioa, Vizcaya, Spain; noelia.ruzafa@ehu.eus (N.R.); xandra.pereiro@gmail.com (X.P.);
    elena.vecino@ehu.eus (E.V.)
4   Association for Innovation and Biomedical Research on Light and Image (AIBILI),
    3000-548 Coimbra, Portugal
*   Correspondence: asantiago@fmed.uc.pt;

Abstract: The retinal ganglion cells (RGCs) are the output cells of the retina into the brain. In mammals, these cells are not able to regenerate their axons after optic nerve injury, leaving the patients with optic neuropathies with permanent visual loss. An effective RGCs-directed therapy could provide a beneficial effect to prevent the progression of the disease. Axonal injury leads to the functional loss of RGCs and subsequently induces neuronal death, and axonal regeneration would be essential to restore the neuronal connectivity, and to reestablish the function of the visual system. The manipulation of several intrinsic and extrinsic factors has been proposed in order to stimulate axonal regeneration and functional repairing of axonal connections in the visual pathway. However, there is a missing point in the process since, until now, there is no therapeutic strategy directed to promote axonal regeneration of RGCs as a therapeutic approach for optic neuropathies.

Keywords: retinal ganglion cells; neurodegeneration; axonal regeneration; neuroprotection; optic neuropathies

1. Introduction

The retina is part of the central nervous system (CNS) and is constituted by neurons, glial cells and blood vessels [1]. The neuronal component of the retina is composed by six types of neurons: photoreceptors (rods and cones), bipolar cells, horizontal cells, amacrine cells and retinal ganglion cells (RGCs). Photoreceptors, whose nuclei is located in the outer nuclear layer (ONL), respond to light and make synapses with second-order neurons. The cell bodies of retinal interneurons (horizontal, bipolar and amacrine cells) are located predominately in the inner nuclear layer (INL) and modify and relay the visual information from the photoreceptors to the RGCs that are located in the innermost layer of the retina, the ganglion cell layer (GCL) (Figure 1). RGCs are the output cells of the retina that convey the visual signals to the brain visual targets. The axons of RGCs run initially in the nerve fiber layer (NFL) and converge into the optic disc, cross the lamina cribrosa at the optic nerve head (ONH), and form the optic nerve (Figure 1) [1].

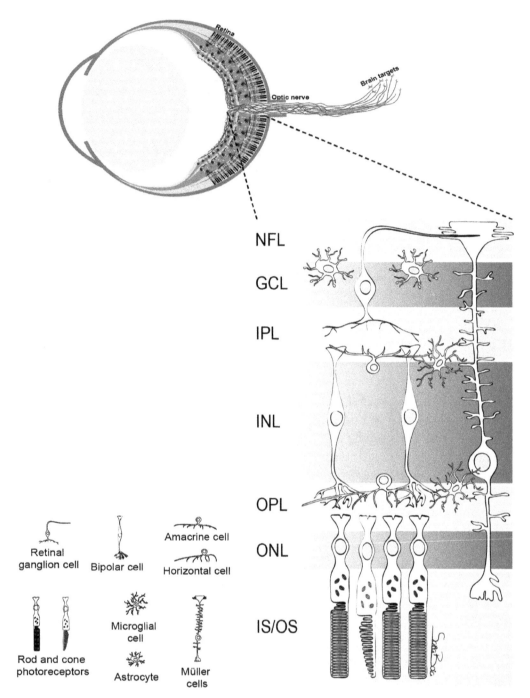

Figure 1. Schematic representation of the neural sensory retina, depicting the organization of the cells into nuclear and plexiform layers. The nuclei of photoreceptors, rods and cones, are located in the outer nuclear layer (ONL) and nuclei of interneurons, amacrine, bipolar and horizontal cells, are located predominately in the inner nuclear layer (INL). The cell bodies of RGCs are in the ganglion cell layer (GCL), and their axons run in the nerve fiber layer (NFL). There are two types of macroglia: Müller cells that span vertically the entire retina and astrocytes that are present in the GCL. Microglial cells are localized predominantly in the inner retina and in the outer plexiform layer (OPL). IPL: inner plexiform layer; IS/OS: inner and outer segments of photoreceptors.

Optic neuropathies comprise a group of ocular diseases, like glaucoma (the most common), anterior ischemic optic neuropathy and retinal ischemia, in which RGCs are the main affected cells [2]. Blindness secondary to optic neuropathies is irreversible since RGCs lack the capacity for self-renewal and have a limited ability for self-repair [3]. The exact mechanism that leads to RGC death and degeneration is still unknown, but axonal injury has been proposed as an early event that culminates in apoptotic death of RGCs [4]. This paper reviews the events that contribute to axonal degeneration and death of RGCs and also the neuroprotective strategies with potential to circumvent this problem.

2. Obstacles to RGC Survival and Regeneration upon Injury: Insights from Development to Disease Models

During development, RGCs extend their axons to synapse in target areas of the brain (reviewed in [5]). After birth, there is a peak in cell death that in rodents occurs between postnatal days 2 and 5 (PND 2-5), ensuring that only cells that reached their targets survive (reviewed in [6]). The ability of RGCs to extend their axons decreases with age and the capacity to regenerate their axons is lost early in development [7]. In fact, cultures of RGCs (Figure 2) prepared at both embryonic day 20 (ED 20) or PND 8 extend their axons with similar calibers; however, after 3 days in culture, ED 20 RGCs extend their axons further and faster than cells isolated at PND 8. The exposure of these cells to conditioned media of superior colliculus cells further potentiates axonal growth of ED 20 RGCs without interfering with PND 8 RGCs, demonstrating that the loss of ability of RGCs axon growth is mediated by retinal maturation [7]. The reason behind the lost in the intrinsic ability of RGCs to regenerate upon injury has been extensively explored. Several players, including cyclic adenosine monophosphate (cAMP), phosphatase and tensin homologue (PTEN)/mammalian target of rapamycin (mTOR) and Krüppel-like family (KLF) transcript factors are implicated in the transition from the rapid axon growth of immature neurons into the poor axon growth of mature neurons in the CNS.

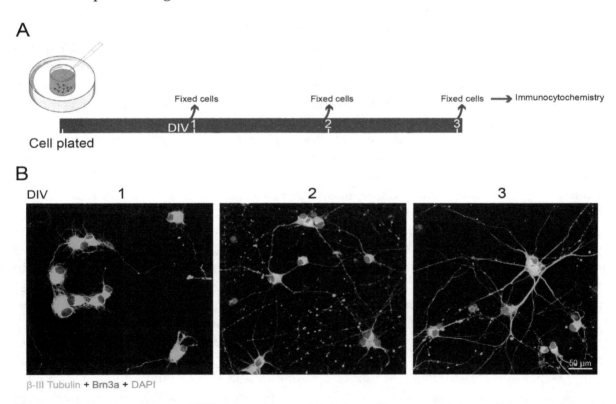

Figure 2. Neurite growth of RGCs in culture. (**A**) Schematic representation of the experimental design. Retinas were dissected from Wistar rats at PND 5 and nearly pure RGC cultures (~93% purity assessed with anti-RBPMS antibody; Abcam, Cat. # ab194213, 1:500) were obtained by sequential immunopanning, as previously described [8,9]. RGCs were cultured for 1 day in vitro (DIV1), DIV2 and DIV3, followed by fixation in paraformaldehyde and processed for immunocytochemistry. (**B**) RGCs were identified by immunolabeling for Brn3a (red, Millipore, Cat. # MAB1585, 1:500), a transcription factor expressed only by these cells in the retina. The neurites, labelled with an antibody that recognizes β-tubulin III (green, BioLegend, Cat. # 802001; 1:1000), extended during the period in culture. Nuclei were stained with DAPI (blue).

cAMP plays an important role in neuronal survival and axon growth and guidance [10]. For example, in the goldfish, the injection of an analogue of cAMP is able to enhance axonal regeneration upon optic nerve crush (ONC) [11]. Moreover, PTEN/mTOR pathway has been implicated in the failure of RGCs axons to regenerate. The deletion of PTEN in RGCs leads to the activation of phosphoinositide 3-kinases (PI3K)/mTOR pathway, increases neuronal survival and promotes robust axon regeneration after optic nerve injury [12,13]. Moreover, it has been reported a coordinated regulation of neurite growth by KLF transcription factors. During development, at least two growth-enhancing KLFs (KLF6 and 7) are down-regulated, and at least two growth-suppressive KLFs (KLF4 and 9) are upregulated [14]. The profile of gene expression from ED 17 through PND 21 RGCs identified the zinc finger transcription factor KLF4 as the most effective suppressor of neurite outgrowth [14]. Indeed, the KLF4 overexpression in ED 20 RGCs reduces their ability to extend axons and, on the other hand, KLF4 knockout enhances axon growth ability by PND 12 RGCs [14]. This decline in the ability of postnatal RGCs to grow axons is associated with KLF-regulated changes in axonal growth cone morphology and protrusive dynamics [15]. The knockout of KLF4 during development increases the regenerative potential of RGCs upon ONC at adulthood [14]. Amacrine cells have been implicated in the process of losing intrinsic growth capability of RGCs [7]. In fact, zinc (Zn^{2+}) increases in amacrine cell processes upon optic nerve injury and is transferred to RGCs via vesicular release [16]. The chelation of Zn^{2+} improves cell survival and axon regeneration [16], raising the possibility that the dysregulation of mobile Zn^{2+} levels is responsible for the loss of axonal growth.

Other transcription factors have been studied for their role in axon growth and regeneration (reviewed in [17]). The tumor suppressor p53 plays a central role in the regulation apoptosis in RGCs. The overstimulation of N-methyl-D-aspartate (NMDA) receptor activates a p53-dependent pathway of cell death [18]. The involvement of p53 in neurite outgrowth and axon regeneration has been explored in CNS injury [19]. However, the deletion of p53 in RGCs fails to promote axonal regeneration, despite the increase in RGC survival upon ONC [12], confirming the hypothesis that inducing neuronal survival is not enough to allow axonal regeneration. The activation of p53 has been implicated in the transcription of several factors responsible for apoptosis, as pro-apoptotic BAX or anti-apoptotic Bcl-2 proteins (reviewed in [20]). It was shown that there is an up-regulation of BAX expression after ONC injury [21], as well as after ischemic retinal damage [22]. BAX deficiency completely prevents RGCs death in a glaucoma animal model [23]. However, deficient BAX expression in not sufficient to hinder axonal degeneration even without RGC death, reinforcing the idea that axon degeneration is not a consequence of RGC death [23]. A down-regulation of the anti-apoptotic protein Bcl-2 was observed in RGCs in the GCL when the onset of regenerative failure of RGCs occurs [24]. Elevating the expression of Bcl-2 maintains neuronal survival even after withdrawing of all trophic factors in cultures of RGCs [3]. However, Bcl-2-overexpressing RGCs fail to elaborate axons or dendrites, unless axon growth-inducing signals are present, clearly demonstrating that axon growth is not a default function of a surviving neuron, but must be specifically signaled [3]. These evidences clearly demonstrate that manipulation of some intrinsic factors could have beneficial effects, not only in the prevention of RGC death but also in promoting axon regeneration upon injury. In the peripheral nervous system (PNS) the injured neurons are able to regenerate, which does not happen in the CNS. However, the observation that CNS neurons, including RGCs, regrow into peripheral nerve grafts [25,26], confirms the possibility that extrinsic factors also have a preponderant role in limiting axonal repair.

Glial scar and myelin that compose the environment of optic nerve particularly at the site of injury inhibit the axonal regeneration (reviewed in [27]). Semaphorin-3 is expressed in the core of the glial scar upon CNS injury [28] and limits regenerating neurons crossing semaphorin-3A (Sema3A)-expressing regions [29]. This raises the hypothesis that semaphorins may have a potential role in the glia inhibiting effect of axonal regeneration. Semaphorins have an important function in neuronal polarity and axonal guidance during RGC development or injury [30]. Sema3A is one of the extracellular factors that is involved in regulating RGC polarity [31,32]. At PND 14, when all RGCs axons reached their targets [33],

Sema3A is elevated [34], and increased expression of Sema3A results in strong axonal inhibition in optic nerve injury model [35]. In line with these findings and corroborating the role of semaphorin in axonal growth, the intravitreous injection of antibodies against the Sema3A-derived peptide to neutralize the function of Sema3A, caused a marked inhibition of RGC loss in an animal model of complete axotomy of the rat optic nerve [36]. Sema5A is a semaphorin produced by oligodendrocytes that also contributes to the inhibitory environment of the injured optic nerve, heralded by the observation that RGC axonal growth increases when blocking Sema5A [37]. It has been demonstrated that myelin proteins inhibit axonal regeneration in adult neurons. Following an insult, nonspecific T cells accumulate at the lesion site on optic nerve [38,39]. Immunization with T cells specifically against myelin proteins (copolymer-1, Cop-1) reduces the post-traumatic neuronal loss after ONC [38,39]. Moreover, it has been shown to be an effective therapy for glutamate-induced toxicity in mice and in a rat model of chronically high intraocular pressure (IOP) [40]. Although these studies were only focused on the survival of RGCs, some years after the authors demonstrated that Cop-1 treatment confer functional protection to RGCs [41]. Other studies led to the identification of several myelin-associated inhibitors of axon growth. Nogo-A is one of the most potent oligodendrocyte-derived inhibitors for axonal regrowth in the injured adult CNS [42,43] that is also expressed by RGCs [44]. In cases of optic nerve injury Nogo-A is upregulated [45], although the overexpression or down-regulation of Nogo-A does not impact the survival of injured RGCs. However, the neuronal knockout of Nogo-A diminishes the axonal growth response, demonstrating a role for Nogo-A in RGCs growth after injury [45]. On the other hand, axonal sprouting is increased in the optic nerves of oligodendrocyte-specific Nogo-A knockout mice [46], demonstrating that the inactivation of Nogo-A in oligodendrocytes appears to be a good strategy to promote axonal regeneration. Moreover, it was reported that neutralizing Nogo-A has beneficial effects on visual recovery and plasticity after retinal injury [47]. Moreover, myelin-associated glycoprotein (MAG) is a component of the myelin-derived inhibition of nerve regeneration [48]. It seems that a possible mechanism underlying synapse degeneration and RGCs death in glaucoma is mediated by Nogo-A [49]. The antagonism of Nogo receptor (NgR) reduces RGCs loss and attenuates synaptic degeneration [50] and the knockout of NgR is effective in enhancing axonal regeneration after ONC [51].

The failure to regenerate has also been attributed to an environment poor in growth-promoting trophic factors. In fact, the importance of trophic factors in promoting viability and axonal regeneration of RGCs has long been recognized [51]. A great variety of neurotrophins were found to induce axon growth, which include nerve growth factor (NGF), brain-derived neurotrophic factor (BDNF) and ciliary neurotrophic factor (CNTF). BDNF plays an important role in RGCs neuroprotection since the levels of BDNF are increased in response to injury [52,53]. BDNF is also highly expressed in the superior colliculus [54,55] and it is retrogradely transported to the retina. However, displaced amacrine cells in the GCL are the main source of BDNF to RGCs [56]. The application of BDNF to the superior colliculus reduces RGC death during development [57]. Moreover, several studies demonstrated that administration of BDNF into the eye increases the survival of RGCs upon injury, and ameliorate their function [58–64].

The survival of RGCs is increased by co-administration of BDNF and CNTF soon after optic nerve injury [65]. Moreover, RGCs extend their axons in response to BDNF and CNTF, but both together induce more axon growth than either alone [3], raising the hypothesis that different factors may be responsible for different facets of axon growth. However, neurotrophins fail to induce axon growth alone. For instance, RGCs fail to survive in the presence of such trophic factors as BDNF or CNTF unless their cAMP levels are elevated [66]. CNTF overexpression promotes long-term survival and regeneration of injured adult RGCs [67]. It was described that exogenously applied CNTF stimulates RGCs partially indirectly via a mechanism that depends on astrocyte-derived CNTF [68]. The NGF has also an important role in promoting RGCs survival, being the Schwann cells the main source of this factor [69]. Intraocular injection of NGF has been previously shown to promote RGC survival [70].

Studying the mechanisms of glaucomatous damage has been a great opportunity to unravel the signaling pathways involved in RGC axonal degeneration and growth. Elevated IOP is the main risk factor of glaucoma and, together with other factors, it has been implicated in RGC degeneration and death [71]. Several in vitro models have been developed [72] and allowed the demonstration that there are pressure-dependent changes in the length of axons and neurites of RGCs [73]. When cultures of RGCs are challenged with elevated pressure there is a severe impact in axon length and in the total neurite length, with a weakened neurite extension (Figure 3), without interfering with cell body area [73]. In glaucoma, the increased IOP perturbs anterograde and retrograde axonal transports that lead to deprivation of RGCs of neurotrophic factors produced by brain targets [74]. In fact, the retrograde transport of BDNF is impaired after IOP elevation, and this may contribute to RGC loss [75,76].

Recently, it was reported that intravitreal injections of BDNF leads to an increase in the levels of synaptic proteins between RGCs and bipolar cells in the IPL, meaning that this could have a beneficial effect in the function of RGCs [77].

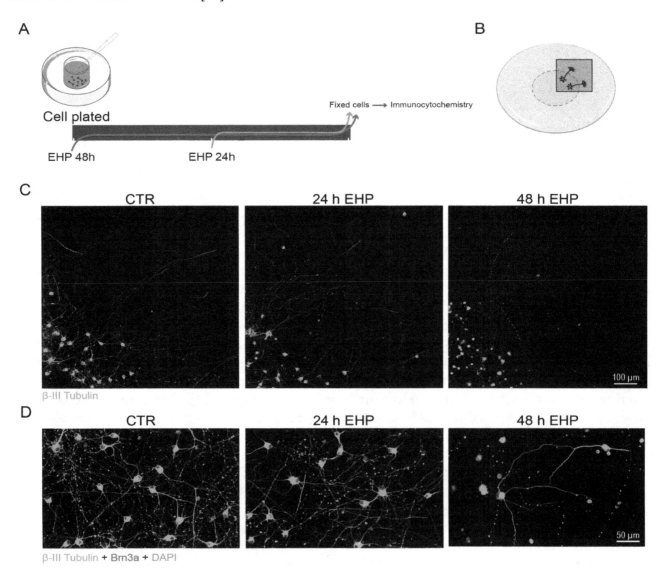

Figure 3. Elevated hydrostatic pressure (EHP) impacts neurite growth of RGCs. (**A**) Schematic representation of the experimental design. RGCs were purified from Wistar rats at PND 5 by sequential

immunopanning, as previously described [8,9] and were cultured for DIV2. RGCs were challenged with EHP (+70 mmHg above atmospheric pressure) [78,79]) for 24 h and 48 h and then processed for immunocytochemistry as described in the legend of Figure 2. (**C**) RGCs were plated in a coverslip with a cloning cylinder and neurite extension was observed beyond the limit established by the cylinder (**B**, grey dashed circle). Exposure to EHP decreased the length of the neurites when compared with the control (CTR) condition (normal pressure). (**D**) Higher magnification. This effect on the neurites of RGCs is dependent on the duration of the exposure to EHP.

3. Potential Therapeutic Targets Aiming RGC Neuroprotection

Several therapeutic strategies have been proposed in order to protect RGCs and restore visual function (Figure 4).

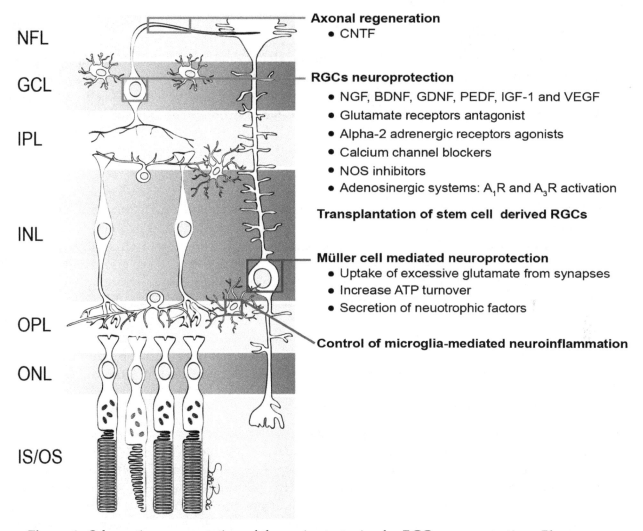

Figure 4. Schematic representation of the main strategies for RGC neuroprotection. Blue squares represent the therapies directed to RGCs and red squares represents the undirected therapies that culminates in RGCs neuroprotection.

3.1. Neuroprotective Therapies

3.1.1. Neurotrophic Factors

Neurotrophic factors are a family of growth factors that regulate the survival, development and differentiation of neurons. Neurotrophic factors generally include the neurotrophin family: NGF, BDNF, neurotrophin-3 (NT-3) and neurotrophin-4/5 (NT-4/5); the glial cell-line derived neurotrophic factor (GDNF) family: GDNF, neurturin (NRTN), artemin (ARTN), and persephin (PSPN); and CNTF [80,81].

It was reported that most of these neurotrophic factors, which can be produced by glial cells, increase RGC survival in different experimental models of injury [53,82–88]. Neurotrophic factors bind to different receptors and transduce diverse intracellular signals. Usually, neurotrophic factors bind to the high affinity receptor tyrosine kinase (Trk family) that promote cell survival. For instance, NGF binds to TrkA, BDNF and NT-4 to TrkB, and NT-3 binds to TrkC. However, they can also bind to the low affinity neurotrophin receptor p75 (p75NTR) and induce programmed cell death. These opposing effects of neurotrophic factors are important for regulating RGCs development [80,81]. The distribution of neurotrophic factors and their receptors in the mammalian retina has been studied in detail in physiology as well as in pathological conditions [52,53]. Of interest, especially when using in vitro models to study these mechanisms, the expression of neurotrophic factors and their receptors is preserved in glial cells and in RGCs even when in culture for 6 days [86] and the factors secreted by Müller cells offer protection to cultured RGCs [89].

Nerve Growth Factor (NGF)

NGF is an important growth factor affecting the survival of nerve cells and their deprivation can lead to apoptosis [90,91]. NGF is produced and utilized by RGCs [92] and protects these cells after injury [93–95]. Furthermore, NGF treatments reduced the progressive loss of RGCs in a glaucoma model [93]. In addition, in patients with glaucoma, NGF eye drops resulted in an improvement of the INL function, neural conduction, visual field, optic nerve function, contrast sensitivity, and visual acuity [96]. However, further studies are required to confirm the therapeutic efficacy of NGF.

Brain-Derived Neurotrophic Factor (BDNF)

BDNF is widely expressed throughout the CNS. RGCs express BDNF and its high affinity receptor TrkB [97]. As mentioned above, it is a powerful neuroprotective agent that promotes the survival and regrowth of RGCs [61,62,98]. The exposure to NMDA induces an increase in BDNF expression in RGCs in the first hours, suggesting that it is an endogenous neuroprotective response of RGCs. However, this effect is not sustained over time, maybe because the cells cannot maintain the synthesis of BDNF or because the activation of the apoptotic mechanism inhibits BDNF synthesis [52,84]. It has been speculated that the therapeutic properties of different neuroprotective agents in promoting RGC survival are related to the induction of retinal BDNF expression [99,100]. Consistently, BDNF levels are reduced in the serum and tears of glaucoma patients, suggesting that deficits in this neurotrophin may participate in RGC death in glaucoma and that BDNF may be a biomarker for glaucoma [101,102].

Glial Cell Line-Derived Neurotrophic Factor (GDNF)

GDNF is secreted by glial cells and binds to the GDNF-α receptor and to the receptor tyrosine kinase in RGCs [103]. GDNF promotes the survival of RGCs after injury [104–106]. Moreover, GDNF treatments, specifically intravitreal injection of microspheres containing GDNF, protect RGCs in glaucoma animal models [107,108]. This neuroprotective property of GDNF may be orchestrated by Müller cells. GDNF upregulates the glutamate/aspartate transporter (GLAST) in Müller cells enhancing glutamate uptake that may indirectly protect RGCs [109]. Another possible mechanism of action could be through osteopontin since activation of Müller cells by GDNF was shown to induce the secretion of osteopontin [110]. Thus, GDNF holds strong therapeutic potential for retinal neurodegenerative diseases.

Ciliary Neurotrophic Factor (CNTF)

CNTF belongs to the interleukin-6 (IL-6) family of cytokines, binds to CNTF receptors (CNTFR) and exerts robust neuroprotection in neurons [81,111]. In the retina, CNTF is expressed by various cell types, particularly by Müller cells [112]. Its neuroprotective effects are mediated especially by these glial cells that directly respond to CNTF by releasing other neurotrophic factors such as basic fibroblast growth factor (bFGF) [113]. The neurotrophic properties of CNTF were tested in several animal models of glaucoma and in ischemic optic neuropathy [60,114–116]. CNTF is also capable of stimulating axonal regeneration [117], which may be mediated by astrocytes [118]. Notably, the concentration of CNTF in the aqueous humor, lacrimal fluid and blood serum is decreased in patients with glaucoma [119]. The results of CNTF in neuroprotection and regeneration suggest a potential for clinical use; however, the pharmacology and administration of CNTF must be optimized.

Other Trophic Factors

Other trophic factors have been described to promote RGCs survival. Pigment epithelium derived factor (PEDF) reduces RGC loss in a mouse model of glaucoma [120] and insulin-like growth factor-1 (IGF-1) also protects RGCs from different injuries [121,122]. Despite the role of vascular endothelial growth factor A (VEGF-A) in neovascularization, VEGF is also a neuronal trophic factor that may play a role in RGC neuroprotection. Indeed, it reduces RGC apoptosis in models of glaucoma and anti-VEGF therapies exacerbate neuronal cell death [123–126].

3.1.2. Glutamate Receptors Antagonists

Despite being the major excitatory neurotransmitter in the retina and involved in the vertical pathway of information [1], excessive glutamate levels have detrimental effects on RGCs [127], a term described as glutamate excitotoxicity [128], due to the activation of a complex apoptotic cascades [128,129]. The fact that intraocular glutamate levels are increased in glaucoma patients [130,131] raised the hypothesis that the blockade of glutamate receptors could be a valuable strategy for RGC neuroprotection, at least for glaucoma. MK801 (dizocilpine maleate) is a potent glutamate receptor antagonist and is a neuroprotective agent of RGCs [132,133], although it could also be neurotoxic [134]. In preclinical studies memantine, a NMDA receptor antagonist, affords robust neuroprotection of RGCs against glutamate toxicity [129,135]. However, memantine had limited efficacy in glaucoma patients [136,137]. More studies are required to clearly evaluate these and other glutamate antagonists as effective neuroprotective therapies for RGCs.

3.1.3. Alpha-2 Adrenergic Receptors Agonists

The presence of alpha-adrenergic receptors in the RGCs has been demonstrated [138]. Additionally, the activation of alpha-2 adrenergic receptors by agonists such as brimonidine has been shown to enhance survival of RGCs after different types of injuries, namely in glaucoma [138–141], ONC [142] and ischemia [143]. Brimonidine can confer protection by reducing the accumulation of extracellular glutamate and by blocking NMDA receptors, independently of the IOP-lowering mechanisms [139,140,142,144]. Several pre-clinical and clinical studies were conducted [139,145–148] to assess the protective properties of brimonidine.

3.1.4. Calcium Channel Blockers

Calcium channel blockers may protect RGCs by preventing cell death mediated by calcium influx secondary to NMDA receptor overactivation and local ischemia [149,150]. Different calcium channel blockers attenuate injury to RGCs [151] and increase the viability of immunopurified RGCs cultures [152]. A randomized clinical trial analyzed the effects of the treatment with nilvadipine, a calcium channel blocker, on visual field performance and ocular circulation in patients with open-angle glaucoma. Nilvadipine slowed visual field progression, maintained the optic disc rim, and increased the posterior choroidal circulation [153]. Although these findings look promising, more studies on the distribution and pharmacology of the several types of calcium channels could help clarifying their therapeutic value [154].

3.1.5. Antioxidants

Oxidative stress occurs when concentrations of reactive oxygen species (ROS) rise above physiological range, and it has been indicated as a potential cause of glaucomatous neurodegeneration [155]. Thus, inhibition of ROS may enhance RGC survival [156–158]. Coenzyme Q10, cofactor of the electron transport chain that inhibits the generation of ROS, protects retinal neurons from damage [159–161]. Moreover, improvement in visual acuity has also been reported in patients with optic neuropathy after treatment with Q10 [162].

Glutathione (GSH) is decreased in glaucoma patients, suggesting a general compromise of the antioxidative defense [163]. The treatment with vitamin E can ameliorate the decrease in the levels of retinal GSH [164,165]. Consequently, vitamin E-deficient diet is associated with an increase of RGC death related to an increase in lipid peroxidation [166]. Moreover, methane increases the activity of several antioxidant enzymes like superoxide dismutase (SOD), catalase (CAT), glutathione peroxidase (GPx), and the expression of anti-apoptotic genes, which culminate in reduced RGC loss [167]. Overexpression of frataxin induces up-regulation of antioxidant enzymes (such as SOD2, CAT, GPx) and increases RGC survival [168]. Other agents, like crocin, increase the levels of GSH and SOD activity, decreasing ROS and promoting RGC survival [169]. Generally, an increase of SOD and alpha-lipoic acid protects RGCs against oxidative stress damage [170,171]. Therefore, evidence demonstrate that antioxidants may be beneficial for neuroprotection of RGCs [148], but further studies are required to investigate their full potential.

3.1.6. Nitric Oxide Synthase Inhibitors

The levels of nitric oxide (NO) are increased in experimental glaucoma, and evidence shows that NO can result in RGCs degeneration [172–175]. Moreover, increased expression of nitric oxide synthase (NOS) was detected in different models of RGCs injury [175–177]. Additionally, in glaucoma patients the astrocytes of ONH become reactive and may produce high amounts of NO causing neurotoxicity to the axons of RGCs [178,179]. This has raised the hypothesis that the inhibition of NOS, in particular inducible NOS (iNOS), could be neuroprotective by delaying RGCs degeneration [180,181]. However, other studies did not identify a relationship between iNOS and RGCs neurodegeneration [182,183]. More studies are necessary to clarify the role of NOS inhibitors in RGCs protection, helping to clarify this "apparent" discrepancy.

3.1.7. Adenosinergic System

Adenosine can exert both neuroprotective and neurodegenerative actions acting through four types of receptors: A_1, A_{2A}, A_{2B} and A_3. Adenosine acting on adenosine A_1 receptor (A_1R) protects cultured retinal neurons from NMDA-induced cell death [184] by blocking calcium channels in RGCs [185], suggesting that agents directed to A_1R could be a good therapeutic strategy. Indeed, the activation of A_1R is neuroprotective against injury induced by ischemia-reperfusion [186], and N(6)-cyclohexyl-adenosine (CHA), an agonist of A_1R, increases RGCs survival mediating the trophic effect of IL-6 [187]. In fact, IL-6 is an interesting cytokine that has been demonstrated to promote RGCs survival [188,189], probably by the modulation of BDNF synthesis [190]. Adenosine A_3 receptor (A_3R) has also been evaluated as a therapeutic target [191]. RGCs are endowed with A_3R [192], and its activation protects RGCs from cell death induced by P2X7 receptor agonist [193,194], possibly by limiting the rise in intracellular calcium [195]. Activation of A_3R promotes RGCs neurite outgrowth and neurite regeneration in an animal model of ONC [196]. Moreover, the activation of A_3R was also demonstrated to afford protection to the retina from excitotoxic-induced cell death, retinal ischemia-reperfusion injury and damage induced by partial optic nerve transection [197].

3.2. Cell-Based Therapies

Beyond neuroprotection, cell replacement may have potential as a strategy for the treatment of optic neuropathies. Replacing the diseased or degenerated cells by stem cell-derived RGCs should provide effective therapeutic treatment in the near future. However, complex circuitry in the retina makes cell replacement challenging and difficult for functional repair [198].

Stem cells are functionally undifferentiated and immature cells of a complex nature. These cells are capable of differentiating into different cell types, indicating that they have the potential to repair tissue and restore function after lesion. Due to this potential, it is believed that stem cells may be able to either replace or repair damaged cells in the retina [199–201].

In the past decade, the capacity to generate retinal cells from pluripotent stem cells using three-dimensional organoid cultures has become well established [202–204]. However, while corneal transplantation is commonly performed with excellent results, many obstacles must be surpassed before retinal transplants can become clinically useful. The major problems are the production of appropriate transplants, functional integration in situ and the survival of the stem cell-derived RGCs.

Various types of stem cells were assessed for retinal differentiation and transplantation such as human embryonic stem cells, induced pluripotent stem cells, isolated retinal stem cells and also from adult stem cells, in particular neural stem cells, mesenchymal stem cells (MSCs) derived from bone marrow, adipose tissues and dental pulp [205].

Various methods to assess the ability of RGCs to survive and integrate with host tissue have been proposed [206,207]. Transplanted RGCs by intravitreal injection acquired the normal morphology of endogenous RGCs, responded to light, and established synaptic contacts with the lateral geniculate nucleus and the superior colliculus [208–210]. These examples show that RGC transplantation is possible, although not very efficient, but further studies will certainly guarantee that transplantation of cells to the retina may become a strategy.

MSCs have been widely demonstrated to afford neuroprotective, immunomodulatory and antioxidant properties, making them a promising strategy for the treatment of neurodegenerative diseases. These cells secrete neurotrophic factors like NGF accelerating the survival of neural cells [211]. The protective properties of MSCs have also been also documented in an animal model of glaucoma and in an animal model of optic nerve injury [212,213]. The protective properties of MSCs extend beyond the cells. Recently, the extracellular vesicles derived by these cells were demonstrated to promote RGCs neuroprotection in rodent models of glaucoma [213,214].

3.3. Glia-Mediated Neuroprotection

The term neuroinflammation comprises a number of events that affects the CNS. In other words, every time the CNS is faced with infectious agents, traumatic injuries or other unknown elements that might cause a disruption of its homeostasis, it will protect itself by the initiation of inflammatory signaling cascades in order to eliminate the pathological factor [215]. Although the main actors in this scenario are astrocytes and microglia [216,217], in the retina, Müller cells can also be activated and get involved in the production of inflammatory cytokines and chemokines, which maintain and enhance the inflammatory condition participating in the progression of several diseases.

Microglial cells have long been recognized as crucial players in the maintenance of retinal homeostasis. During development, microglial cells are involved in synaptic pruning and in retinal wiring [218] and throughout the life of the organism these cells screen the parenchyma searching for alterations in the environment, including cell interactions and external threats [219,220]. In pathological conditions, microglia have been shown to interfere with neural and glial cell function contributing to retinal degeneration and RGC loss [221]. Indeed, several reports show that abnormally responsive microglia can directly reduce the survival of RGCs. For example, even though microglial cells are not endowed with NMDA receptors, upon intravitreal NMDA injection, these cells detect the alterations in calcium and adenosine triphosphate (ATP) signaling in other retinal cells, including RGCs, by increasing the inflammatory response [222]. Interestingly, the report that isolated RGCs are resistant to

NMDA excitotoxicity [223], while in the retina NMDA exposure leads to RGCs degeneration triggered by increased production of tumor necrosis factor (TNF) and abnormal behavior of microglial cells [222] is another evidence of the role of microglial cells shaping RGCs degeneration.

The pivotal role of microglia in RGCs degeneration has been mostly explored in glaucoma. Historically, reactive microglial cells have been associated with human glaucomatous ONH lesion, mainly by their spatial distribution along the damaged fibers and expression of activation markers as well as pro-inflammatory mediators [224,225]. Indeed, enlarged reactive microglial cells were found in the retina of human post-mortem donors with glaucoma manifestations [224]. Nevertheless, this finding may raise the question of whether microgliosis might be a cause or a consequence of the retinal degeneration. This question was very elegantly addressed using the DBA/2J mouse model of glaucoma when microglia activation in the ONH was visualized before the detection of RGC loss [226,227]. Furthermore, microglial cell response initiates in the unmyelinated region of the ONH and further develops along the retina, correlating with the progression of the neurodegenerative process [227]. In accordance with these findings, microglia reactivity was shown to impact RGCs survival in different experimental models of glaucoma [78,79,228]. Altered ROS signalling has been associated with glaucomatous damage both in animal models and in human glaucoma [179,229], and reactive microglial cells may be the main cellular source [79]. In a model of induced ocular hypertension (OHT), microglia were shown to be reactive as detected by the increased expression of translocator protein (TSPO), major histocompatibility complex class II (MHC-II) and pro-inflammatory mediators in the retina early after OHT induction [230]. Even when exposed to elevated hydrostatic pressure (EHP) an in vitro model of elevated IOP, microglia become reactive, release pro-inflammatory mediators and increase ATP and adenosine secretion [78,231]. Alterations in ATP levels are determinant to propagate microglial cell response by acting as a "call for action" [232]. In addition, adenosine mainly acting through the activation of A_{2A} receptor ($A_{2A}R$) may propel microglia deleterious response overtime [233]. The $A_{2A}R$ has been described to control microglia reactivity. Its expression increases in microglia in models of glaucoma [78,79], and $A_{2A}R$ antagonists were shown to confer protection to retinal neurons, including RGCs, through the control of microglia reactivity [78,79,228]. Caffeine, a non-selective adenosine antagonist, also protects RGCs by hampering microglial cell response and controlling the neuroinflammatory environment in models of transient retinal ischemia and ocular hypertension [230,234,235]. KW6002, another $A_{2A}R$ antagonist with good oral bioavailability, confers protection to the retina, including RGCs, through the control of microglia-mediated neuroinflammation [234]. Recently, the potential of $A_{2A}R$ antagonists was further confirmed as a strategy for the human retina [78]. By using human retinal organotypic cultures, the $A_{2A}R$ antagonist was able to reduce microglia alterations and the production of ROS, suggesting that microglia-mediated inflammation in the human retina also involves $A_{2A}R$ [78]. The neutralization of the actions of TNF and interleukin-1β (IL-1β) in the retinal organotypic cultures was able to prevent the loss of RGCs triggered by EHP, reinforcing the role of retinal inflammation in neurodegeneration in glaucoma [79]. The central role of microglia causing RGCs loss was further demonstrated with a strategy to deplete microglia from primary retinal cultures following exposure to EHP [78]. In such case, the effect of EHP on cell death was abrogated, showing that microglia are indeed the main triggers and propellants of neuroinflammation-mediated glaucomatous damage [78].

The secretion of TNF by microglial cells was shown to contribute to RGC degeneration as its receptor is highly increased in glaucoma in RGCs, astrocytes, microglia and Müller cells, triggering a cascade of events that culminates in RGC demise [236,237]. Indeed, simple experiments neutralizing the actions of TNF were able to restore axon function and decrease the loss of RGCs in glaucoma [238].

Recently it has been shown that chronic OHT promotes the expression of P2X7 receptor in the retina leading to the activation of NLRP3 (NOD-, LRR- and pyrin domain-containing protein 3) inflammasome [239]. The activation of P2X7R-dependent NLRP3 inflammasome in microglia increases the production of pro-inflammatory cytokines and caspase activation that leads to RGC death [239]. In accordance with the role of purine receptors in microglia reactivity, the inhibition of P2X7 receptor in microglial cells confers protection to RGCs in vitro upon exposure to conditioned media from microglia exposed to BzATP by decreasing NLRP3 inflammasome activation [239]. Furthermore, in a model of OHT the oral administration of a saffron extract reduced retinal microglia inflammation and the loss of RGCs, while decreasing the expression of the adenosine diphosphate P2Y12 receptor [240].

Microglial cells also modulate retinal cell function by expressing complement molecules. In fact, in human and experimental glaucoma the expression of complement factors is increased in conditions of elevated IOP [241–243]. The complement proteins C1q and C3 are crucial during retinal development by allowing the targeting of dysfunctional or unnecessary synapses to prune by microglial cells [244,245]. However, in glaucoma the inadequate targeting of synapses by increased expression of complement factors by microglia leads to indiscriminate pruning of healthy neurons, which might contribute to disease progression [246]. In addition, in glaucoma, microglia were found to actively phagocyte functional RGCs increasing the loss of visual capacity [246]. Furthermore, if neuron-microglia communication is impaired by interfering with the fractalkine receptor (CX3C chemokine receptor 1, Cx3cr1) in microglia, this would aggravate RGC loss in disease models such the ischemia-reperfusion [247] and glaucoma DBA/2J mouse [248], with no alterations in uninjured retinas [247]. These findings suggest that in the context of disease although the control of microglia response might be beneficial, it is important to preserve cell communication to restrain microglial cell response. Therefore, a strategy to confer protection to retinal cells might be to block the over targeting of retinal neurons by microglia through the complement system [241].

In the model of ischemia-reperfusion, treatment with minocycline, which decreases microglia reactivity, was able to protect RGCs [247]. Moreover, in the DBA/2J mouse model of glaucoma, minocycline decreases the number of ameboid microglia increasing their ramification and reducing the neuroinflammatory milieu [249]. Moreover, minocycline also improved axonal transport in RGCs and overall retinal integrity in the glaucoma model [249], providing evidence that the control of microglia-mediated neuroinflammation can have potential in RGC neuroprotection.

Müller cells are the main glial cells in the retina. In addition to structural support, among other functions, Müller cells are involved in metabolism, phagocytosis of neuronal debris and in the release of trophic factors. These cells can enhance the survival of RGCs [89,250–252].

Müller cells are crucial to protect neurons against toxic molecules (Figure 5). They can uptake excessive glutamate from the synapses, preventing glutamate-induced RGC death [253,254]. Some studies have demonstrated this function of Müller cells in vivo as well as in vitro [255–258]. The glutamate transporter GLAST contributes to the uptake of excess of glutamate from the medium protecting against the excitotoxic effect of glutamate [254,256]. Moreover, it has been shown that in some ocular diseases, the expression of GLAST is altered, including in an animal model of glaucoma [259]. Moreover, Müller cells are implicated in maintaining the retinal extracellular levels of other neurotransmitters, such as gamma-aminobutyric acid (GABA), contributing to neuronal protection [260].

Müller cells are also involved in the regulation of glycogen and glucose metabolism and during metabolic stress can provide lactate to retinal neurons [261]. For instance, in early phases of diabetic retinopathy, Müller glia may afford neuroprotection against high glucose [262]. In addition, due to their energy metabolism, Müller cells may protect neurons towards toxic stress by increasing ATP turnover [263]. Furthermore, they play a role in water and ion regulation, buffering the retina and inducing neuroprotection [250,264]. It is worth highlighting the important antioxidant role of Müller cells. One crucial molecule that protects the retina against reactive oxygen species is GSH, which can be synthesized by Müller cells [254,265]. In addition, GSH can prevent RGC degeneration in an experimental model of glaucoma [266].

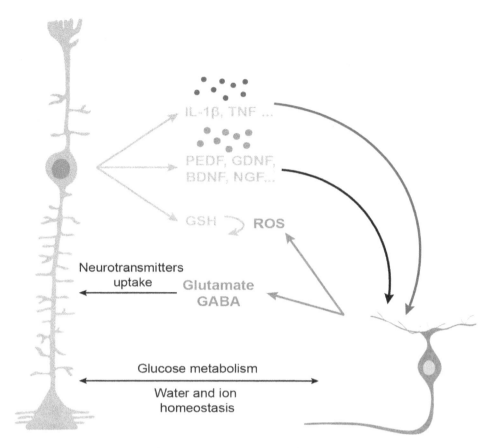

Figure 5. Diagram summarizing the main interactions of Müller cells (blue) with RGCs (orange). Scheme showing the roles of Müller cells in RGC neuroprotection, such as glucose metabolism regulation, water and ion homeostasis, neurotransmitters uptake, antioxidant defense systems (GSH) against ROS, secretion of trophic factors. The role of Müller cells in inflammation by secretion of cytokines that may be detrimental for RGCs is also depicted (red arrow).

Müller cells secrete a great number of factors in response to injury that can protect retinal neurons. Müller cells are known to synthesize neurotrophins and growth factors that can increase RGC survival [53,86,252,254], such as PEDF [267] or GDNF [105] among others. Moreover, Müller cells produce selective neurotrophins under different conditions, for instance, in response to glutamate, these cells upregulate the secretion of BDNF, NGF, NT-3, NT-4, and GDNF [268]. Müller cells are not only a source of neurotrophins, they also respond to neurotrophins as they express neurotrophin receptors [53,269] (see the neurotrophic factors functions protecting RGCs above).

Furthermore, Müller glial cells can release several inflammatory factors and cytokines [270], and some cytokines are even known to stimulate the production of other cytokines by Müller glia [271] in response to different stressors. Müller cells are a major source of retinal IL-1β [272,273] and they also secrete TNF, facilitating the apoptotic death of RGCs in response to damage [274,275]. In addition, Müller cells express toll-like receptors (TLRs) [276] and receptors for advanced glycation end-products (RAGE) [277] that induce the production of pro-inflammatory cytokines, chemokines and neuroprotective growth factors by these cells. In the beginning, this process acts as a protective mechanism to prevent further damage to the retina and to promote tissue repair. However, in the adult mammalian retina it does not appear to be beneficial since the release of pro-inflammatory cytokines and growth factors from Müller cells can lead to further degeneration [278]. For these reasons, understanding the processes in which Müller cells are involved and how these processes differ between pathological conditions and finding strategies to circumvent these barriers represent major challenges to the advancement of many ocular therapies.

4. Clinical Trials Targeting RGCs Neuroprotection

A therapeutic strategy to optic neuropathies should protect RGCs from death but should also manipulate axonal regeneration in order to repair the visual function that was lost due to the disease. However, there is still no effective therapy for optic neuropathies. Innovative study designs and integrating therapeutic testing with biomarkers have advanced several neuroprotective and neuroenhancement compounds to clinical trials. Numerous neuroprotection strategies have been investigated for optic neuropathies, including peripheral nerve grafting, electrical stimulation, and in agreement with their well-known role in maintaining neuronal homeostasis, neurotrophic factors have been proposed as a novel therapy. However, the outcomes of the completed clinical trials were not completely satisfactory, presenting only partial or no expected effects [198,279–281].

There are several drugs in clinical trials that are currently being developed focused on RGC neuroprotection (Table 1). In the context of neurotrophic factors some clinical trials are available. NT-501 encapsulated cell therapy (NT-501 ECT) is a device produced by Neurotech that consists of an intravitreal implant with a capsule filled with human cells genetically modified to secrete CNTF. NT-501 ECT is in phase 2 for glaucoma (ClinicalTrials.gov Identifier: NCT02862938) and in phase 1 for ischemic optic neuropathy (ClinicalTrials.gov Identifier: NCT01411657). For glaucoma, other therapies have been proposed such as the use of recombinant human NGF (rhNGF) (ClinicalTrials.gov Identifier: NCT02855450). In this phase 1 clinical trial the safety and tolerability of an 8-week treatment with 180 μg/mL of rhNGF eye drop solution will be determined. Additionally, the study wants to assess the changes in best corrected distance visual acuity (BCDVA), visual field, electroretinography (ERG) and structural changes in GCL and NFL thickness measured by optical coherence tomography (OCT) at 1, 4 and 8 weeks of therapy, and at 4 and 24 weeks after therapy cessation. In another clinical trial the safety of treatment with single and multiple ascending doses of rhNGF (0.5–180 μg/mL) was tested in healthy patients (ClinicalTrials.gov Identifier: NCT01744704), and the results demonstrated that rhNGF eye drops were well tolerated by the patients [282].

The only modifiable risk factor for glaucoma development is elevated IOP. Brimonidine is a non-selective α2-adrenergic receptor agonist and is currently used as a treatment option in glaucoma to lower IOP [283]. Preclinical studies demonstrated the neuroprotective properties of brimonidine [143,284], leading to the hypothesis that an implant with brimonidine can have beneficial properties for glaucoma patients. Indeed, this device is being evaluated in patients with glaucomatous optic neuropathy (ClinicalTrials.gov Identifier: NCT00693485). Moreover, cytidine-5'-diphosphocholine (citicoline) is also in a phase 4 clinical trial for glaucoma (ClinicalTrials.gov Identifier: NCT00404729). Citicoline is an endogenous molecule that has a role in the biosynthesis of phospholipids of cell membranes and increases the levels of neurotransmitters, like acetylcholine, in the CNS [285]. The neuroprotective properties of citicoline in glaucoma have been tested [286,287]. Intramuscular treatment of citicoline improves glaucomatous visual defects [286], RGC function (assessed by pattern ERG) and neural conduction along postretinal visual pathways (assessed by visual-evoked potential) [288]. That way, the phase 4 clinical trial aims to assess the effects of oral citicoline treatment in visual function outcomes in glaucoma patients. Memantine, a NMDA subtype of glutamate receptor antagonist, is already being used for Alzheimer's disease, and has undergone phase 3 clinical trials for glaucoma (ClinicalTrials.gov Identifier: NCT00141882 and NCT00168350). However, the drug did not show significant efficacy in preserving visual function in glaucoma patients [289].

Table 1. Drug-based therapies in clinical trials for optic neuropathies.

Condition or Disease	Intervention	ClinicalTrials.gov Identifier	Phase	Starting Date
Glaucoma	NT-501 ECT implant	NCT02862938	2	2016
Glaucoma	rhNGF	NCT02855450	1	2016
Glaucoma, Primary Open Angle	NT-501 CNTF Implant	NCT01408472	1	2011
Glaucoma, Open-Angle	Brimonidine Implant	NCT00693485	2	2008
Glaucoma and Ischemic optic neuropathy	Citicoline	NCT00404729	4	2006
Open-Angle Glaucoma	Memantine	NCT00141882	3	2005
Open-Angle Glaucoma	Memantine	NCT00168350	3	2005
Ischemic Optic Neuropathy	Alprostadil (prostaglandin E1)	NCT03851562	2	2019
Ischemic Optic Neuropathy	Bosentan	NCT02377271	3	2015
Ischemic Optic Neuropathy	Triamcinolone Acetonide	NCT02329288	3	2014
Ischemic Optic Neuropathy	NT-501 CNTF Implant	NCT01411657	1	2011
Non-arteritic Anterior Ischemic Optic Neuropathy	Prednisolone and Erythropoietin	NCT03715881	2	2018
Non-arteritic Ischemic Optic Neuropathy	RPh201	NCT03547206	3	2018
Non-arteritic Anterior Ischemic Optic Neuropathy	Citicoline	NCT03046693	4	2017
Non-arteritic Anterior Ischemic Optic Neuropathy	Methylprednisolone	NCT02439866	3	2015
Non-arteritic Ischemic Optic Neuropathy	RPh201	NCT02045212	2	2014
Non-arteritic Ischemic Optic Neuropathy	Dalfampridine	NCT01975324	4	2013
Non-arteritic Anterior Ischemic Optic Neuropathy	Avastin and Triamcinolone	NCT01330524	1 and 2	2011
Non-arteritic Anterior Ischemic Optic Neuropathy	Bevacizumab	NCT00813059	2	2008
Non-arteritic Anterior Ischemic Optic Neuropathy	Ranibizumab	NCT00561834	1	2007
Non-arteritic Anterior Ischemic Optic Neuropathy	Levodopa-carbidopa	NCT00432393	4	2007

Table 1. *Cont.*

Condition or Disease	Intervention	ClinicalTrials.gov Identifier	Phase	Starting Date
Traumatic Optic Neuropathy	Recombinant human erythropoietin	NCT03308448	3	2017
Traumatic Optic Neuropathy	Recombinant human erythropoietin	NCT01783847	1 and 2	2013
Optic Nerve Diseases (methanol associated optic neuropathy)	Erythropoietin	NCT02376881	3	2015
Leber's Hereditary Optic Neuropathy	Idebenone	NCT02774005	4	2016
Leber's Hereditary Optic Neuropathy	Cyclosporine	NCT02176733	2	2014
Leber's Hereditary Optic Neuropathy	Idebenone	NCT00747487	2	2008

Moreover, prostaglandin E1 (alprostadil) administered by intravenous infusion, is very recently in phase 2 clinical trial (ClinicalTrials.gov Identifier: NCT03851562). Prostaglandin E1 is a potent vasodilator of the microcirculation [290], and may correct the deficits in the perfusion pressure of the microcirculation that supplies the optic nerve in patients with ischemic optic neuropathy, improving visual function. In fact, intravenous prostaglandin E1 is an effective treatment for ocular and optic nerve ischemia leading to immediate visual improvement [290]. On the other hand, due to the role of endothelin in glaucoma as a potent vasoconstrictor [291], the antagonism of its signaling seems to be a good therapeutic strategy for optic neuropathies. Bosentan, an endothelin receptor antagonist, is in phase 3 clinical trial for ischemic optic neuropathy in order to assess if the treatment could recover anatomical (NFL in OCT, optic atrophy) and functional (visual acuity, visual field) criteria (ClinicalTrials.gov Identifier: NCT02377271). The last drug-based therapy for ischemic optic neuropathy, the retrobulbar injection of triamcinolone acetonide to halt the progression of the visual acuity and visual field loss in patients improving their chances of avoiding blindness, is in phase 3 clinical trial (ClinicalTrials.gov Identifier: NCT02329288). In preclinical studies, besides the neuroprotective effects to RGCs conferred by triamcinolone acetonide, it was demonstrated that this drug also decreases the activation of retinal microglia [292]. For non-arteritic ischemic optic neuropathy there are several clinical trials targeting neuroprotection. EPO administered by intravenous injection started recently in phase 2 clinical trial, in order to assess visual field and thickness of the retinal NFL by OCT in glaucoma patients (ClinicalTrials.gov Identifier: NCT03715881). In the same clinical trial, another aim is to assess the potential retinal neuroprotective effect of prednisolone. Moreover, methylprednisolone is also in phase 3 clinical trial (ClinicalTrials.gov Identifier: NCT02439866). Preclinical studies demonstrated that methylprednisolone inhibits the apoptosis of RGCs after ONC, probably through an up-regulation of Bcl-2 expression and a down-regulation of Bax expression [293], two of the intrinsic factors that limit the axon regeneration described previously. Moreover, citicoline is in clinical trials for non-arteritic ischemic optic neuropathy (ClinicalTrials.gov Identifier: NCT03046693) in order to assess the function of RGCs by pattern ERG, thickness of GCL and visual field test.

RPh201 is a drug extracted from a botanical source and it has been produced by Regenera Pharma. RPh201 started recently the phase 3 clinical trial for non-arteritic ischemic optic neuropathy (ClinicalTrials.gov Identifier: NCT03547206). The results of the phase 2 clinical trial (ClinicalTrials.gov Identifier: NCT02045212) are already available. Patients showed an improvement in visual function after the treatment [294]. Dalfampridine is used to improve the walking ability in multiple sclerosis patients and is in a phase 4 clinical trial for non-arteritic ischemic optic neuropathy (ClinicalTrials.gov Identifier: NCT01975324).

Anti-VEGF antibodies (bevacizumab, avastin or ranibizumab) are used for the treatment of macular edema and neovascular age-related macular degeneration. However, they have also been tested for neuroprotection in optic neuropathies, and they are in three different clinical trials for non-arteritic anterior ischemic optic neuropathy (ClinicalTrials.gov Identifier: NCT01330524, NCT00813059 and NCT00561834) in order to halt the progression of visual acuity and visual field loss due to the disease. The thickness of GCL increased after the treatment with bevacizumab in diabetic macular edema [295]. Moreover, levodopa-carbidopa is used to treat the symptoms of Parkinson's disease and it is in a phase 4 clinical trial for non-arteritic anterior ischemic optic neuropathy (ClinicalTrials.gov Identifier: NCT00432393).

A phase 1 and 2 clinical trial (ClinicalTrials.gov Identifier: NCT01783847) assessing the effect of erythropoietin (EPO) demonstrated an improvement in visual function [296,297]. These beneficial effects can be due to the protection conferred to RGCs by EPO previously demonstrated in animal models of retinal degeneration [298]. Moreover, it has been tested whether EPO could improve optic nerve function and help patients to recover visual function after methanol associated optic neuropathy (ClinicalTrials.gov Identifier: NCT02376881). EPO is currently in phase 3 clinical trial for traumatic optic neuropathy (ClinicalTrials.gov Identifier: NCT03308448).

Leber's hereditary optic neuropathy is an inherited optic neuropathy characterized by mitochondrial dysfunction that leads to vision loss due to RGCs loss [299]. Idebenone was in clinical trials for the treatment of vision loss due to Leber's hereditary optic neuropathy (ClinicalTrials.gov Identifier: NCT02774005 and NCT00747487). The beneficial effects of idebenone are due to its antioxidant properties and its ability to act as an electron carrier in the mitochondrial respiratory chain, thus resulting in the restoration of cellular energy (ATP) generation and contributing to the recovery of visual function in patients (reviewed in [300]). That way, idebenone (Raxone®) is the first, and currently the only disease-specific treatment for Leber's hereditary optic neuropathy and the only approved for optic neuropathies aiming RGCs neuroprotection. Moreover, cyclosporine is also in a phase 2 clinical trial for Leber's hereditary optic neuropathy (ClinicalTrials.gov Identifier: NCT02176733), due to protective properties against ischemic injury-mediated mitochondrial dysfunction in RGCs [301].

Currently, there are two clinical trials involving stem-cell based therapies targeting RGCs (Table 2). One trial aims to assess the safety and efficacy of the transplantation of autologous purified stem cells (ClinicalTrials.gov Identifier: NCT02638714) on restoring function in damaged optic nerves using autologous purified populations of bone-marrow derived stem cells in optic neuropathy. The intravitreal injection of MSCs (ClinicalTrials.gov Identifier: NCT03173638) aims to evaluate if the treatment may reduce the progression of axonal degeneration caused by non-arteritic ischemic optic neuropathy, but this clinical trial is focused in the evaluation of the safety of cell therapy as a new treatment for these patients.

Table 2. Stem cell-based therapies in clinical trials for optic neuropathies.

Condition or Disease	Intervention	ClinicalTrials.gov Identifier	Phase	Starting Date
Optic Neuropathy	Transplantation of autologous purified stem cells	NCT02638714	1 and 2	2015
Non-arteritic Ischemic Optic Neuropathy	Intravitreal injection of mesenchymal stem cells	NCT03173638	2	2017

5. Different Types of RGCs and their Susceptibility after Retinal Damage

The complexity of the CNS is due to the great number of specialized neuronal types and subtypes that give rise to a complex connectome [302]. However, due to the heterogeneity and complexity of the mammalian neuronal types, neuronal classification has been challenging and many cell subtypes have not yet been characterized [303]. Just like neurons in the brain, in the retina, although most RGCs serve a similar function, it was proven that these RGCs are highly diverse. The total RGC population develops from a common precursor into different subtypes of RGCs, with that they may differ in their physiological roles generating varied responses to visual stimuli [304]. RGCs have been classified based on differences in size, morphology, dendritic arborization, electrophysiological functions, susceptibility to degeneration, regenerative capacity and expression of specific molecular signatures, and more than thirty different subtypes of RGCs subtypes have been identified to date in the mammalian retina [305]. In 1953, the first classifications were made and the ON- and OFF-center RGCs were distinguished [305]. In recent works, combining different criteria, RGCs were classified into four types of ON-OFF directionally selective ganglion cells (DS-RGCs), three types of ON DS-RGCs, three types of alpha RGCs (sustained ON, sustained OFF, and transient OFF αRGCs), five types of intrinsically photosensitive melanopsin-containing RGCs (ipRGCs), three types of JamB expressing RGCs (J-RGCs), two types of beta cells (βRGCs), chromatically sensitive ganglion cells, orientation-sensitive cells, and suppressed-by-contrast cells, among others [306].

The major requirement to properly characterize and classify RGCs is to distinguish selectively each specific subtype. Thus, recently, a number of molecular subtype-specific markers have been described to further classify different subtypes of RGCs [307]. Several markers are being proposed, but most of them sign more than a single RGC subtype. Four types of ON–OFF DS-RGCs have been described, depending on the direction of the moving object to which they respond. They all have similar dendritic stratification and express CART (cocaine and amphetamine-regulated transcript) [308]. DS-RGCs have been also identified by the expression of specific molecular markers, such as CDH6 and FSTL4 [307]. Moreover, the ON DS-RGCs can be identified by the expression of the secretory protein SPIG1 [309]. In addition, three types of α-RGCs express similar markers, including neurofilaments, spp1 and kcng4, among others [310], although they differ in their physiological properties, dendritic arborization and stratification in the IPL [306]. On the other hand, the ipRGCs mediate many relevant non-image forming functions of the eye and they are identified by the expression of the photopigment melanopsin [311].

Another molecular marker, Tbr2, identifies RGCs that are hardwired during developmental stages and they could be precursors of ipRGCs [312]. Other single subtype of RGCs appears to be uniquely marked by the transcription factor Prdm16. However, the precise identity of these RGCs is unclear, but they most resemble the G9 subtype described by Völgyi and colleagues in 2009 [313].

Moreover, mouse transgenic lines have been also used to label and identify specific subsets of RGCs [314]. For instance, the line CB2-GFP labels transient OFF αRGCs [315] and the line Isl2-GFP labels αRGCs but not ON-OFF DS-RGCs [316]. In addition, using single cell transcriptome profiling of RGCs, specific markers for cellular subtypes have been identified, such as Zic1, Runx1 and Fst [317]. This capacity to successfully identify RGCs subtypes hopefully will help to understand the different susceptibility of certain RGCs to progression of pathologies like glaucoma.

In order to understand the pathophysiology of neurodegenerative diseases in which the RGCs death is implicated, it is important to analyze the response of these RGCs subtypes individually rather than studying them as a single entity. RGCs are susceptible to various injuries in a type-specific manner. Thereby, their type-specific vulnerability has been extensively studied [318]. The identification and characterization of the loss of specific RGCs subtypes in axotomy [310], ONC [319] and glaucoma [320] models has been analyzed, suggesting subtype specific responses to injury. The importance of studying the response of these subtypes individually rather than studying them as a single entity could help us understand the pathophysiology of diseases in which RGCs are affected. For instance, it was found that a greater loss of large RGCs in the peripheral retina occur in a pig glaucoma model resembling what was described in glaucoma patients [321]. However, in the periphery of the retina, some cells are resistant to damage, and it will be very important to know the nature of the cells that possess the capacity to recover after an insult. The αRGCs seem to be the least susceptible RGCs subtype to optic nerve injury [310]. The αRGCs are also the most resistant RGCs to NMDA excitotoxicity, while the J-RGCs are the most sensitive to the same damage [322]. Nevertheless, αRGCs seem to be the more susceptible RGCs subtype in other studies, such as in autoimmune optic neuritis, where αRGCs are more vulnerable to degeneration than ON αRGCs [323], and after ONC injury, where OFF-transient αRGCs are the most susceptible to injury followed by ON-OFF DS-RGCs [319]. In experimental models of OHT, OFF-transient RGCs exhibited a faster decline on survival when compared to ON RGCs, and they were also the first to undergo structural alterations [318]. Similarly, after ONC injury, functional responses and receptive fields of OFF cells were also impaired earlier than ON cells, and ON sustained RGCs seem to be more susceptible than ON transient RGCs [324]. In another model of OHT, the mono-laminated ON RGCs were more susceptible to chronic OHT than bi-laminated ON-OFF cells [325].

It has been shown that non-image forming ipRGCs exhibited a preferential survival following injury compared to image forming RGCs. This fact was observed in different injury and disease models, demonstrating the resilience to damage of this subtype of RGCs [326]. ipRGCs have the ability to respond to light using the photopigment melanopsin, and they play a role in circadian rhythms and pupillary reflexes through their projections to the suprachiasmatic nucleus and the olivary pretectal nucleus [327]. This unique feature may be the basis of their resistance to insult, as these cells are not necessary for the formation of images in the visual transduction pathway [328].

All these studies clearly imply that RGCs respond in a subtype specific manner to injury. Moreover, each subtype of RGCs can have a unique gene expression pattern [306,329], this differential gene expression may protect some types of RGCs and facilitate the death of others [330]. Therefore, the analysis of the type-specific vulnerability of RGCs based on their gene expression may provide insights of the selective vulnerability of RGCs to pathological insults and to better understand disease mechanisms [322]. Moreover, further studies are needed to determine how the molecular differences between RGCs subtypes underlie their electrophysiological functions, and it is necessary to investigate whether they differ in morphology, retinal spatial distribution, target cell connectivity, and associated visual parameters. These studies could provide a new opportunity to the development of strategies to target specific subtypes of RGCs for diagnostic and therapeutic approaches to treat optic neuropathies, such as glaucoma.

6. Potential Pitfalls in Translating Preclinical Studies into the Clinics

The main goal in finding new therapeutic strategies for optic neuropathies is to preserve the function of RGCs in order to maintain visual pathways. Therefore, besides the neuroprotection of RGCs and axon regeneration, the re-integration of RGC axons into the appropriate visual circuity is also important. Despite that several therapeutic strategies have demonstrated promising results in this field, there are significant issues affecting their translation to clinical practice.

Much work has been done in order to identify the inhibitors of axonal growth in the CNS as well as to isolate neurotrophic factors, with the hope that one day these factors could be applied to protect and regenerate the optic nerve. From what was described above, it seems that we are getting closer to a therapeutic strategy focused on RGC neuroprotection for optic neuropathies. However, we can discuss the example of memantine that, despite the convincing neuroprotective effects in animal models of glaucoma, in clinical trials the drug did not reveal significant effects in preventing the progression of visual field loss in patients with glaucoma [289].

Several issues contributing to the lack of success of drugs in clinical trials could be suggested, but in the case of glaucoma, the lack of an animal model that fully mimics the human disease is an important factor that adds to this failure [331]. Another issue is that, in preclinical trials, several studies use a preventive strategy to assess the effect of a specific drug, as opposed to the human condition in which the treatment starts after diagnosis. Moreover, in most of the animal studies the evaluation of the drug beneficial effects occurs by histopathological methodologies, and this is not possible in human studies. The increasingly use of OCT and ERG in preclinical studies will benefit the translation of what is observed in an animal models of disease into human.

Besides the protection of RGCs from death and degeneration, one of the goals in RGCs regeneration therapies should be to allow the reintegration of the regenerating axons into visual circuity reaching the appropriate brain targets. However, there are few studies that focus on this issue [26]. Moreover, the identification of different types of RGCs and the characterization of their different susceptibility to disease [306,324] may also contribute to the failure of the therapeutic strategies with high potential of success in the clinical trials phase.

It is fundamental a better characterization of the beneficial effects of drugs in the preclinical phase, meaning that the observation of the loss of RGCs is not enough as it is not enough to observe potential regenerative events of the axons of RGCs. It is essential to clearly and more deeply evaluate the beneficial effects of a specific new drug also in visual function.

The research in the field of neuroprotection in glaucoma has been difficult, but new animal models of disease and techniques will help to bridge the gap between preclinical and clinical studies, with clear beneficial outcomes in the forthcoming years. Many of the approaches outlined in this review are applicable not only to RGC neuroprotection in glaucoma but also to other pathologies of the optic nerve and retina. Gene therapy may have also a therapeutic potential especially for Leber's hereditary optic neuropathy, an optic neuropathy caused by mitochondrial mutation G11778A in NADH dehydrogenase subunit 4 (ND4) gene [332]. It was conducted in patients and the recombinant adeno-associated virus 2 (AAV2) carrying ND4 (rAAV2-ND4) demonstrated to improve patients visual acuity [333–335]. In addition, CRISPR/Cas9-based therapies are starting to be applied making significant progress in mammalian preclinical models of eye disease such as blind rodents [336] or in the disruption of mutant genes that cause certain forms of glaucoma [337]. Applications of CRISPR/Cas9 technology and other gene therapies may soon be available, not only as research tools but also as therapies to treat retinal diseases.

Author Contributions: Conceptualization, R.B. and A.R.S.; writing—original draft, R.B., N.R., I.D.A. and X.P.; writing—review and editing, R.B., N.R., I.D.A., X.P., A.F.A., E.V. and A.R.S. All authors have read and agreed to the published version of the manuscript.

Acknowledgments: We thank Sara Boia for providing the illustration in Figure 1.

Abbreviations

A_1	Adenosine A_1 receptor
A_{2A}	Adenosine A_{2A} receptor
A_{2B}	Adenosine A_{2B} receptor
A_3	Adenosine A_3 receptor
ARTN	Artemin
ATP	Adenosine triphosphate
BCDVA	Best corrected distance visual acuity
BDNF	Brain-derived neurotrophic factor
bFGF	Basic fibroblast growth factor
cAMP	Cyclic adenosine monophosphate
CART	Cocaine and amphetamine-regulated transcript
CAT	Catalase
CHA	N(6)-cyclohexyl-adenosine
CNS	Central nervous system
CNTF	Ciliary neurotrophic factor
CNTFR	CNTF receptors
Cop-1	Copolymer-1
Cx3cr1	CX3C chemokine receptor 1
DS-RGCs	Directionally selective ganglion cells
ED	Embryonic day
EHP	Elevated hydrostatic pressure
EPO	Erythropoietin
ERG	Electroretinography
GCL	Ganglion cell layer
GDNF	Glial cell-line derived neurotrophic factor
GLAST	Glutamate/aspartate transporter
GPx	Glutathione peroxidase
GSH	Glutathione
IGF-1	Insulin-like growth factor-1
IL-1β	Interleukin-1β
IL-6	Interleukin-6
INL	Inner nuclear layer
iNOS	Inducible nitric oxide synthase

IOP	Intraocular pressure
ipRGCs	Intrinsically photosensitive melanopsin-containing RGCs
J-RGCs	JamB expressing RGCs
KLF	Krüppel-like family
MAG	Myelin-associated glycoprotein
MHC-II	Major histocompatibility complex class II
mTOR	Mammalian target of rapamycin
ND4	NADH dehydrogenase subunit 4
NFL	Nerve fiber layer
NGF	Nerve growth factor
NgR	Nogo receptor
NLRP3	NOD-, LRR- and pyrin domain-containing protein 3
NMDA	N-methyl-D-aspartate
NO	Nitric oxide
NOS	Nitric oxide synthase
NRTN	Neurturin
NT-3	Neurotrophin-3
NT-4/5	Neurotrophin-4/5
OCT	Optical coherence tomography
OHT	Ocular hypertension
ONC	Optic nerve crush
ONH	Optic nerve head
ONL	Outer nuclear layer
PEDF	Pigment epithelium derived factor
PI3K	Phosphoinositide 3-kinases
PND	Postnatal day
PNS	Peripheral nervous system
PSPN	Persephin
PTEN	Phosphatase and tensin homologue
RAGE	Receptors for advanced glycation end-products
RGCs	Retinal ganglion cells
rhNGF	Recombinant human nerve growth factor
ROS	Reactive oxygen species
Sema3A	Semaphorin-3A
Sema5A	Semaphorin-5A
SOD	Superoxide dismutase
TLRs	Toll-like receptors
TNF	Tumour necrosis factor
TrK	Tyrosine kinase
TSPO	Translocator protein
VEGF-A	Vascular endothelial growth factor A
Zn^{2+}	Zinc
αRGCs	alpha retinal ganglion cells
βRGCs	beta retinal ganglion cells

References

1. Kolb, H.; Fernandez, E.; Nelson, R. Webvision: The Organization of the Retina and Visual System. In *Webvision: The Organization of the Retina and Visual System*; Kolb, H., Fernandez, E., Nelson, R., Eds.; University of Utah Health Sciences Center: Salt Lake City, UT, USA, 1995.

2. Carelli, V.; La Morgia, C.; Ross-Cisneros, F.N.; Sadun, A.A. Optic neuropathies: The tip of the neurodegeneration iceberg. *Hum. Mol. Genet.* **2017**, *26*, R139–R150. [CrossRef] [PubMed]

3. Goldberg, J.L.; Espinosa, J.S.; Xu, Y.; Davidson, N.; Kovacs, G.T.; Barres, B.A. Retinal ganglion cells do not extend axons by default: Promotion by neurotrophic signaling and electrical activity. *Neuron* **2002**, *33*, 689–702. [CrossRef]

4.   Dratviman-Storobinsky, O.; Hasanreisoglu, M.; Offen, D.; Barhum, Y.; Weinberger, D.; Goldenberg-Cohen, N. Progressive damage along the optic nerve following induction of crush injury or rodent anterior ischemic optic neuropathy in transgenic mice. *Mol. Vis.* **2008**, *14*, 2171–2179. [PubMed]

5.   Kutsarova, E.; Munz, M.; Ruthazer, E.S. Rules for shaping neural connections in the developing brain. *Front. Neural Circuits* **2016**, *10*, 111. [CrossRef]

6.   Guerin, M.B.; McKernan, D.P.; O'Brien, C.J.; Cotter, T.G. Retinal ganglion cells: Dying to survive. *Int. J. Dev. Biol.* **2006**, *50*, 665–674. [CrossRef]

7.   Goldberg, J.L.; Klassen, M.P.; Hua, Y.; Barres, B.A. Amacrine-signaled loss of intrinsic axon growth ability by retinal ganglion cells. *Science* **2002**, *296*, 1860–1864. [CrossRef]

8.   Martins, J.; Elvas, F.; Brudzewsky, D.; Martins, T.; Kolomiets, B.; Tralhao, P.; Gotzsche, C.R.; Cavadas, C.; Castelo-Branco, M.; Woldbye, D.P.; et al. Activation of neuropeptide y receptors modulates retinal ganglion cell physiology and exerts neuroprotective actions in vitro. *ASN Neuro* **2015**, *7*. [CrossRef]

9.   Barres, B.A.; Silverstein, B.E.; Corey, D.P.; Chun, L.L. Immunological, morphological, and electrophysiological variation among retinal ganglion cells purified by panning. *Neuron* **1988**, *1*, 791–803. [CrossRef]

10. Ming, G.L.; Song, H.J.; Berninger, B.; Holt, C.E.; Tessier-Lavigne, M.; Poo, M.M. cAMP-dependent growth cone guidance by netrin-1. *Neuron* **1997**, *19*, 1225–1235. [CrossRef]

11. Rodger, J.; Goto, H.; Cui, Q.; Chen, P.B.; Harvey, A.R. cAMP regulates axon outgrowth and guidance during optic nerve regeneration in goldfish. *Mol. Cell. Neurosci.* **2005**, *30*, 452–464. [CrossRef]

12. Park, K.K.; Liu, K.; Hu, Y.; Smith, P.D.; Wang, C.; Cai, B.; Xu, B.; Connolly, L.; Kramvis, I.; Sahin, M.; et al. Promoting axon regeneration in the adult CNS by modulation of the PTEN/mTOR pathway. *Science* **2008**, *322*, 963–966. [CrossRef] [PubMed]

13. Huang, Z.R.; Chen, H.Y.; Hu, Z.Z.; Xie, P.; Liu, Q.H. PTEN knockdown with the Y444F mutant AAV2 vector promotes axonal regeneration in the adult optic nerve. *Neural Regen. Res.* **2018**, *13*, 135–144. [CrossRef] [PubMed]

14. Moore, D.L.; Blackmore, M.G.; Hu, Y.; Kaestner, K.H.; Bixby, J.L.; Lemmon, V.P.; Goldberg, J.L. KLF family members regulate intrinsic axon regeneration ability. *Science* **2009**, *326*, 298–301. [CrossRef] [PubMed]

15. Steketee, M.B.; Oboudiyat, C.; Daneman, R.; Trakhtenberg, E.; Lamoureux, P.; Weinstein, J.E.; Heidemann, S.; Barres, B.A.; Goldberg, J.L. Regulation of intrinsic axon growth ability at retinal ganglion cell growth cones. *Investig. Ophthalmol. Vis. Sci.* **2014**, *55*, 4369–4377. [CrossRef] [PubMed]

16. Li, Y.; Andereggen, L.; Yuki, K.; Omura, K.; Yin, Y.; Gilbert, H.Y.; Erdogan, B.; Asdourian, M.S.; Shrock, C.; de Lima, S.; et al. Mobile zinc increases rapidly in the retina after optic nerve injury and regulates ganglion cell survival and optic nerve regeneration. *Proc. Natl. Acad. Sci. USA* **2017**, *114*, E209–E218. [CrossRef]

17. Moore, D.L.; Goldberg, J.L. Multiple transcription factor families regulate axon growth and regeneration. *Dev. Neurobiol.* **2011**, *71*, 1186–1211. [CrossRef]

18. Li, Y.; Schlamp, C.L.; Poulsen, G.L.; Jackson, M.W.; Griep, A.E.; Nickells, R.W. p53 regulates apoptotic retinal ganglion cell death induced by N-methyl-D-aspartate. *Mol. Vis.* **2002**, *8*, 341–350.

19. Di Giovanni, S.; Knights, C.D.; Rao, M.; Yakovlev, A.; Beers, J.; Catania, J.; Avantaggiati, M.L.; Faden, A.I. The tumor suppressor protein p53 is required for neurite outgrowth and axon regeneration. *EMBO J.* **2006**, *25*, 4084–4096. [CrossRef]

20. Maes, M.E.; Schlamp, C.L.; Nickells, R.W. BAX to basics: How the BCL2 gene family controls the death of retinal ganglion cells. *Prog. Retin. Eye Res.* **2017**, *57*, 1–25. [CrossRef]

21. Isenmann, S.; Wahl, C.; Krajewski, S.; Reed, J.C.; Bahr, M. Up-regulation of Bax protein in degenerating retinal ganglion cells precedes apoptotic cell death after optic nerve lesion in the rat. *Eur. J. Neurosci.* **1997**, *9*, 1763–1772. [CrossRef]

22. Kaneda, K.; Kashii, S.; Kurosawa, T.; Kaneko, S.; Akaike, A.; Honda, Y.; Minami, M.; Satoh, M. Apoptotic DNA fragmentation and upregulation of Bax induced by transient ischemia of the rat retina. *Brain Res.* **1999**, *815*, 11–20. [CrossRef]

23. Libby, R.T.; Li, Y.; Savinova, O.V.; Barter, J.; Smith, R.S.; Nickells, R.W.; John, S.W. Susceptibility to neurodegeneration in a glaucoma is modified by Bax gene dosage. *PLoS Genet.* **2005**, *1*, 17–26. [CrossRef] [PubMed]

24. Chen, D.F.; Schneider, G.E.; Martinou, J.C.; Tonegawa, S. Bcl-2 promotes regeneration of severed axons in mammalian CNS. *Nature* **1997**, *385*, 434–439. [CrossRef] [PubMed]

25. Richardson, P.M.; McGuinness, U.M.; Aguayo, A.J. Axons from CNS neurones regenerate into PNS grafts. *Nature* **1980**, *284*, 264–265. [CrossRef]

26. Vidal-Sanz, M.; Bray, G.M.; Villegas-Perez, M.P.; Thanos, S.; Aguayo, A.J. Axonal regeneration and synapse formation in the superior colliculus by retinal ganglion cells in the adult rat. *J. Neurosci. Off. J. Soc. Neurosci.* **1987**, *7*, 2894–2909. [CrossRef]

27. Yiu, G.; He, Z. Glial inhibition of CNS axon regeneration. *Nat. Rev. Neurosci.* **2006**, *7*, 617–627. [CrossRef]

28. Pasterkamp, R.J.; Giger, R.J.; Ruitenberg, M.J.; Holtmaat, A.J.; De Wit, J.; De Winter, F.; Verhaagen, J. Expression of the gene encoding the chemorepellent semaphorin III is induced in the fibroblast component of neural scar tissue formed following injuries of adult but not neonatal CNS. *Mol. Cell. Neurosci.* **1999**, *13*, 143–166. [CrossRef]

29. Pasterkamp, R.J.; Anderson, P.N.; Verhaagen, J. Peripheral nerve injury fails to induce growth of lesioned ascending dorsal column axons into spinal cord scar tissue expressing the axon repellent Semaphorin3A. *Eur. J. Neurosci.* **2001**, *13*, 457–471. [CrossRef]

30. Van Horck, F.P.G.; Weinl, C.; Holt, C.E. Retinal axon guidance: Novel mechanisms for steering. *Curr. Opin. Neurobiol.* **2004**, *14*, 61–66. [CrossRef]

31. Tillo, M.; Ruhrberg, C.; Mackenzie, F. Emerging roles for semaphorins and VEGFs in synaptogenesis and synaptic plasticity. *Cell Adhes. Migr.* **2012**, *6*, 541–546. [CrossRef]

32. Chan-Juan, H.; Sen, L.; Li-Qianyu, A.; Jian, Y.; Rong-Di, Y. MicroRNA-30b regulates the polarity of retinal ganglion cells by inhibiting semaphorin-3A. *Mol. Vis.* **2019**, *25*, 722–730. [PubMed]

33. Dallimore, E.J.; Cui, Q.; Beazley, L.D.; Harvey, A.R. Postnatal innervation of the rat superior colliculus by axons of late-born retinal ganglion cells. *Eur. J. Neurosci.* **2002**, *16*, 1295–1304. [CrossRef] [PubMed]

34. De Winter, F.; Cui, Q.; Symons, N.; Verhaagen, J.; Harvey, A.R. Expression of class-3 semaphorins and their receptors in the neonatal and adult rat retina. *Investig. Ophthalmol. Vis. Sci.* **2004**, *45*, 4554–4562. [CrossRef]

35. Zylbersztejn, K.; Petkovic, M.; Burgo, A.; Deck, M.; Garel, S.; Marcos, S.; Bloch-Gallego, E.; Nothias, F.; Serini, G.; Bagnard, D.; et al. The vesicular SNARE Synaptobrevin is required for Semaphorin 3A axonal repulsion. *J. Cell Biol.* **2012**, *196*, 37–46. [CrossRef]

36. Shirvan, A.; Kimron, M.; Holdengreber, V.; Ziv, I.; Ben-Shaul, Y.; Melamed, S.; Melamed, E.; Barzilai, A.; Solomon, A.S. Anti-semaphorin 3A antibodies rescue retinal ganglion cells from cell death following optic nerve axotomy. *J. Biol. Chem.* **2002**, *277*, 49799–49807. [CrossRef]

37. Goldberg, J.L.; Vargas, M.E.; Wang, J.T.; Mandemakers, W.; Oster, S.F.; Sretavan, D.W.; Barres, B.A. An oligodendrocyte lineage-specific semaphorin, Sema5A, inhibits axon growth by retinal ganglion cells. *J. Neurosci. Off. J. Soc. Neurosci.* **2004**, *24*, 4989–4999. [CrossRef]

38. Fisher, J.; Levkovitch-Verbin, H.; Schori, H.; Yoles, E.; Butovsky, O.; Kaye, J.F.; Ben-Nun, A.; Schwartz, M. Vaccination for neuroprotection in the mouse optic nerve: Implications for optic neuropathies. *J. Neurosci.* **2001**, *21*, 136–142. [CrossRef]

39. Kipnis, J.; Yoles, E.; Porat, Z.; Cohen, A.; Mor, F.; Sela, M.; Cohen, I.R.; Schwartz, M. T cell immunity to copolymer 1 confers neuroprotection on the damaged optic nerve: Possible therapy for optic neuropathies. *Proc. Natl. Acad. Sci. USA* **2000**, *97*, 7446–7451. [CrossRef]

40. Schori, H.; Kipnis, J.; Yoles, E.; WoldeMussie, E.; Ruiz, G.; Wheeler, L.A.; Schwartz, M. Vaccination for protection of retinal ganglion cells against death from glutamate cytotoxicity and ocular hypertension: Implications for glaucoma. *Proc. Natl. Acad. Sci. USA* **2001**, *98*, 3398–3403. [CrossRef]

41. Bakalash, S.; Ben-Shlomo, G.; Aloni, E.; Shaked, I.; Wheeler, L.; Ofri, R.; Schwartz, M. T-cell-based vaccination for morphological and functional neuroprotection in a rat model of chronically elevated intraocular pressure. *J. Mol. Med.* **2005**, *83*, 904–916. [CrossRef]

42. Pernet, V.; Joly, S.; Christ, F.; Dimou, L.; Schwab, M.E. Nogo-A and myelin-associated glycoprotein differently regulate oligodendrocyte maturation and myelin formation. *J. Neurosci. Off. J. Soc. Neurosci.* **2008**, *28*, 7435–7444. [CrossRef] [PubMed]

43. Pernet, V. Nogo-A in the visual system development and in ocular diseases. *Biochim. Biophys. Acta Mol. Basis Dis.* **2017**, *1863*, 1300–1311. [CrossRef] [PubMed]

44. Solomon, A.M.; Westbrook, T.; Field, G.D.; McGee, A.W. Nogo receptor 1 is expressed by nearly all retinal ganglion cells. *PLoS ONE* **2018**, *13*, e0196565. [CrossRef] [PubMed]

45. Pernet, V.; Joly, S.; Dalkara, D.; Schwarz, O.; Christ, F.; Schaffer, D.; Flannery, J.G.; Schwab, M.E. Neuronal Nogo-A upregulation does not contribute to ER stress-associated apoptosis but participates in the regenerative response in the axotomized adult retina. *Cell Death Differ.* **2012**, *19*, 1096–1108. [CrossRef] [PubMed]

46. Vajda, F.; Jordi, N.; Dalkara, D.; Joly, S.; Christ, F.; Tews, B.; Schwab, M.E.; Pernet, V. Cell type-specific Nogo-A gene ablation promotes axonal regeneration in the injured adult optic nerve. *Cell Death Differ.* **2015**, *22*, 323–335. [CrossRef] [PubMed]

47. Mdzomba, J.B.; Jordi, N.; Rodriguez, L.; Joly, S.; Bretzner, F.; Pernet, V. Nogo-A inactivation improves visual plasticity and recovery after retinal injury. *Cell Death Dis.* **2018**, *9*, 727. [CrossRef]

48. Wong, E.V.; David, S.; Jacob, M.H.; Jay, D.G. Inactivation of myelin-associated glycoprotein enhances optic nerve regeneration. *J. Neurosci. Off. J. Soc. Neurosci.* **2003**, *23*, 3112–3117. [CrossRef]

49. Liao, X.-X.; Chen, D.; Shi, J.; Sun, Y.-Q.; Sun, S.-J.; So, K.-F.; Fu, Q.-L. The expression patterns of Nogo-A, Myelin Associated Glycoprotein and Oligodendrocyte Myelin Glycoprotein in the Retina After Ocular hypertension. *Neurochem. Res.* **2011**, *36*, 1955–1961. [CrossRef]

50. Fu, Q.-L.; Liao, X.-X.; Li, X.; Chen, D.; Shi, J.; Wen, W.; Lee, D.H.S.; So, K.-F. Soluble Nogo-66 receptor prevents synaptic dysfunction and rescues retinal ganglion cell loss in chronic glaucoma. *Investig. Opthalmol. Vis. Sci.* **2011**, *52*, 8374. [CrossRef]

51. Su, Y.; Wang, F.; Teng, Y.; Zhao, S.G.; Cui, H.; Pan, S.H. Axonal regeneration of optic nerve after crush in Nogo66 receptor knockout mice. *Neurosci. Lett.* **2009**, *460*, 223–226. [CrossRef]

52. Vecino, E.; Ugarte, M.; Nash, M.S.; Osborne, N.N. NMDA induces BDNF expression in the albino rat retina in vivo. *Neuroreport* **1999**, *10*, 1103–1106. [CrossRef] [PubMed]

53. Vecino, E.; Caminos, E.; Ugarte, M.; Martin-Zanca, D.; Osborne, N.N. Immunohistochemical distribution of neurotrophins and their receptors in the rat retina and the effects of ischemia and reperfusion. *Gen. Pharmacol.* **1998**, *30*, 305–314. [CrossRef]

54. Hofer, M.; Pagliusi, S.R.; Hohn, A.; Leibrock, J.; Barde, Y.A. Regional distribution of brain-derived neurotrophic factor mRNA in the adult mouse brain. *EMBO J.* **1990**, *9*, 2459–2464. [CrossRef] [PubMed]

55. Wetmore, C.; Ernfors, P.; Persson, H.; Olson, L. Localization of brain-derived neurotrophic factor mRNA to neurons in the brain by in situ hybridization. *Exp. Neurol.* **1990**, *109*, 141–152. [CrossRef]

56. Herzog, K.H.; von Bartheld, C.S. Contributions of the optic tectum and the retina as sources of brain-derived neurotrophic factor for retinal ganglion cells in the chick embryo. *J. Neurosci. Off. J. Soc. Neurosci.* **1998**, *18*, 2891–2906. [CrossRef]

57. Ma, Y.T.; Hsieh, T.; Forbes, M.E.; Johnson, J.E.; Frost, D.O. BDNF injected into the superior colliculus reduces developmental retinal ganglion cell death. *J. Neurosci. Off. J. Soc. Neurosci.* **1998**, *18*, 2097–2107. [CrossRef]

58. Di Polo, A.; Aigner, L.J.; Dunn, R.J.; Bray, G.M.; Aguayo, A.J. Prolonged delivery of brain-derived neurotrophic factor by adenovirus-infected Muller cells temporarily rescues injured retinal ganglion cells. *Proc. Natl. Acad. Sci. USA* **1998**, *95*, 3978–3983. [CrossRef]

59. Chen, H.; Weber, A.J. BDNF enhances retinal ganglion cell survival in cats with optic nerve damage. *Investig. Ophthalmol. Vis. Sci.* **2001**, *42*, 966–974.

60. Mey, J.; Thanos, S. Intravitreal injections of neurotrophic factors support the survival of axotomized retinal ganglion cells in adult rats in vivo. *Brain Res.* **1993**, *602*, 304–317. [CrossRef]

61. Mansour-Robaey, S.; Clarke, D.B.; Wang, Y.C.; Bray, G.M.; Aguayo, A.J. Effects of ocular injury and administration of brain-derived neurotrophic factor on survival and regrowth of axotomized retinal ganglion cells. *Proc. Natl. Acad. Sci. USA* **1994**, *91*, 1632–1636. [CrossRef]

62. Peinado-Ramon, P.; Salvador, M.; Villegas-Perez, M.P.; Vidal-Sanz, M. Effects of axotomy and intraocular administration of NT-4, NT-3, and brain-derived neurotrophic factor on the survival of adult rat retinal ganglion cells. A quantitative in vivo study. *Investig. Ophthalmol. Vis. Sci.* **1996**, *37*, 489–500.

63. Domenici, L.; Origlia, N.; Falsini, B.; Cerri, E.; Barloscio, D.; Fabiani, C.; Sanso, M.; Giovannini, L. Rescue of retinal function by BDNF in a mouse model of glaucoma. *PLoS ONE* **2014**, *9*, e115579. [CrossRef] [PubMed]

64. Galindo-Romero, C.; Valiente-Soriano, F.J.; Jimenez-Lopez, M.; Garcia-Ayuso, D.; Villegas-Perez, M.P.; Vidal-Sanz, M.; Agudo-Barriuso, M. Effect of brain-derived neurotrophic factor on mouse axotomized retinal ganglion cells and phagocytic microglia. *Investig. Ophthalmol. Vis. Sci.* **2013**, *54*, 974–985. [CrossRef] [PubMed]

65. Zhang, C.-W.; Lu, Q.; You, S.-W.; Zhi, Y.; Yip, H.K.; Wu, W.; So, K.-F.; Cui, Q. CNTF and BDNF have similar effects on retinal ganglion cell survival but differential effects on nitric oxide synthase expression soon after optic nerve injury. *Investig. Opthalmol. Vis. Sci.* **2005**, *46*, 1497. [CrossRef]

66. Meyer-Franke, A.; Kaplan, M.R.; Pfrieger, F.W.; Barres, B.A. Characterization of the signaling interactions that promote the survival and growth of developing retinal ganglion cells in culture. *Neuron* **1995**, *15*, 805–819. [CrossRef]

67. Leaver, S.G.; Cui, Q.; Plant, G.W.; Arulpragasam, A.; Hisheh, S.; Verhaagen, J.; Harvey, A.R. AAV-mediated expression of CNTF promotes long-term survival and regeneration of adult rat retinal ganglion cells. *Gene Ther.* **2006**, *13*, 1328–1341. [CrossRef]

68. Muller, A.; Hauk, T.G.; Leibinger, M.; Marienfeld, R.; Fischer, D. Exogenous CNTF stimulates axon regeneration of retinal ganglion cells partially via endogenous CNTF. *Mol. Cell. Neurosci.* **2009**, *41*, 233–246. [CrossRef]

69. Maffei, L.; Carmignoto, G.; Perry, V.H.; Candeo, P.; Ferrari, G. Schwann cells promote the survival of rat retinal ganglion cells after optic nerve section. *Proc. Natl. Acad. Sci. USA* **1990**, *87*, 1855–1859. [CrossRef]

70. Carmignoto, G.; Maffei, L.; Candeo, P.; Canella, R.; Comelli, C. Effect of NGF on the survival of rat retinal ganglion cells following optic nerve section. *J. Neurosci. Off. J. Soc. Neurosci.* **1989**, *9*, 1263–1272. [CrossRef]

71. Morgan, J.E. Retina ganglion cell degeneration in glaucoma: An opportunity missed? A review. *Clin. Exp. Ophthalmol.* **2012**, *40*, 364–368. [CrossRef]

72. Aires, I.D.; Ambrosio, A.F.; Santiago, A.R. Modeling human glaucoma: Lessons from the in vitro models. *Ophthalmic Res.* **2017**, *57*, 77–86. [CrossRef] [PubMed]

73. Wu, J.; Mak, H.K.; Chan, Y.K.; Lin, C.; Kong, C.; Leung, C.K.S.; Shum, H.C. An in vitro pressure model towards studying the response of primary retinal ganglion cells to elevated hydrostatic pressures. *Sci. Rep.* **2019**, *9*, 9057. [CrossRef] [PubMed]

74. Quigley, H.A.; Guy, J.; Anderson, D.R. Blockade of rapid axonal transport. Effect of intraocular pressure elevation in primate optic nerve. *Arch. Ophthalmol.* **1979**, *97*, 525–531. [CrossRef]

75. Quigley, H.A.; McKinnon, S.J.; Zack, D.J.; Pease, M.E.; Kerrigan-Baumrind, L.A.; Kerrigan, D.F.; Mitchell, R.S. Retrograde axonal transport of BDNF in retinal ganglion cells is blocked by acute IOP elevation in rats. *Investig. Ophthalmol. Vis. Sci.* **2000**, *41*, 3460–3466.

76. Pease, M.E.; McKinnon, S.J.; Quigley, H.A.; Kerrigan-Baumrind, L.A.; Zack, D.J. Obstructed axonal transport of BDNF and its receptor TrkB in experimental glaucoma. *Investig. Ophthalmol. Vis. Sci.* **2000**, *41*, 764–774.

77. Park, H.L.; Kim, S.W.; Kim, J.H.; Park, C.K. Increased levels of synaptic proteins involved in synaptic plasticity after chronic intraocular pressure elevation and modulation by brain-derived neurotrophic factor in a glaucoma animal model. *Dis. Models Mech.* **2019**, *12*. [CrossRef]

78. Aires, I.D.; Boia, R.; Rodrigues-Neves, A.C.; Madeira, M.H.; Marques, C.; Ambrosio, A.F.; Santiago, A.R. Blockade of microglial adenosine A2A receptor suppresses elevated pressure-induced inflammation, oxidative stress, and cell death in retinal cells. *Glia* **2019**, *67*, 896–914. [CrossRef]

79. Madeira, M.H.; Elvas, F.; Boia, R.; Goncalves, F.Q.; Cunha, R.A.; Ambrosio, A.F.; Santiago, A.R. Adenosine A2AR blockade prevents neuroinflammation-induced death of retinal ganglion cells caused by elevated pressure. *J. Neuroinflamm.* **2015**, *12*, 115. [CrossRef]

80. Harada, T.; Harada, C.; Parada, L.F. Molecular regulation of visual system development: More than meets the eye. *Genes Dev.* **2007**, *21*, 367–378. [CrossRef]

81. Kimura, A.; Namekata, K.; Guo, X.; Harada, C.; Harada, T. Neuroprotection, growth factors and BDNF-TrkB signalling in retinal degeneration. *Int. J. Mol. Sci.* **2016**, *17*, 1584. [CrossRef]

82. Johnson, T.V.; Bull, N.D.; Martin, K.R. Neurotrophic factor delivery as a protective treatment for glaucoma. *Exp. Eye Res.* **2011**, *93*, 196–203. [CrossRef] [PubMed]

83. Guo, X.J.; Tian, X.S.; Ruan, Z.; Chen, Y.T.; Wu, L.; Gong, Q.; Wang, W.; Zhang, H.Y. Dysregulation of neurotrophic and inflammatory systems accompanied by decreased CREB signaling in ischemic rat retina. *Exp. Eye Res.* **2014**, *125*, 156–163. [CrossRef] [PubMed]

84. Johnson, E.C.; Deppmeier, L.M.; Wentzien, S.K.; Hsu, I.; Morrison, J.C. Chronology of optic nerve head and retinal responses to elevated intraocular pressure. *Investig. Ophthalmol. Vis. Sci.* **2000**, *41*, 431–442.

85. Pietrucha-Dutczak, M.; Amadio, M.; Govoni, S.; Lewin-Kowalik, J.; Smedowski, A. The Role of endogenous neuroprotective mechanisms in the prevention of retinal ganglion cells degeneration. *Front. Neurosci.* **2018**, *12*, 834. [CrossRef]

86.   Garcia, M.; Forster, V.; Hicks, D.; Vecino, E. In vivo expression of neurotrophins and neurotrophin receptors is conserved in adult porcine retina in vitro. *Investig. Ophthalmol. Vis. Sci.* **2003**, *44*, 4532–4541. [CrossRef]

87.   Ruiz-Ederra, J.; Hitchcock, P.F.; Vecino, E. Two classes of astrocytes in the adult human and pig retina in terms of their expression of high affinity NGF receptor (TrkA). *Neurosci. Lett.* **2003**, *337*, 127–130. [CrossRef]

88.   Vecino, E.; Caminos, E.; Becker, E.; Martín-Zanca, D.; Osborne, N.N. Expression of neurotrophins and their receptors within the glial cells of retina and optic nerve. In *Understanding glial cells*; Springer: Boston, MA, USA, 1998; pp. 149–166. [CrossRef]

89.   Garcia, M.; Forster, V.; Hicks, D.; Vecino, E. Effects of muller glia on cell survival and neuritogenesis in adult porcine retina in vitro. *Investig. Ophthalmol. Vis. Sci.* **2002**, *43*, 3735–3743.

90.   Freeman, R.S.; Burch, R.L.; Crowder, R.J.; Lomb, D.J.; Schoell, M.C.; Straub, J.A.; Xie, L. NGF deprivation-induced gene expression: After ten years, where do we stand? *Prog. Brain Res.* **2004**, *146*, 111–126. [CrossRef]

91.   Lomb, D.J.; Desouza, L.A.; Franklin, J.L.; Freeman, R.S. Prolyl hydroxylase inhibitors depend on extracellular glucose and hypoxia-inducible factor (HIF)-2alpha to inhibit cell death caused by nerve growth factor (NGF) deprivation: Evidence that HIF-2alpha has a role in NGF-promoted survival of sympathetic neurons. *Mol. Pharmacol.* **2009**, *75*, 1198–1209. [CrossRef]

92.   Roberti, G.; Mantelli, F.; Macchi, I.; Massaro-Giordano, M.; Centofanti, M. Nerve growth factor modulation of retinal ganglion cell physiology. *J. Cell. Physiol.* **2014**, *229*, 1130–1133. [CrossRef]

93.   Colafrancesco, V.; Parisi, V.; Sposato, V.; Rossi, S.; Russo, M.A.; Coassin, M.; Lambiase, A.; Aloe, L. Ocular application of nerve growth factor protects degenerating retinal ganglion cells in a rat model of glaucoma. *J. Glaucoma* **2011**, *20*, 100–108. [CrossRef] [PubMed]

94.   Aloe, L.; Rocco, M.L.; Balzamino, B.O.; Micera, A. Nerve growth factor: A focus on neuroscience and therapy. *Curr. Neuropharmacol.* **2015**, *13*, 294–303. [CrossRef] [PubMed]

95.   Chen, Q.; Wang, H.; Liao, S.; Gao, Y.; Liao, R.; Little, P.J.; Xu, J.; Feng, Z.P.; Zheng, Y.; Zheng, W. Nerve growth factor protects retinal ganglion cells against injury induced by retinal ischemia-reperfusion in rats. *Growth Factors* **2015**, *33*, 149–159. [CrossRef] [PubMed]

96.   Lambiase, A.; Aloe, L.; Centofanti, M.; Parisi, V.; Bao, S.N.; Mantelli, F.; Colafrancesco, V.; Manni, G.L.; Bucci, M.G.; Bonini, S.; et al. Experimental and clinical evidence of neuroprotection by nerve growth factor eye drops: Implications for glaucoma. *Proc. Natl. Acad. Sci. USA* **2009**, *106*, 13469–13474. [CrossRef]

97.   Vecino, E.; Garcia-Crespo, D.; Garcia, M.; Martinez-Millan, L.; Sharma, S.C.; Carrascal, E. Rat retinal ganglion cells co-express brain derived neurotrophic factor (BDNF) and its receptor TrkB. *Vis. Res.* **2002**, *42*, 151–157. [CrossRef]

98.   Pernet, V.; Di Polo, A. Synergistic action of brain-derived neurotrophic factor and lens injury promotes retinal ganglion cell survival, but leads to optic nerve dystrophy in vivo. *Brain A J. Neurol.* **2006**, *129*, 1014–1026. [CrossRef]

99.   Pietrucha-Dutczak, M.; Smedowski, A.; Liu, X.; Matuszek, I.; Varjosalo, M.; Lewin-Kowalik, J. Candidate proteins from predegenerated nerve exert time-specific protection of retinal ganglion cells in glaucoma. *Sci. Rep.* **2017**, *7*, 14540. [CrossRef]

100. Bai, Y.; Xu, J.; Brahimi, F.; Zhuo, Y.; Sarunic, M.V.; Saragovi, H.U. An agonistic TrkB mAb causes sustained TrkB activation, delays RGC death, and protects the retinal structure in optic nerve axotomy and in glaucoma. *Investig. Ophthalmol. Vis. Sci.* **2010**, *51*, 4722–4731. [CrossRef]

101. Ghaffariyeh, A.; Honarpisheh, N.; Shakiba, Y.; Puyan, S.; Chamacham, T.; Zahedi, F.; Zarrineghbal, M. Brain-derived neurotrophic factor in patients with normal-tension glaucoma. *Optometry* **2009**, *80*, 635–638. [CrossRef]

102. Oddone, F.; Roberti, G.; Micera, A.; Busanello, A.; Bonini, S.; Quaranta, L.; Agnifili, L.; Manni, G. Exploring serum levels of brain derived neurotrophic factor and nerve growth factor across glaucoma stages. *PLoS ONE* **2017**, *12*, e0168565. [CrossRef]

103. Airaksinen, M.S.; Saarma, M. The GDNF family: Signalling, biological functions and therapeutic value. *Nat. Rev. Neurosci.* **2002**, *3*, 383–394. [CrossRef]

104. Koeberle, P.D.; Ball, A.K. Effects of GDNF on retinal ganglion cell survival following axotomy. *Vis. Res.* **1998**, *38*, 1505–1515. [CrossRef]

105. Yan, Q.; Wang, J.; Matheson, C.R.; Urich, J.L. Glial cell line-derived neurotrophic factor (GDNF) promotes the survival of axotomized retinal ganglion cells in adult rats: Comparison to and combination with brain-derived neurotrophic factor (BDNF). *J. Neurobiol.* **1999**, *38*, 382–390. [CrossRef]

106. Kyhn, M.V.; Klassen, H.; Johansson, U.E.; Warfvinge, K.; Lavik, E.; Kiilgaard, J.F.; Prause, J.U.; Scherfig, E.; Young, M.; la Cour, M. Delayed administration of glial cell line-derived neurotrophic factor (GDNF) protects retinal ganglion cells in a pig model of acute retinal ischemia. *Exp. Eye Res.* **2009**, *89*, 1012–1020. [CrossRef] [PubMed]

107. Checa-Casalengua, P.; Jiang, C.; Bravo-Osuna, I.; Tucker, B.A.; Molina-Martinez, I.T.; Young, M.J.; Herrero-Vanrell, R. Retinal ganglion cells survival in a glaucoma model by GDNF/Vit E PLGA microspheres prepared according to a novel microencapsulation procedure. *J. Control. Release Off. J. Control. Release Soc.* **2011**, *156*, 92–100. [CrossRef] [PubMed]

108. Ward, M.S.; Khoobehi, A.; Lavik, E.B.; Langer, R.; Young, M.J. Neuroprotection of retinal ganglion cells in DBA/2J mice with GDNF-loaded biodegradable microspheres. *J. Pharm. Sci.* **2007**, *96*, 558–568. [CrossRef]

109. Koeberle, P.D.; Bahr, M. The upregulation of GLAST-1 is an indirect antiapoptotic mechanism of GDNF and neurturin in the adult CNS. *Cell Death Differ.* **2008**, *15*, 471–483. [CrossRef]

110. Del Rio, P.; Irmler, M.; Arango-Gonzalez, B.; Favor, J.; Bobe, C.; Bartsch, U.; Vecino, E.; Beckers, J.; Hauck, S.M.; Ueffing, M. GDNF-induced osteopontin from Muller glial cells promotes photoreceptor survival in the Pde6brd1 mouse model of retinal degeneration. *Glia* **2011**, *59*, 821–832. [CrossRef]

111. Ernst, M.; Jenkins, B.J. Acquiring signalling specificity from the cytokine receptor gp130. *Trends Genet. TIG* **2004**, *20*, 23–32. [CrossRef]

112. Kirsch, M.; Lee, M.Y.; Meyer, V.; Wiese, A.; Hofmann, H.D. Evidence for multiple, local functions of ciliary neurotrophic factor (CNTF) in retinal development: Expression of CNTF and its receptors and in vitro effects on target cells. *J. Neurochem.* **1997**, *68*, 979–990. [CrossRef]

113. Wen, R.; Song, Y.; Liu, Y.; Li, Y.; Zhao, L.; Laties, A.M. CNTF negatively regulates the phototransduction machinery in rod photoreceptors: Implication for light-induced photostasis plasticity. *Adv. Exp. Med. Biol.* **2008**, *613*, 407–413. [CrossRef] [PubMed]

114. Mathews, M.K.; Guo, Y.; Langenberg, P.; Bernstein, S.L. Ciliary neurotrophic factor (CNTF)-mediated ganglion cell survival in a rodent model of non-arteritic anterior ischaemic optic neuropathy (NAION). *Br. J. Ophthalmol.* **2015**, *99*, 133–137. [CrossRef] [PubMed]

115. Pease, M.E.; Zack, D.J.; Berlinicke, C.; Bloom, K.; Cone, F.; Wang, Y.; Klein, R.L.; Hauswirth, W.W.; Quigley, H.A. Effect of CNTF on retinal ganglion cell survival in experimental glaucoma. *Investig. Ophthalmol. Vis. Sci.* **2009**, *50*, 2194–2200. [CrossRef] [PubMed]

116. Maier, K.; Rau, C.R.; Storch, M.K.; Sattler, M.B.; Demmer, I.; Weissert, R.; Taheri, N.; Kuhnert, A.V.; Bahr, M.; Diem, R. Ciliary neurotrophic factor protects retinal ganglion cells from secondary cell death during acute autoimmune optic neuritis in rats. *Brain Pathol.* **2004**, *14*, 378–387. [CrossRef]

117. Fischer, D.; Leibinger, M. Promoting optic nerve regeneration. *Prog. Retin. Eye Res.* **2012**, *31*, 688–701. [CrossRef]

118. Muller, A.; Hauk, T.G.; Fischer, D. Astrocyte-derived CNTF switches mature RGCs to a regenerative state following inflammatory stimulation. *Brain A J. Neurol.* **2007**, *130*, 3308–3320. [CrossRef]

119. Shpak, A.A.; Guekht, A.B.; Druzhkova, T.A.; Kozlova, K.I.; Gulyaeva, N.V. Ciliary neurotrophic factor in patients with primary open-angle glaucoma and age-related cataract. *Mol. Vis.* **2017**, *23*, 799–809.

120. Zhou, X.; Li, F.; Kong, L.; Chodosh, J.; Cao, W. Anti-inflammatory effect of pigment epithelium-derived factor in DBA/2J mice. *Mol. Vis.* **2009**, *15*, 438–450.

121. Yang, X.; Wei, A.; Liu, Y.; He, G.; Zhou, Z.; Yu, Z. IGF-1 protects retinal ganglion cells from hypoxia-induced apoptosis by activating the Erk-1/2 and Akt pathways. *Mol. Vis.* **2013**, *19*, 1901–1912.

122. Kermer, P.; Klocker, N.; Labes, M.; Bahr, M. Insulin-like growth factor-I protects axotomized rat retinal ganglion cells from secondary death via PI3-K-dependent Akt phosphorylation and inhibition of caspase-3 in vivo. *J. Neurosci. Off. J. Soc. Neurosci.* **2000**, *20*, 2–8. [CrossRef]

123. Foxton, R.H.; Finkelstein, A.; Vijay, S.; Dahlmann-Noor, A.; Khaw, P.T.; Morgan, J.E.; Shima, D.T.; Ng, Y.S. VEGF-A is necessary and sufficient for retinal neuroprotection in models of experimental glaucoma. *Am. J. Pathol.* **2013**, *182*, 1379–1390. [CrossRef] [PubMed]

124. Lv, B.; Wang, R.; Gao, X.; Dong, X.; Ji, X. Effect of vascular endothelial growth factor on retinal ganglion cells of rats with chronic intraocular hypertension. *Int. J. Clin. Exp. Pathol.* **2014**, *7*, 5717–5724. [PubMed]

125. Brar, V.S.; Sharma, R.K.; Murthy, R.K.; Chalam, K.V. Bevacizumab neutralizes the protective effect of vascular endothelial growth factor on retinal ganglion cells. *Mol. Vis.* **2010**, *16*, 1848–1853. [PubMed]

126. Lee, W.J.; Kim, Y.K.; Kim, Y.W.; Jeoung, J.W.; Kim, S.H.; Heo, J.W.; Yu, H.G.; Park, K.H. Rate of macular ganglion cell-inner plexiform layer thinning in glaucomatous eyes with vascular endothelial growth factor inhibition. *J. Glaucoma* **2017**, *26*, 980–986. [CrossRef] [PubMed]

127. Sisk, D.R.; Kuwabara, T. Histologic changes in the inner retina of albino rats following intravitreal injection of monosodium L-glutamate. *Graefes Arch. Clin. Exp. Ophthalmol.* **1985**, *223*, 250–258. [CrossRef]

128. Sucher, N.J.; Lipton, S.A.; Dreyer, E.B. Molecular basis of glutamate toxicity in retinal ganglion cells. *Vis. Res.* **1997**, *37*, 3483–3493. [CrossRef]

129. Vorwerk, C.K.; Lipton, S.A.; Zurakowski, D.; Hyman, B.T.; Sabel, B.A.; Dreyer, E.B. Chronic low-dose glutamate is toxic to retinal ganglion cells. Toxicity blocked by memantine. *Investig. Ophthalmol. Vis. Sci.* **1996**, *37*, 1618–1624.

130. Dreyer, E.B.; Zurakowski, D.; Schumer, R.A.; Podos, S.M.; Lipton, S.A. Elevated glutamate levels in the vitreous body of humans and monkeys with glaucoma. *Arch. Ophthalmol.* **1996**, *114*, 299–305. [CrossRef]

131. Brooks, D.E.; Garcia, G.A.; Dreyer, E.B.; Zurakowski, D.; Franco-Bourland, R.E. Vitreous body glutamate concentration in dogs with glaucoma. *Am. J. Vet. Res.* **1997**, *58*, 864–867.

132. Chaudhary, P.; Ahmed, F.; Sharma, S.C. MK801-a neuroprotectant in rat hypertensive eyes. *Brain Res.* **1998**, *792*, 154–158. [CrossRef]

133. Guo, L.; Salt, T.E.; Maass, A.; Luong, V.; Moss, S.E.; Fitzke, F.W.; Cordeiro, M.F. Assessment of neuroprotective effects of glutamate modulation on glaucoma-related retinal ganglion cell apoptosis in vivo. *Investig. Ophthalmol. Vis. Sci.* **2006**, *47*, 626–633. [CrossRef] [PubMed]

134. Lipton, S.A. Prospects for clinically tolerated NMDA antagonists: Open-channel blockers and alternative redox states of nitric oxide. *Trends Neurosci.* **1993**, *16*, 527–532. [CrossRef]

135. Lagreze, W.A.; Knorle, R.; Bach, M.; Feuerstein, T.J. Memantine is neuroprotective in a rat model of pressure-induced retinal ischemia. *Investig. Ophthalmol. Vis. Sci.* **1998**, *39*, 1063–1066.

136. Hare, W.A.; WoldeMussie, E.; Lai, R.K.; Ton, H.; Ruiz, G.; Chun, T.; Wheeler, L. Efficacy and safety of memantine treatment for reduction of changes associated with experimental glaucoma in monkey, I: Functional measures. *Investig. Ophthalmol. Vis. Sci.* **2004**, *45*, 2625–2639. [CrossRef] [PubMed]

137. Danesh-Meyer, H.V.; Levin, L.A. Neuroprotection: Extrapolating from neurologic diseases to the eye. *Am. J. Ophthalmol.* **2009**, *148*, 186–191.e2. [CrossRef] [PubMed]

138. Wheeler, L.A.; Gil, D.W.; WoldeMussie, E. Role of alpha-2 adrenergic receptors in neuroprotection and glaucoma. *Surv. Ophthalmol.* **2001**, *45* (Suppl. 3), S290–S294, discussion S295–S296. [CrossRef]

139. Hernandez, M.; Urcola, J.H.; Vecino, E. Retinal ganglion cell neuroprotection in a rat model of glaucoma following brimonidine, latanoprost or combined treatments. *Exp. Eye Res.* **2008**, *86*, 798–806. [CrossRef]

140. Pinar-Sueiro, S.; Urcola, H.; Rivas, M.A.; Vecino, E. Prevention of retinal ganglion cell swelling by systemic brimonidine in a rat experimental glaucoma model. *Clin. Exp. Ophthalmol.* **2011**, *39*, 799–807. [CrossRef]

141. Ahmed, F.A.; Hegazy, K.; Chaudhary, P.; Sharma, S.C. Neuroprotective effect of alpha(2) agonist (brimonidine) on adult rat retinal ganglion cells after increased intraocular pressure. *Brain Res.* **2001**, *913*, 133–139. [CrossRef]

142. Yoles, E.; Wheeler, L.A.; Schwartz, M. Alpha2-adrenoreceptor agonists are neuroprotective in a rat model of optic nerve degeneration. *Investig. Ophthalmol. Vis. Sci.* **1999**, *40*, 65–73.

143. Donello, J.E.; Padillo, E.U.; Webster, M.L.; Wheeler, L.A.; Gil, D.W. alpha(2)-Adrenoceptor agonists inhibit vitreal glutamate and aspartate accumulation and preserve retinal function after transient ischemia. *J. Pharmacol. Exp. Ther.* **2001**, *296*, 216–223. [PubMed]

144. Kalapesi, F.B.; Coroneo, M.T.; Hill, M.A. Human ganglion cells express the alpha-2 adrenergic receptor: Relevance to neuroprotection. *Br. J. Ophthalmol.* **2005**, *89*, 758–763. [CrossRef] [PubMed]

145. Aung, T.; Oen, F.T.; Wong, H.T.; Chan, Y.H.; Khoo, B.K.; Liu, Y.P.; Ho, C.L.; See, J.; Thean, L.H.; Viswanathan, A.C.; et al. Randomised controlled trial comparing the effect of brimonidine and timolol on visual field loss after acute primary angle closure. *Br. J. Ophthalmol.* **2004**, *88*, 88–94. [CrossRef] [PubMed]

146. Lambert, W.S.; Ruiz, L.; Crish, S.D.; Wheeler, L.A.; Calkins, D.J. Brimonidine prevents axonal and somatic degeneration of retinal ganglion cell neurons. *Mol. Neurodegener.* **2011**, *6*, 4. [CrossRef]

147. Tsai, J.C.; Chang, H.W. Comparison of the effects of brimonidine 0.2% and timolol 0.5% on retinal nerve fiber layer thickness in ocular hypertensive patients: A prospective, unmasked study. *J. Ocul. Pharmacol. Ther.* **2005**, *21*, 475–482. [CrossRef]

148. Doozandeh, A.; Yazdani, S. Neuroprotection in glaucoma. *J. Ophthalmic Vis. Res.* **2016**, *11*, 209–220. [CrossRef]
149. Crish, S.D.; Calkins, D.J. Neurodegeneration in glaucoma: Progression and calcium-dependent intracellular mechanisms. *Neuroscience* **2011**, *176*, 1–11. [CrossRef]
150. Stout, A.K.; Raphael, H.M.; Kanterewicz, B.I.; Klann, E.; Reynolds, I.J. Glutamate-induced neuron death requires mitochondrial calcium uptake. *Nat. Neurosci.* **1998**, *1*, 366–373. [CrossRef]
151. Osborne, N.N.; Wood, J.P.; Cupido, A.; Melena, J.; Chidlow, G. Topical flunarizine reduces IOP and protects the retina against ischemia-excitotoxicity. *Investig. Ophthalmol. Vis. Sci.* **2002**, *43*, 1456–1464.
152. Yamada, H.; Chen, Y.N.; Aihara, M.; Araie, M. Neuroprotective effect of calcium channel blocker against retinal ganglion cell damage under hypoxia. *Brain Res.* **2006**, *1071*, 75–80. [CrossRef]
153. Koseki, N.; Araie, M.; Tomidokoro, A.; Nagahara, M.; Hasegawa, T.; Tamaki, Y.; Yamamoto, S. A placebo-controlled 3-year study of a calcium blocker on visual field and ocular circulation in glaucoma with low-normal pressure. *Ophthalmology* **2008**, *115*, 2049–2057. [CrossRef] [PubMed]
154. Mayama, C. Calcium channels and their blockers in intraocular pressure and glaucoma. *Eur. J. Pharmacol.* **2014**, *739*, 96–105. [CrossRef] [PubMed]
155. Izzotti, A.; Bagnis, A.; Sacca, S.C. The role of oxidative stress in glaucoma. *Mutat. Res.* **2006**, *612*, 105–114. [CrossRef] [PubMed]
156. Geiger, L.K.; Kortuem, K.R.; Alexejun, C.; Levin, L.A. Reduced redox state allows prolonged survival of axotomized neonatal retinal ganglion cells. *Neuroscience* **2002**, *109*, 635–642. [CrossRef]
157. Caprioli, J.; Munemasa, Y.; Kwong, J.M.; Piri, N. Overexpression of thioredoxins 1 and 2 increases retinal ganglion cell survival after pharmacologically induced oxidative stress, optic nerve transection, and in experimental glaucoma. *Trans. Am. Ophthalmol. Soc.* **2009**, *107*, 161–165.
158. Swanson, K.I.; Schlieve, C.R.; Lieven, C.J.; Levin, L.A. Neuroprotective effect of sulfhydryl reduction in a rat optic nerve crush model. *Investig. Ophthalmol. Vis. Sci.* **2005**, *46*, 3737–3741. [CrossRef]
159. Nucci, C.; Tartaglione, R.; Cerulli, A.; Mancino, R.; Spano, A.; Cavaliere, F.; Rombola, L.; Bagetta, G.; Corasaniti, M.T.; Morrone, L.A. Retinal damage caused by high intraocular pressure-induced transient ischemia is prevented by coenzyme Q10 in rat. *Int. Rev. Neurobiol.* **2007**, *82*, 397–406. [CrossRef]
160. Russo, R.; Cavaliere, F.; Rombola, L.; Gliozzi, M.; Cerulli, A.; Nucci, C.; Fazzi, E.; Bagetta, G.; Corasaniti, M.T.; Morrone, L.A. Rational basis for the development of coenzyme Q10 as a neurotherapeutic agent for retinal protection. *Prog. Brain Res.* **2008**, *173*, 575–582. [CrossRef]
161. Nakajima, Y.; Inokuchi, Y.; Nishi, M.; Shimazawa, M.; Otsubo, K.; Hara, H. Coenzyme Q10 protects retinal cells against oxidative stress in vitro and in vivo. *Brain Res.* **2008**, *1226*, 226–233. [CrossRef]
162. Pinar-Sueiro, S.; Martinez-Fernandez, R.; Lage-Medina, S.; Aldamiz-Echevarria, L.; Vecino, E. Optic neuropathy in methylmalonic acidemia: The role of neuroprotection. *J. Inherit. Metab. Dis.* **2010**, *33* (Suppl. 3), S199–S203. [CrossRef]
163. Gherghel, D.; Griffiths, H.R.; Hilton, E.J.; Cunliffe, I.A.; Hosking, S.L. Systemic reduction in glutathione levels occurs in patients with primary open-angle glaucoma. *Investig. Ophthalmol. Vis. Sci.* **2005**, *46*, 877–883. [CrossRef]
164. Aydemir, O.; Naziroglu, M.; Celebi, S.; Yilmaz, T.; Kukner, A.S. Antioxidant effects of alpha-, gamma- and succinate-tocopherols in guinea pig retina during ischemia-reperfusion injury. *Pathophysiol. Off. J. Int. Soc. Pathophysiol.* **2004**, *11*, 167–171. [CrossRef]
165. Dilsiz, N.; Sahaboglu, A.; Yildiz, M.Z.; Reichenbach, A. Protective effects of various antioxidants during ischemia-reperfusion in the rat retina. *Graefes Arch. Clin. Exp. Ophthalmol.* **2006**, *244*, 627–633. [CrossRef]
166. Ko, M.L.; Peng, P.H.; Hsu, S.Y.; Chen, C.F. Dietary deficiency of vitamin E aggravates retinal ganglion cell death in experimental glaucoma of rats. *Curr. Eye Res.* **2010**, *35*, 842–849. [CrossRef] [PubMed]
167. Liu, L.; Sun, Q.; Wang, R.; Chen, Z.; Wu, J.; Xia, F.; Fan, X.Q. Methane attenuates retinal ischemia/reperfusion injury via anti-oxidative and anti-apoptotic pathways. *Brain Res.* **2016**, *1646*, 327–333. [CrossRef] [PubMed]
168. Schultz, R.; Witte, O.W.; Schmeer, C. Increased frataxin levels protect retinal ganglion cells after acute ischemia/reperfusion in the mouse retina in vivo. *Investig. Ophthalmol. Vis. Sci.* **2016**, *57*, 4115–4124. [CrossRef] [PubMed]
169. Chen, L.; Qi, Y.; Yang, X. Neuroprotective effects of crocin against oxidative stress induced by ischemia/reperfusion injury in rat retina. *Ophthalmic Res.* **2015**, *54*, 157–168. [CrossRef]
170. Nebbioso, M.; Scarsella, G.; Tafani, M.; Pescosolido, N. Mechanisms of ocular neuroprotection by antioxidant molecules in animal models. *J. Biol. Regul. Homeost. Agents* **2013**, *27*, 197–209.

171. Jiang, W.; Tang, L.; Zeng, J.; Chen, B. Adeno-associated virus mediated SOD gene therapy protects the retinal ganglion cells from chronic intraocular pressure elevation induced injury via attenuating oxidative stress and improving mitochondrial dysfunction in a rat model. *Am. J. Transl. Res.* **2016**, *8*, 799–810.

172. Park, S.H.; Kim, J.H.; Kim, Y.H.; Park, C.K. Expression of neuronal nitric oxide synthase in the retina of a rat model of chronic glaucoma. *Vis. Res.* **2007**, *47*, 2732–2740. [CrossRef]

173. Aslan, M.; Cort, A.; Yucel, I. Oxidative and nitrative stress markers in glaucoma. *Free Radic. Biol. Med.* **2008**, *45*, 367–376. [CrossRef] [PubMed]

174. Siu, A.W.; Leung, M.C.; To, C.H.; Siu, F.K.; Ji, J.Z.; So, K.F. Total retinal nitric oxide production is increased in intraocular pressure-elevated rats. *Exp. Eye Res.* **2002**, *75*, 401–406. [CrossRef] [PubMed]

175. Shareef, S.; Sawada, A.; Neufeld, A.H. Isoforms of nitric oxide synthase in the optic nerves of rat eyes with chronic moderately elevated intraocular pressure. *Investig. Ophthalmol. Vis. Sci.* **1999**, *40*, 2884–2891.

176. Hangai, M.; Yoshimura, N.; Hiroi, K.; Mandai, M.; Honda, Y. Inducible nitric oxide synthase in retinal ischemia-reperfusion injury. *Exp. Eye Res.* **1996**, *63*, 501–509. [CrossRef] [PubMed]

177. Neufeld, A.H.; Kawai, S.; Das, S.; Vora, S.; Gachie, E.; Connor, J.R.; Manning, P.T. Loss of retinal ganglion cells following retinal ischemia: The role of inducible nitric oxide synthase. *Exp. Eye Res.* **2002**, *75*, 521–528. [CrossRef] [PubMed]

178. Liu, B.; Neufeld, A.H. Expression of nitric oxide synthase-2 (NOS-2) in reactive astrocytes of the human glaucomatous optic nerve head. *Glia* **2000**, *30*, 178–186. [CrossRef]

179. Neufeld, A.H.; Hernandez, M.R.; Gonzalez, M. Nitric oxide synthase in the human glaucomatous optic nerve head. *Arch. Ophthalmol.* **1997**, *115*, 497–503. [CrossRef]

180. Neufeld, A.H.; Sawada, A.; Becker, B. Inhibition of nitric-oxide synthase 2 by aminoguanidine provides neuroprotection of retinal ganglion cells in a rat model of chronic glaucoma. *Proc. Natl. Acad. Sci. USA* **1999**, *96*, 9944–9948. [CrossRef]

181. Geyer, O.; Almog, J.; Lupu-Meiri, M.; Lazar, M.; Oron, Y. Nitric oxide synthase inhibitors protect rat retina against ischemic injury. *FEBS Lett.* **1995**, *374*, 399–402. [CrossRef]

182. Libby, R.T.; Howell, G.R.; Pang, I.H.; Savinova, O.V.; Mehalow, A.K.; Barter, J.W.; Smith, R.S.; Clark, A.F.; John, S.W. Inducible nitric oxide synthase, Nos2, does not mediate optic neuropathy and retinopathy in the DBA/2J glaucoma model. *BMC Neurosci.* **2007**, *8*, 108. [CrossRef]

183. Pang, I.H.; Johnson, E.C.; Jia, L.; Cepurna, W.O.; Shepard, A.R.; Hellberg, M.R.; Clark, A.F.; Morrison, J.C. Evaluation of inducible nitric oxide synthase in glaucomatous optic neuropathy and pressure-induced optic nerve damage. *Investig. Ophthalmol. Vis. Sci.* **2005**, *46*, 1313–1321. [CrossRef] [PubMed]

184. Oku, H.; Goto, W.; Kobayashi, T.; Okuno, T.; Hirao, M.; Sugiyama, T.; Yoneda, S.; Hara, H.; Ikeda, T. Adenosine protects cultured retinal neurons against NMDA-induced cell death through A1 receptors. *Curr. Eye Res.* **2004**, *29*, 449–455. [CrossRef] [PubMed]

185. Sun, X.; Barnes, S.; Baldridge, W.H. Adenosine inhibits calcium channel currents via A1 receptors on salamander retinal ganglion cells in a mini-slice preparation. *J. Neurochem.* **2002**, *81*, 550–556. [CrossRef] [PubMed]

186. Larsen, A.K.; Osborne, N.N. Involvement of adenosine in retinal ischemia. Studies on the rat. *Investig. Ophthalmol. Vis. Sci.* **1996**, *37*, 2603–2611.

187. Perigolo-Vicente, R.; Ritt, K.; Pereira, M.R.; Torres, P.M.; Paes-de-Carvalho, R.; Giestal-de-Araujo, E. IL-6 treatment increases the survival of retinal ganglion cells in vitro: The role of adenosine A1 receptor. *Biochem. Biophys. Res. Commun.* **2013**, *430*, 512–518. [CrossRef]

188. Mendonca Torres, P.M.; de Araujo, E.G. Interleukin-6 increases the survival of retinal ganglion cells in vitro. *J. Neuroimmunol.* **2001**, *117*, 43–50. [CrossRef]

189. Sappington, R.M.; Chan, M.; Calkins, D.J. Interleukin-6 protects retinal ganglion cells from pressure-induced death. *Investig. Ophthalmol. Vis. Sci.* **2006**, *47*, 2932–2942. [CrossRef]

190. Murphy, P.G.; Borthwick, L.A.; Altares, M.; Gauldie, J.; Kaplan, D.; Richardson, P.M. Reciprocal actions of interleukin-6 and brain-derived neurotrophic factor on rat and mouse primary sensory neurons. *Eur. J. Neurosci.* **2000**, *12*, 1891–1899. [CrossRef]

191. Mailavaram, R.P.; Al-Attraqchi, O.H.A.; Kar, S.; Ghosh, S. Current status in the design and development of agonists and antagonists of adenosine A3 receptor as potential therapeutic agents. *Curr. Pharm. Des.* **2019**, *25*, 2772–2787. [CrossRef]

192. Zhang, M.; Budak, M.T.; Lu, W.; Khurana, T.S.; Zhang, X.; Laties, A.M.; Mitchell, C.H. Identification of the A3 adenosine receptor in rat retinal ganglion cells. *Mol. Vis.* **2006**, *12*, 937–948.

193. Hu, H.; Lu, W.; Zhang, M.; Zhang, X.; Argall, A.J.; Patel, S.; Lee, G.E.; Kim, Y.C.; Jacobson, K.A.; Laties, A.M.; et al. Stimulation of the P2X7 receptor kills rat retinal ganglion cells in vivo. *Exp. Eye Res.* **2010**, *91*, 425–432. [CrossRef] [PubMed]

194. Zhang, X.; Zhang, M.; Laties, A.M.; Mitchell, C.H. Balance of purines may determine life or death of retinal ganglion cells as A3 adenosine receptors prevent loss following P2X7 receptor stimulation. *J. Neurochem.* **2006**, *98*, 566–575. [CrossRef] [PubMed]

195. Zhang, M.; Hu, H.; Zhang, X.; Lu, W.; Lim, J.; Eysteinsson, T.; Jacobson, K.A.; Laties, A.M.; Mitchell, C.H. The A3 adenosine receptor attenuates the calcium rise triggered by NMDA receptors in retinal ganglion cells. *Neurochem. Int.* **2010**, *56*, 35–41. [CrossRef] [PubMed]

196. Nakashima, K.I.; Iwao, K.; Inoue, T.; Haga, A.; Tsutsumi, T.; Mochita, M.I.; Fujimoto, T.; Tanihara, H. Stimulation of the adenosine A3 receptor, not the A1 or A2 receptors, promote neurite outgrowth of retinal ganglion cells. *Exp. Eye Res.* **2018**, *170*, 160–168. [CrossRef]

197. Galvao, J.; Elvas, F.; Martins, T.; Cordeiro, M.F.; Ambrosio, A.F.; Santiago, A.R. Adenosine A3 receptor activation is neuroprotective against retinal neurodegeneration. *Exp. Eye Res.* **2015**, *140*, 65–74. [CrossRef]

198. Cen, L.P.; Ng, T.K. Stem cell therapy for retinal ganglion cell degeneration. *Neural Regen. Res.* **2018**, *13*, 1352–1353. [CrossRef]

199. Bennicelli, J.L.; Bennett, J. Stem cells set their sights on retinitis pigmentosa. *eLife* **2013**, *2*, e01291. [CrossRef]

200. Siqueira, R.C. Stem cell therapy for retinal diseases: Update. *Stem Cell Res. Ther.* **2011**, *2*, 50. [CrossRef]

201. Zarbin, M. Cell-based therapy for degenerative retinal disease. *Trends Mol. Med.* **2016**, *22*, 115–134. [CrossRef]

202. Eiraku, M.; Takata, N.; Ishibashi, H.; Kawada, M.; Sakakura, E.; Okuda, S.; Sekiguchi, K.; Adachi, T.; Sasai, Y. Self-organizing optic-cup morphogenesis in three-dimensional culture. *Nature* **2011**, *472*, 51–56. [CrossRef]

203. Nakano, T.; Ando, S.; Takata, N.; Kawada, M.; Muguruma, K.; Sekiguchi, K.; Saito, K.; Yonemura, S.; Eiraku, M.; Sasai, Y. Self-formation of optic cups and storable stratified neural retina from human ESCs. *Cell Stem Cell* **2012**, *10*, 771–785. [CrossRef] [PubMed]

204. Eiraku, M.; Sasai, Y. Mouse embryonic stem cell culture for generation of three-dimensional retinal and cortical tissues. *Nat. Protoc.* **2011**, *7*, 69–79. [CrossRef] [PubMed]

205. Mead, B.; Berry, M.; Logan, A.; Scott, R.A.; Leadbeater, W.; Scheven, B.A. Stem cell treatment of degenerative eye disease. *Stem Cell Res.* **2015**, *14*, 243–257. [CrossRef] [PubMed]

206. Hankin, M.H.; Lund, R.D. Directed early axonal outgrowth from retinal transplants into host rat brains. *J. Neurobiol.* **1990**, *21*, 1202–1218. [CrossRef] [PubMed]

207. Lund, R.D.; Hankin, M.H. Pathfinding by retinal ganglion cell axons: Transplantation studies in genetically and surgically blind mice. *J. Comp. Neurol.* **1995**, *356*, 481–489. [CrossRef]

208. Hertz, J.; Qu, B.; Hu, Y.; Patel, R.D.; Valenzuela, D.A.; Goldberg, J.L. Survival and integration of developing and progenitor-derived retinal ganglion cells following transplantation. *Cell Transplant.* **2014**, *23*, 855–872. [CrossRef]

209. Venugopalan, P.; Wang, Y.; Nguyen, T.; Huang, A.; Muller, K.J.; Goldberg, J.L. Transplanted neurons integrate into adult retinas and respond to light. *Nat. Commun.* **2016**, *7*, 10472. [CrossRef]

210. Tang, R.; Jing, L.; Willard, V.P.; Wu, C.L.; Guilak, F.; Chen, J.; Setton, L.A. Differentiation of human induced pluripotent stem cells into nucleus pulposus-like cells. *Stem Cell Res. Ther.* **2018**, *9*, 61. [CrossRef]

211. Razavi, S.; Razavi, M.R.; Zarkesh Esfahani, H.; Kazemi, M.; Mostafavi, F.S. Comparing brain-derived neurotrophic factor and ciliary neurotrophic factor secretion of induced neurotrophic factor secreting cells from human adipose and bone marrow-derived stem cells. *Dev. Growth Differ.* **2013**, *55*, 648–655. [CrossRef]

212. Hu, Y.; Tan, H.B.; Wang, X.M.; Rong, H.; Cui, H.P.; Cui, H. Bone marrow mesenchymal stem cells protect against retinal ganglion cell loss in aged rats with glaucoma. *Clin. Interv. Aging* **2013**, *8*, 1467–1470. [CrossRef]

213. Osborne, A.; Sanderson, J.; Martin, K.R. Neuroprotective Effects of Human Mesenchymal Stem Cells and Platelet-Derived Growth Factor on Human Retinal Ganglion Cells. *Stem Cells* **2018**, *36*, 65–78. [CrossRef]

214. Mead, B.; Amaral, J.; Tomarev, S. Mesenchymal stem cell-derived small extracellular vesicles promote neuroprotection in rodent models of glaucoma. *Investig. Ophthalmol. Vis. Sci.* **2018**, *59*, 702–714. [CrossRef]

215. Sochocka, M.; Diniz, B.S.; Leszek, J. Inflammatory response in the CNS: Friend or foe? *Mol. Neurobiol.* **2017**, *54*, 8071–8089. [CrossRef]

216. Kreutzberg, G.W. Microglia: A sensor for pathological events in the CNS. *Trends Neurosci.* **1996**, *19*, 312–318. [CrossRef]

217. O'Callaghan, J.P.; Sriram, K. Glial fibrillary acidic protein and related glial proteins as biomarkers of neurotoxicity. *Expert Opin. Drug Saf.* **2005**, *4*, 433–442. [CrossRef]

218. Silverman, S.M.; Wong, W.T. Microglia in the retina: Roles in development, maturity, and disease. *Ann. Rev. Vis. Sci.* **2018**, *4*, 45–77. [CrossRef]

219. Karlstetter, M.; Ebert, S.; Langmann, T. Microglia in the healthy and degenerating retina: Insights from novel mouse models. *Immunobiology* **2010**, *215*, 685–691. [CrossRef]

220. Karlstetter, M.; Langmann, T. Microglia in the aging retina. *Adv. Exp. Med. Biol.* **2014**, *801*, 207–212. [CrossRef]

221. Rashid, K.; Akhtar-Schaefer, I.; Langmann, T. Microglia in retinal degeneration. *Front. Immunol.* **2019**, *10*, 1975. [CrossRef]

222. Takeda, A.; Shinozaki, Y.; Kashiwagi, K.; Ohno, N.; Eto, K.; Wake, H.; Nabekura, J.; Koizumi, S. Microglia mediate non-cell-autonomous cell death of retinal ganglion cells. *Glia* **2018**, *66*, 2366–2384. [CrossRef]

223. Ullian, E.M.; Barkis, W.B.; Chen, S.; Diamond, J.S.; Barres, B.A. Invulnerability of retinal ganglion cells to NMDA excitotoxicity. *Mol. Cell. Neurosci.* **2004**, *26*, 544–557. [CrossRef]

224. Neufeld, A.H. Microglia in the optic nerve head and the region of parapapillary chorioretinal atrophy in glaucoma. *Arch. Ophthalmol.* **1999**, *117*, 1050–1056. [CrossRef]

225. Yuan, L.; Neufeld, A.H. Activated microglia in the human glaucomatous optic nerve head. *J. Neurosci. Res.* **2001**, *64*, 523–532. [CrossRef]

226. Bosco, A.; Steele, M.R.; Vetter, M.L. Early microglia activation in a mouse model of chronic glaucoma. *J. Comp. Neurol.* **2011**, *519*, 599–620. [CrossRef]

227. Bosco, A.; Romero, C.O.; Breen, K.T.; Chagovetz, A.A.; Steele, M.R.; Ambati, B.K.; Vetter, M.L. Neurodegeneration severity can be predicted from early microglia alterations monitored in vivo in a mouse model of chronic glaucoma. *Dis. Models Mech.* **2015**, *8*, 443–455. [CrossRef]

228. Madeira, M.H.; Boia, R.; Elvas, F.; Martins, T.; Cunha, R.A.; Ambrosio, A.F.; Santiago, A.R. Selective A2A receptor antagonist prevents microglia-mediated neuroinflammation and protects retinal ganglion cells from high intraocular pressure-induced transient ischemic injury. *Transl. Res. J. Lab. Clin. Med.* **2016**, *169*, 112–128. [CrossRef]

229. Cho, K.J.; Kim, J.H.; Park, H.Y.; Park, C.K. Glial cell response and iNOS expression in the optic nerve head and retina of the rat following acute high IOP ischemia-reperfusion. *Brain Res.* **2011**, *1403*, 67–77. [CrossRef]

230. Madeira, M.H.; Ortin-Martinez, A.; Nadal-Nicolas, F.; Ambrosio, A.F.; Vidal-Sanz, M.; Agudo-Barriuso, M.; Santiago, A.R. Caffeine administration prevents retinal neuroinflammation and loss of retinal ganglion cells in an animal model of glaucoma. *Sci. Rep.* **2016**, *6*, 27532. [CrossRef]

231. Rodrigues-Neves, A.C.; Aires, I.D.; Vindeirinho, J.; Boia, R.; Madeira, M.H.; Goncalves, F.Q.; Cunha, R.A.; Santos, P.F.; Ambrosio, A.F.; Santiago, A.R. Elevated Pressure Changes the Purinergic System of Microglial Cells. *Front. Pharmacol.* **2018**, *9*, 16. [CrossRef]

232. Davalos, D.; Grutzendler, J.; Yang, G.; Kim, J.V.; Zuo, Y.; Jung, S.; Littman, D.R.; Dustin, M.L.; Gan, W.B. ATP mediates rapid microglial response to local brain injury in vivo. *Nat. Neurosci.* **2005**, *8*, 752–758. [CrossRef]

233. Santiago, A.R.; Baptista, F.I.; Santos, P.F.; Cristovao, G.; Ambrosio, A.F.; Cunha, R.A.; Gomes, C.A. Role of microglia adenosine A(2A) receptors in retinal and brain neurodegenerative diseases. *Mediat. Inflamm.* **2014**, *2014*, 465694. [CrossRef]

234. Boia, R.; Elvas, F.; Madeira, M.H.; Aires, I.D.; Rodrigues-Neves, A.C.; Tralhao, P.; Szabo, E.C.; Baqi, Y.; Muller, C.E.; Tome, A.R.; et al. Treatment with A2A receptor antagonist KW6002 and caffeine intake regulate microglia reactivity and protect retina against transient ischemic damage. *Cell Death Dis.* **2017**, *8*, e3065. [CrossRef]

235. Boia, R.; Ambrosio, A.F.; Santiago, A.R. Therapeutic opportunities for caffeine and A2A receptor antagonists in retinal diseases. *Ophthalmic Res.* **2016**, *55*, 212–218. [CrossRef]

236. Tezel, G. TNF-alpha signaling in glaucomatous neurodegeneration. *Prog. Brain Res.* **2008**, *173*, 409–421. [CrossRef]

237. Yuan, L.; Neufeld, A.H. Tumor necrosis factor-alpha: A potentially neurodestructive cytokine produced by glia in the human glaucomatous optic nerve head. *Glia* **2000**, *32*, 42–50. [CrossRef]

238. Roh, M.; Zhang, Y.; Murakami, Y.; Thanos, A.; Lee, S.C.; Vavvas, D.G.; Benowitz, L.I.; Miller, J.W. Etanercept, a widely used inhibitor of tumor necrosis factor-alpha (TNF-alpha), prevents retinal ganglion cell loss in a rat model of glaucoma. *PLoS ONE* **2012**, *7*, e40065. [CrossRef]

239. Zhang, Y.; Xu, Y.; Sun, Q.; Xue, S.; Guan, H.; Ji, M. Activation of P2X7R- NLRP3 pathway in Retinal microglia contribute to Retinal Ganglion Cells death in chronic ocular hypertension (COH). *Exp. Eye Res.* **2019**, *188*, 107771. [CrossRef]

240. Fernandez-Albarral, J.A.; Ramirez, A.I.; de Hoz, R.; Lopez-Villarin, N.; Salobrar-Garcia, E.; Lopez-Cuenca, I.; Licastro, E.; Inarejos-Garcia, A.M.; Almodovar, P.; Pinazo-Duran, M.D.; et al. Neuroprotective and Anti-Inflammatory Effects of a Hydrophilic Saffron Extract in a Model of Glaucoma. *Int. J. Mol. Sci.* **2019**, *20*, 4110. [CrossRef]

241. Howell, G.R.; Macalinao, D.G.; Sousa, G.L.; Walden, M.; Soto, I.; Kneeland, S.C.; Barbay, J.M.; King, B.L.; Marchant, J.K.; Hibbs, M.; et al. Molecular clustering identifies complement and endothelin induction as early events in a mouse model of glaucoma. *J. Clin. Investig.* **2011**, *121*, 1429–1444. [CrossRef]

242. Mirzaei, M.; Gupta, V.B.; Chick, J.M.; Greco, T.M.; Wu, Y.; Chitranshi, N.; Wall, R.V.; Hone, E.; Deng, L.; Dheer, Y.; et al. Age-related neurodegenerative disease associated pathways identified in retinal and vitreous proteome from human glaucoma eyes. *Sci. Rep.* **2017**, *7*, 12685. [CrossRef]

243. Tezel, G.; Yang, X.; Luo, C.; Kain, A.D.; Powell, D.W.; Kuehn, M.H.; Kaplan, H.J. Oxidative stress and the regulation of complement activation in human glaucoma. *Investig. Ophthalmol. Vis. Sci.* **2010**, *51*, 5071–5082. [CrossRef]

244. Tyler, C.M.; Boulanger, L.M. Complement-mediated microglial clearance of developing retinal ganglion cell axons. *Neuron* **2012**, *74*, 597–599. [CrossRef]

245. Schafer, D.P.; Lehrman, E.K.; Kautzman, A.G.; Koyama, R.; Mardinly, A.R.; Yamasaki, R.; Ransohoff, R.M.; Greenberg, M.E.; Barres, B.A.; Stevens, B. Microglia sculpt postnatal neural circuits in an activity and complement-dependent manner. *Neuron* **2012**, *74*, 691–705. [CrossRef]

246. Rosen, A.M.; Stevens, B. The role of the classical complement cascade in synapse loss during development and glaucoma. *Adv. Exp. Med. Biol.* **2010**, *703*, 75–93. [CrossRef]

247. Wang, K.; Peng, B.; Lin, B. Fractalkine receptor regulates microglial neurotoxicity in an experimental mouse glaucoma model. *Glia* **2014**, *62*, 1943–1954. [CrossRef]

248. Breen, K.T.; Anderson, S.R.; Steele, M.R.; Calkins, D.J.; Bosco, A.; Vetter, M.L. Loss of fractalkine signaling exacerbates axon transport dysfunction in a chronic model of glaucoma. *Front. Neurosci.* **2016**, *10*, 526. [CrossRef]

249. Bosco, A.; Inman, D.M.; Steele, M.R.; Wu, G.; Soto, I.; Marsh-Armstrong, N.; Hubbard, W.C.; Calkins, D.J.; Horner, P.J.; Vetter, M.L. Reduced retina microglial activation and improved optic nerve integrity with minocycline treatment in the DBA/2J mouse model of glaucoma. *Investig. Ophthalmol. Vis. Sci.* **2008**, *49*, 1437–1446. [CrossRef]

250. Vecino, E.; Rodriguez, F.D.; Ruzafa, N.; Pereiro, X.; Sharma, S.C. Glia-neuron interactions in the mammalian retina. *Prog. Retin. Eye Res.* **2016**, *51*, 1–40. [CrossRef]

251. Ruzafa, N.; Vecino, E. Effect of Muller cells on the survival and neuritogenesis in retinal ganglion cells. *Arch. Soc. Esp. Oftalmol.* **2015**, *90*, 522–526. [CrossRef]

252. Ruzafa, N.; Pereiro, X.; Lepper, M.F.; Hauck, S.M.; Vecino, E. A proteomics approach to identify candidate proteins secreted by muller glia that protect ganglion cells in the retina. *Proteomics* **2018**, *18*, e1700321. [CrossRef]

253. Bringmann, A.; Pannicke, T.; Biedermann, B.; Francke, M.; Iandiev, I.; Grosche, J.; Wiedemann, P.; Albrecht, J.; Reichenbach, A. Role of retinal glial cells in neurotransmitter uptake and metabolism. *Neurochem. Int.* **2009**, *54*, 143–160. [CrossRef]

254. Garcia, M.; Vecino, E. Role of Muller glia in neuroprotection and regeneration in the retina. *Histol. Histopathol.* **2003**, *18*, 1205–1218. [CrossRef]

255. Heidinger, V.; Hicks, D.; Sahel, J.; Dreyfus, H. Ability of retinal Muller glial cells to protect neurons against excitotoxicity in vitro depends upon maturation and neuron-glial interactions. *Glia* **1999**, *25*, 229–239. [CrossRef]

256. Kawasaki, A.; Otori, Y.; Barnstable, C.J. Muller cell protection of rat retinal ganglion cells from glutamate and nitric oxide neurotoxicity. *Investig. Ophthalmol. Vis. Sci.* **2000**, *41*, 3444–3450.

257. Kitano, S.; Morgan, J.; Caprioli, J. Hypoxic and excitotoxic damage to cultured rat retinal ganglion cells. *Exp. Eye Res.* **1996**, *63*, 105–112. [CrossRef]

258. Izumi, Y.; Kirby, C.O.; Benz, A.M.; Olney, J.W.; Zorumski, C.F. Muller cell swelling, glutamate uptake, and excitotoxic neurodegeneration in the isolated rat retina. *Glia* **1999**, *25*, 379–389. [CrossRef]

259. Carter-Dawson, L.; Crawford, M.L.; Harwerth, R.S.; Smith, E.L., 3rd; Feldman, R.; Shen, F.F.; Mitchell, C.K.; Whitetree, A. Vitreal glutamate concentration in monkeys with experimental glaucoma. *Investig. Ophthalmol. Vis. Sci.* **2002**, *43*, 2633–2637.

260. Biedermann, B.; Bringmann, A.; Franze, K.; Faude, F.; Wiedemann, P.; Reichenbach, A. GABA(A) receptors in Muller glial cells of the human retina. *Glia* **2004**, *46*, 302–310. [CrossRef]

261. Hurley, J.B.; Lindsay, K.J.; Du, J. Glucose, lactate, and shuttling of metabolites in vertebrate retinas. *J. Neurosci. Res.* **2015**, *93*, 1079–1092. [CrossRef]

262. Matteucci, A.; Gaddini, L.; Villa, M.; Varano, M.; Parravano, M.; Monteleone, V.; Cavallo, F.; Leo, L.; Mallozzi, C.; Malchiodi-Albedi, F.; et al. Neuroprotection by rat Muller glia against high glucose-induced neurodegeneration through a mechanism involving ERK1/2 activation. *Exp. Eye Res.* **2014**, *125*, 20–29. [CrossRef]

263. Vohra, R.; Kolko, M. Neuroprotection of the inner retina: Muller cells and lactate. *Neural Regen. Res.* **2018**, *13*, 1741–1742. [CrossRef]

264. Eastlake, K.; Luis, J.; Limb, G.A. Potential of muller glia for retina neuroprotection. *Curr. Eye Res.* **2020**, *45*, 339–348. [CrossRef]

265. Reichelt, W.; Stabel-Burow, J.; Pannicke, T.; Weichert, H.; Heinemann, U. The glutathione level of retinal Muller glial cells is dependent on the high-affinity sodium-dependent uptake of glutamate. *Neuroscience* **1997**, *77*, 1213–1224. [CrossRef]

266. Harada, T.; Harada, C.; Nakamura, K.; Quah, H.M.; Okumura, A.; Namekata, K.; Saeki, T.; Aihara, M.; Yoshida, H.; Mitani, A.; et al. The potential role of glutamate transporters in the pathogenesis of normal tension glaucoma. *J. Clin. Investig.* **2007**, *117*, 1763–1770. [CrossRef]

267. Eichler, W.; Savkovic-Cvijic, H.; Burger, S.; Beck, M.; Schmidt, M.; Wiedemann, P.; Reichenbach, A.; Unterlauft, J.D. Muller cell-derived PEDF mediates neuroprotection via STAT3 activation. *Cell. Physiol. Biochem.* **2017**, *44*, 1411–1424. [CrossRef]

268. Taylor, S.; Srinivasan, B.; Wordinger, R.J.; Roque, R.S. Glutamate stimulates neurotrophin expression in cultured Muller cells. *Brain Res. Mol. Brain Res.* **2003**, *111*, 189–197. [CrossRef]

269. Harada, T.; Harada, C.; Nakayama, N.; Okuyama, S.; Yoshida, K.; Kohsaka, S.; Matsuda, H.; Wada, K. Modification of glial-neuronal cell interactions prevents photoreceptor apoptosis during light-induced retinal degeneration. *Neuron* **2000**, *26*, 533–541. [CrossRef]

270. Eastlake, K.; Banerjee, P.J.; Angbohang, A.; Charteris, D.G.; Khaw, P.T.; Limb, G.A. Muller glia as an important source of cytokines and inflammatory factors present in the gliotic retina during proliferative vitreoretinopathy. *Glia* **2016**, *64*, 495–506. [CrossRef]

271. Yoshida, S.; Sotozono, C.; Ikeda, T.; Kinoshita, S. Interleukin-6 (IL-6) production by cytokine-stimulated human Muller cells. *Curr. Eye Res.* **2001**, *22*, 341–347. [CrossRef]

272. Busik, J.V.; Mohr, S.; Grant, M.B. Hyperglycemia-induced reactive oxygen species toxicity to endothelial cells is dependent on paracrine mediators. *Diabetes* **2008**, *57*, 1952–1965. [CrossRef]

273. Mohr, S.; Xi, X.; Tang, J.; Kern, T.S. Caspase activation in retinas of diabetic and galactosemic mice and diabetic patients. *Diabetes* **2002**, *51*, 1172–1179. [CrossRef]

274. Tezel, G.; Wax, M.B. Increased production of tumor necrosis factor-alpha by glial cells exposed to simulated ischemia or elevated hydrostatic pressure induces apoptosis in cocultured retinal ganglion cells. *J. Neurosci. Off. J. Soc. Neurosci.* **2000**, *20*, 8693–8700. [CrossRef]

275. Pereiro, X.; Ruzafa, N.; Acera, A.; Fonollosa, A.; Rodriguez, F.D.; Vecino, E. Dexamethasone protects retinal ganglion cells but not Muller glia against hyperglycemia in vitro. *PLoS ONE* **2018**, *13*, e0207913. [CrossRef]

276. Kumar, A.; Pandey, R.K.; Miller, L.J.; Singh, P.K.; Kanwar, M. Muller glia in retinal innate immunity: A perspective on their roles in endophthalmitis. *Crit. Rev. Immunol.* **2013**, *33*, 119–135. [CrossRef]

277. Zong, H.; Ward, M.; Madden, A.; Yong, P.H.; Limb, G.A.; Curtis, T.M.; Stitt, A.W. Hyperglycaemia-induced pro-inflammatory responses by retinal Muller glia are regulated by the receptor for advanced glycation end-products (RAGE). *Diabetologia* **2010**, *53*, 2656–2666. [CrossRef]

278. Bringmann, A.; Wiedemann, P. Muller glial cells in retinal disease. *Ophthalmologica* **2012**, *227*, 1–19. [CrossRef]

279. Greenberg, M.E.; Xu, B.; Lu, B.; Hempstead, B.L. New insights in the biology of BDNF synthesis and release: Implications in CNS function. *J. Neurosci. Off. J. Soc. Neurosci.* **2009**, *29*, 12764–12767. [CrossRef]

280. Allen, S.J.; Watson, J.J.; Shoemark, D.K.; Barua, N.U.; Patel, N.K. GDNF, NGF and BDNF as therapeutic options for neurodegeneration. *Pharmacol. Ther.* **2013**, *138*, 155–175. [CrossRef]

281. Shruthi, S.; Sumitha, R.; Varghese, A.M.; Ashok, S.; Chandrasekhar Sagar, B.K.; Sathyaprabha, T.N.; Nalini, A.; Kramer, B.W.; Raju, T.R.; Vijayalakshmi, K.; et al. Brain-Derived Neurotrophic Factor Facilitates Functional Recovery from ALS-Cerebral Spinal Fluid-Induced Neurodegenerative Changes in the NSC-34 Motor Neuron Cell Line. *Neuro Degener. Dis.* **2017**, *17*, 44–58. [CrossRef]

282. Ferrari, M.P.; Mantelli, F.; Sacchetti, M.; Antonangeli, M.I.; Cattani, F.; D'Anniballe, G.; Sinigaglia, F.; Ruffini, P.A.; Lambiase, A. Safety and pharmacokinetics of escalating doses of human recombinant nerve growth factor eye drops in a double-masked, randomized clinical trial. *BioDrugs Clin. Immunother. Biopharm. Gene Ther.* **2014**, *28*, 275–283. [CrossRef]

283. Cantor, L.B. Brimonidine in the treatment of glaucoma and ocular hypertension. *Ther. Clin. Risk Manag.* **2006**, *2*, 337–346. [CrossRef]

284. WoldeMussie, E.; Ruiz, G.; Wijono, M.; Wheeler, L.A. Neuroprotection of retinal ganglion cells by brimonidine in rats with laser-induced chronic ocular hypertension. *Investig. Ophthalmol. Vis. Sci.* **2001**, *42*, 2849–2855.

285. Grieb, P. Neuroprotective properties of citicoline: Facts, doubts and unresolved issues. *CNS Drugs* **2014**, *28*, 185–193. [CrossRef]

286. Parisi, V.; Manni, G.; Colacino, G.; Bucci, M.G. Cytidine-5′-diphosphocholine (citicoline) improves retinal and cortical responses in patients with glaucoma. *Ophthalmology* **1999**, *106*, 1126–1134. [CrossRef]

287. Parisi, V.; Oddone, F.; Ziccardi, L.; Roberti, G.; Coppola, G.; Manni, G. Citicoline and retinal ganglion cells: Effects on morphology and function. *Curr. Neuropharmacol.* **2018**, *16*, 919–932. [CrossRef]

288. Parisi, V. Electrophysiological assessment of glaucomatous visual dysfunction during treatment with cytidine-5′-diphosphocholine (citicoline): A study of 8 years of follow-up. *Doc. Ophthalmol. Adv. Ophthalmol.* **2005**, *110*, 91–102. [CrossRef]

289. Weinreb, R.N.; Liebmann, J.M.; Cioffi, G.A.; Goldberg, I.; Brandt, J.D.; Johnson, C.A.; Zangwill, L.M.; Schneider, S.; Badger, H.; Bejanian, M. Oral memantine for the treatment of glaucoma. *Ophthalmology* **2018**, *125*, 1874–1885. [CrossRef]

290. Steigerwalt, R.D., Jr.; Cesarone, M.R.; Pascarella, A.; De Angelis, M.; Nebbioso, M.; Belcaro, G.; Feragalli, B. Ocular and optic nerve ischemia: Recognition and treatment with intravenous prostaglandin E1. *Panminerva Med.* **2011**, *53*, 119–124.

291. Rosenthal, R.; Fromm, M. Endothelin antagonism as an active principle for glaucoma therapy. *Br. J. Pharmacol.* **2011**, *162*, 806–816. [CrossRef]

292. Wang, J.; Chen, S.; Zhang, X.; Huang, W.; Jonas, J.B. Intravitreal triamcinolone acetonide, retinal microglia and retinal ganglion cell apoptosis in the optic nerve crush model. *Acta Ophthalmol.* **2016**, *94*, e305–e311. [CrossRef]

293. Sheng, Y.; Zhu, Y.; Wu, L. Effect of high dosage of methylprednisolone on rat retinal ganglion cell apoptosis after optic nerve crush. *Yan Ke Xue Bao Eye Sci.* **2004**, *20*, 181–186.

294. Rath, E.Z.; Hazan, Z.; Adamsky, K.; Solomon, A.; Segal, Z.I.; Levin, L.A. Randomized controlled phase 2a study of RPh201 in previous nonarteritic anterior ischemic optic neuropathy. *J. Neuroophthalmol.* **2019**, *39*, 291–298. [CrossRef] [PubMed]

295. Shaheer, M.; Amjad, A.; Saleem, Z. Retinal ganglion cell complex changes after intravitreal bevacizumab for diabetic macular edema. *J. Coll. Phys. Surg. Pak. JCPSP* **2019**, *29*, 426–429. [CrossRef] [PubMed]

296. Entezari, M.; Esmaeili, M.; Yaseri, M. A pilot study of the effect of intravenous erythropoietin on improvement of visual function in patients with recent indirect traumatic optic neuropathy. *Graefes Arch. Clin. Exp. Ophthalmol.* **2014**, *252*, 1309–1313. [CrossRef]

297. Kashkouli, M.B.; Pakdel, F.; Sanjari, M.S.; Haghighi, A.; Nojomi, M.; Homaee, M.H.; Heirati, A. Erythropoietin: A novel treatment for traumatic optic neuropathy—A pilot study. *Graefes Arch. Clin. Exp. Ophthalmol.* **2011**, *249*, 731–736. [CrossRef]

298. Kilic, U.; Kilic, E.; Soliz, J.; Bassetti, C.I.; Gassmann, M.; Hermann, D.M. Erythropoietin protects from axotomy-induced degeneration of retinal ganglion cells by activating ERK-1/-2. *FASEB J. Off. Publ. Fed. Am. Soc. Exp. Biol.* **2005**, *19*, 249–251. [CrossRef]

299. Meyerson, C.; Van Stavern, G.; McClelland, C. Leber hereditary optic neuropathy: Current perspectives. *Clin. Ophthalmol.* **2015**, *9*, 1165–1176. [CrossRef]

300. Lyseng-Williamson, K.A. Idebenone: A Review in leber's hereditary optic neuropathy. *Drugs* **2016**, *76*, 805–813. [CrossRef]

301. Kim, S.Y.; Shim, M.S.; Kim, K.Y.; Weinreb, R.N.; Wheeler, L.A.; Ju, W.K. Inhibition of cyclophilin D by cyclosporin A promotes retinal ganglion cell survival by preventing mitochondrial alteration in ischemic injury. *Cell Death Dis.* **2014**, *5*, e1105. [CrossRef]

302. Medvedev, Z.A. An attempt at a rational classification of theories of ageing. *Biol. Rev. Camb. Philos. Soc.* **1990**, *65*, 375–398. [CrossRef]

303. Zeng, H.; Sanes, J.R. Neuronal cell-type classification: Challenges, opportunities and the path forward. *Nat. Rev. Neurosci.* **2017**, *18*, 530–546. [CrossRef] [PubMed]

304. Diao, L.; Sun, W.; Deng, Q.; He, S. Development of the mouse retina: Emerging morphological diversity of the ganglion cells. *J. Neurobiol.* **2004**, *61*, 236–249. [CrossRef] [PubMed]

305. Fukuda, Y. A three-group classification of rat retinal ganglion cells: Histological and physiological studies. *Brain Res.* **1977**, *119*, 327–334. [CrossRef]

306. Sanes, J.R.; Masland, R.H. The types of retinal ganglion cells: Current status and implications for neuronal classification. *Ann. Rev. Neurosci.* **2015**, *38*, 221–246. [CrossRef] [PubMed]

307. Langer, K.B.; Ohlemacher, S.K.; Phillips, M.J.; Fligor, C.M.; Jiang, P.; Gamm, D.M.; Meyer, J.S. Retinal ganglion cell diversity and subtype specification from human pluripotent stem cells. *Stem Cell Rep.* **2018**, *10*, 1282–1293. [CrossRef]

308. Kay, J.N.; De la Huerta, I.; Kim, I.J.; Zhang, Y.; Yamagata, M.; Chu, M.W.; Meister, M.; Sanes, J.R. Retinal ganglion cells with distinct directional preferences differ in molecular identity, structure, and central projections. *J. Neurosci. Off. J. Soc. Neurosci.* **2011**, *31*, 7753–7762. [CrossRef]

309. Yonehara, K.; Shintani, T.; Suzuki, R.; Sakuta, H.; Takeuchi, Y.; Nakamura-Yonehara, K.; Noda, M. Expression of SPIG1 reveals development of a retinal ganglion cell subtype projecting to the medial terminal nucleus in the mouse. *PLoS ONE* **2008**, *3*, e1533. [CrossRef]

310. Duan, X.; Qiao, M.; Bei, F.; Kim, I.J.; He, Z.; Sanes, J.R. Subtype-specific regeneration of retinal ganglion cells following axotomy: Effects of osteopontin and mTOR signaling. *Neuron* **2015**, *85*, 1244–1256. [CrossRef]

311. Hattar, S.; Liao, H.W.; Takao, M.; Berson, D.M.; Yau, K.W. Melanopsin-containing retinal ganglion cells: Architecture, projections, and intrinsic photosensitivity. *Science* **2002**, *295*, 1065–1070. [CrossRef]

312. Mao, C.A.; Li, H.; Zhang, Z.; Kiyama, T.; Panda, S.; Hattar, S.; Ribelayga, C.P.; Mills, S.L.; Wang, S.W. T-box transcription regulator Tbr2 is essential for the formation and maintenance of Opn4/melanopsin-expressing intrinsically photosensitive retinal ganglion cells. *J. Neurosci. Off. J. Soc. Neurosci.* **2014**, *34*, 13083–13095. [CrossRef]

313. Volgyi, B.; Chheda, S.; Bloomfield, S.A. Tracer coupling patterns of the ganglion cell subtypes in the mouse retina. *J. Comp. Neurol.* **2009**, *512*, 664–687. [CrossRef] [PubMed]

314. Kim, I.J.; Zhang, Y.; Meister, M.; Sanes, J.R. Laminar restriction of retinal ganglion cell dendrites and axons: Subtype-specific developmental patterns revealed with transgenic markers. *J. Neurosci. Off. J. Soc. Neurosci.* **2010**, *30*, 1452–1462. [CrossRef] [PubMed]

315. Huberman, A.D.; Manu, M.; Koch, S.M.; Susman, M.W.; Lutz, A.B.; Ullian, E.M.; Baccus, S.A.; Barres, B.A. Architecture and activity-mediated refinement of axonal projections from a mosaic of genetically identified retinal ganglion cells. *Neuron* **2008**, *59*, 425–438. [CrossRef] [PubMed]

316. Triplett, J.W.; Wei, W.; Gonzalez, C.; Sweeney, N.T.; Huberman, A.D.; Feller, M.B.; Feldheim, D.A. Dendritic and axonal targeting patterns of a genetically-specified class of retinal ganglion cells that participate in image-forming circuits. *Neural Dev.* **2014**, *9*, 2. [CrossRef]

317. Rheaume, B.A.; Jereen, A.; Bolisetty, M.; Sajid, M.S.; Yang, Y.; Renna, K.; Sun, L.; Robson, P.; Trakhtenberg, E.F. Single cell transcriptome profiling of retinal ganglion cells identifies cellular subtypes. *Nat. Commun.* **2018**, *9*, 2759. [CrossRef]

318. Ou, Y.; Jo, R.E.; Ullian, E.M.; Wong, R.O.; Della Santina, L. Selective vulnerability of specific retinal ganglion cell types and synapses after transient ocular hypertension. *J. Neurosci. Off. J. Soc. Neurosci.* **2016**, *36*, 9240–9252. [CrossRef] [PubMed]

319. Daniel, S.; Clark, A.F.; McDowell, C.M. Subtype-specific response of retinal ganglion cells to optic nerve crush. *Cell Death Discov.* **2018**, *4*, 7. [CrossRef]

320. Cui, Q.; Ren, C.; Sollars, P.J.; Pickard, G.E.; So, K.F. The injury resistant ability of melanopsin-expressing intrinsically photosensitive retinal ganglion cells. *Neuroscience* **2015**, *284*, 845–853. [CrossRef]

321. Ruiz-Ederra, J.; Garcia, M.; Hernandez, M.; Urcola, H.; Hernandez-Barbachano, E.; Araiz, J.; Vecino, E. The pig eye as a novel model of glaucoma. *Exp. Eye Res.* **2005**, *81*, 561–569. [CrossRef]

322. Christensen, I.; Lu, B.; Yang, N.; Huang, K.; Wang, P.; Tian, N. The susceptibility of retinal ganglion cells to glutamatergic excitotoxicity is type-specific. *Front. Neurosci.* **2019**, *13*, 219. [CrossRef]

323. Mayer, C.; Bruehl, C.; Salt, E.L.; Diem, R.; Draguhn, A.; Fairless, R. Selective vulnerability of alphaOFF retinal ganglion cells during onset of autoimmune optic neuritis. *Neuroscience* **2018**, *393*, 258–272. [CrossRef] [PubMed]

324. Puyang, Z.; Gong, H.Q.; He, S.G.; Troy, J.B.; Liu, X.; Liang, P.J. Different functional susceptibilities of mouse retinal ganglion cell subtypes to optic nerve crush injury. *Exp. Eye Res.* **2017**, *162*, 97–103. [CrossRef] [PubMed]

325. Feng, L.; Zhao, Y.; Yoshida, M.; Chen, H.; Yang, J.F.; Kim, T.S.; Cang, J.; Troy, J.B.; Liu, X. Sustained ocular hypertension induces dendritic degeneration of mouse retinal ganglion cells that depends on cell type and location. *Investig. Ophthalmol. Vis. Sci.* **2013**, *54*, 1106–1117. [CrossRef] [PubMed]

326. Vidal-Sanz, M.; Galindo-Romero, C.; Valiente-Soriano, F.J.; Nadal-Nicolas, F.M.; Ortin-Martinez, A.; Rovere, G.; Salinas-Navarro, M.; Lucas-Ruiz, F.; Sanchez-Migallon, M.C.; Sobrado-Calvo, P.; et al. Shared and Differential Retinal Responses against Optic Nerve Injury and Ocular Hypertension. *Front. Neurosci.* **2017**, *11*, 235. [CrossRef] [PubMed]

327. La Morgia, C.; Carelli, V.; Carbonelli, M. Melanopsin retinal ganglion cells and pupil: Clinical implications for neuro-ophthalmology. *Front. Neurol.* **2018**, *9*, 1047. [CrossRef]

328. VanderWall, K.B.; Lu, B.; Wang, S.; Meyer, J.S. Differential susceptibility of rat retinal ganglion cells following optic nerve crush. *bioRxiv* **2018**, 429282. [CrossRef]

329. Siegert, S.; Scherf, B.G.; Del Punta, K.; Didkovsky, N.; Heintz, N.; Roska, B. Genetic address book for retinal cell types. *Nat. Neurosci.* **2009**, *12*, 1197–1204. [CrossRef]

330. Norsworthy, M.W.; Bei, F.; Kawaguchi, R.; Wang, Q.; Tran, N.M.; Li, Y.; Brommer, B.; Zhang, Y.; Wang, C.; Sanes, J.R.; et al. Sox11 Expression Promotes Regeneration of Some Retinal Ganglion Cell Types but Kills Others. *Neuron* **2017**, *94*, 1112–1120.e4. [CrossRef]

331. Harada, C.; Kimura, A.; Guo, X.; Namekata, K.; Harada, T. Recent advances in genetically modified animal models of glaucoma and their roles in drug repositioning. *Br. J. Ophthalmol.* **2019**, *103*, 161–166. [CrossRef]

332. DeBusk, A.; Moster, M.L. Gene therapy in optic nerve disease. *Curr. Opin. Ophthalmol.* **2018**, *29*, 234–238. [CrossRef]

333. Yang, S.; Ma, S.Q.; Wan, X.; He, H.; Pei, H.; Zhao, M.J.; Chen, C.; Wang, D.W.; Dong, X.Y.; Yuan, J.J.; et al. Long-term outcomes of gene therapy for the treatment of Leber's hereditary optic neuropathy. *EBioMedicine* **2016**, *10*, 258–268. [CrossRef] [PubMed]

334. Feuer, W.J.; Schiffman, J.C.; Davis, J.L.; Porciatti, V.; Gonzalez, P.; Koilkonda, R.D.; Yuan, H.; Lalwani, A.; Lam, B.L.; Guy, J. Gene therapy for leber hereditary optic neuropathy: Initial results. *Ophthalmology* **2016**, *123*, 558–570. [CrossRef] [PubMed]

335. Wan, X.; Pei, H.; Zhao, M.J.; Yang, S.; Hu, W.K.; He, H.; Ma, S.Q.; Zhang, G.; Dong, X.Y.; Chen, C.; et al. Efficacy and safety of rAAV2-ND4 treatment for leber's hereditary optic neuropathy. *Sci. Rep.* **2016**, *6*, 21587. [CrossRef] [PubMed]

336. Suzuki, K.; Tsunekawa, Y.; Hernandez-Benitez, R.; Wu, J.; Zhu, J.; Kim, E.J.; Hatanaka, F.; Yamamoto, M.; Araoka, T.; Li, Z.; et al. In vivo genome editing via CRISPR/Cas9 mediated homology-independent targeted integration. *Nature* **2016**, *540*, 144–149. [CrossRef] [PubMed]

337. Jain, A.; Zode, G.; Kasetti, R.B.; Ran, F.A.; Yan, W.; Sharma, T.P.; Bugge, K.; Searby, C.C.; Fingert, J.H.; Zhang, F.; et al. CRISPR-Cas9-based treatment of myocilin-associated glaucoma. *Proc. Natl. Acad. Sci. USA* **2017**, *114*, 11199–11204. [CrossRef] [PubMed]

2

From Rust to Quantum Biology: The Role of Iron in Retina Physiopathology

Emilie Picard [1,*], Alejandra Daruich [1,2], Jenny Youale [1], Yves Courtois [1] and Francine Behar-Cohen [1,3]

[1] Centre de Recherche des Cordeliers, INSERM, Sorbonne Université, USPC, Université Paris Descartes, Team 17, F-75006 Paris, France; adaruich.matet@gmail.com (A.D.); youale.j@hotmail.fr (J.Y.); courtois.yves@numericable.com (Y.C.); francine.behar@gmail.com (F.B.-C.)

[2] Ophthalmology Department, Necker-Enfants Malades University Hospital, APHP, 75015 Paris, France

[3] Ophtalmopole, Cochin Hospital, AP-HP, Assistance Publique Hôpitaux de Paris, 24 rue du Faubourg Saint-Jacques, 75014 Paris, France

[*] Correspondence: picardemilie@gmail.com;

Abstract: Iron is essential for cell survival and function. It is a transition metal, that could change its oxidation state from Fe^{2+} to Fe^{3+} involving an electron transfer, the key of vital functions but also organ dysfunctions. The goal of this review is to illustrate the primordial role of iron and local iron homeostasis in retinal physiology and vision, as well as the pathological consequences of iron excess in animal models of retinal degeneration and in human retinal diseases. We summarize evidence of the potential therapeutic effect of iron chelation in retinal diseases and especially the interest of transferrin, a ubiquitous endogenous iron-binding protein, having the ability to treat or delay degenerative retinal diseases.

Keywords: iron; retina; transferrin

1. Introduction

Iron is a major element in biology. Besides its well-known role in prebiotic conditions after the rise of oxygen in the atmosphere, its insolubility led to the development of many mechanisms to allow the primitive cells and organisms to use it. They are driven by the transition of ferrous iron (Fe^{2+}) to ferric iron (Fe^{3+}) involving an electron which is particularly available and is the basis of vital functions and dysfunctions in the organs.

In this review, we analyze several of the well-known or recently discovered functions of iron in the eye, mainly in the retina, and the most promising approaches to regulate it and improve a large number of its negative side effects which can lead to vision impairment. We will focus on the main functions of transferrin (TF) as a partner in the systemic and cellular mechanisms that underlie the regulation of iron homeostasis and its disorders.

2. The Retina Structure and Retinal Oxygen Supply

The eye is a complex and confined organ formed by different compartments and structures essential for the transmission and focus of photons from the cornea to the photoreceptors (PRs), which convert them into an electrical signal transmitted to the brain. The neural retina comprises the PRs, cones, rods, the interneurons, the ganglion cells, the glial cells such as retinal Müller's glial cells (MGC), astrocytes, and microglia (Figure 1). The retina is vascularized by two separate vascular systems, the retinal vessels, branches of the central retinal artery that vascularize the inner retinal layers, and the choroidal vessels, branches of the ciliary arteries that supply the avascular PR layer through the retinal pigment epithelium (RPE) cells. In primates and human, visual acuity, photopic vision, and color vision are ensured by the macula, a highly specialized retinal area that comprises less than 5% of the total retinal surface, located at the center of the visual axis. The center of the macula, the fovea, is devoid of retinal vessels and composed exclusively of cones and MGC cells.

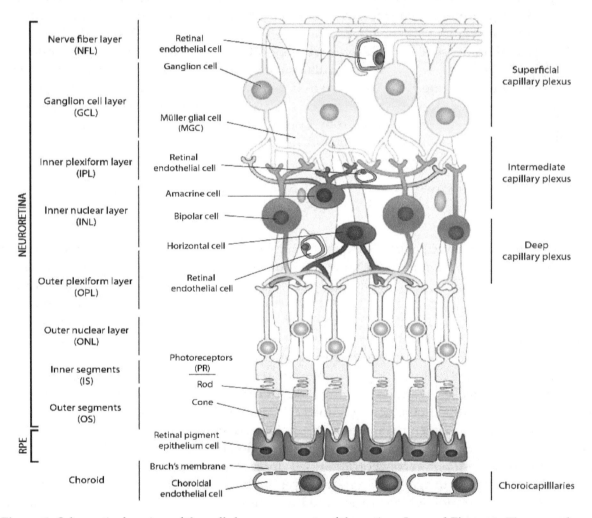

Figure 1. Schematic drawing of the cellular components of the retina. **Legend Figure 1:** There are three retinal vascular plexuses tightly coordinated with retinal neurons and a choroid plexus underlying RPE. GCL: Ganglion cell layer; NFL: Nerve fiber layer; INL: Inner nuclear layer; IPL: Inner plexiform layer; MGC: Müller glial cell; ONL: Outer nuclear layer; OPL: Outer plexiform layer; OS: Outer segments; IS: Inner segments; PR: Photoreceptors; RPE, retinal pigment epithelium.

The retina is separated from the circulation by two blood-retinal barriers (BRB). The inner BRB consists of a neuro-glio-vascular complex formed by tight junctions between endothelial cells of the retinal capillaries, pericytes, astrocytes, MGC, and microglia [1]. The outer BRB is formed by the tight-junction monolayer of RPE cells that are in close contact with the choriocapillaries, which control exchanges through diaphragmed fenestrations [1]. Oxygen is the most supply-limited metabolite in the retina [2]. Its supply to the retina is ensured by the choroid, which provides oxygen to the outer retina, whilst the retinal circulation provides the oxygen requirements of the inner retina. In normal condition, the level of oxygen tension (Po_2) in the outer retina is ten times lower than in the inner retina [3]. Oxygen and glucose consumption are metabolized to lactate, while aerobic glycolysis dominates energy production in the outer retina. Several factors modify Po_2 level and utilization at the cellular level: the retinal depth, the light, and hyperoxia [4,5]. PRs have almost all mitochondria in their inner segments far from blood vessels. Light decreases oxygen utilization on the outer retina as much as by a factor of two and increase Po_2. Hyperoxia dramatically increases Po_2 in the retina with the increase higher in outer retina compared to inner retina. The development and maintenance of retinal vasculature is regulated by α subunits of hypoxia-inducible factor (HIF), which induce genes required for retinal homeostasis, such as vascular endothelial growth factor (VEGF) under hypoxic conditions [6]. HIF proteins, which act as regulators of oxygen homeostasis, also depend on iron for their activity, and they regulate genes involved in iron metabolism [7]. Hyperoxia is deleterious to the outer retina as the oxygen leads to the formation of reactive oxygen species (ROS) according to the Fenton and Haber–Weiss reaction catalyzed by iron to generate $RO°$ radical (review in [3]). Iron and oxygen are thus closely linked in retinal metabolism in health and disease conditions.

3. Iron Homeostasis in the Retina

3.1. Distribution of Iron in the Retina

Iron is widely and unevenly distributed throughout the adult rat retina. The highest concentrations of iron were observed by proton-induced X-ray emission in the choroid, the RPE, and the inner segments of the PR. PR outer segments also contain iron, as inclusions inside the discs [8]. Iron and iron-related parameter (total iron binding capacity, TF and TF saturation percentage) distribution in the eye are different between diurnal and nocturnal animals. In cow and pig retina, iron concentration is higher than in rat retina, suggesting that the nocturnal habit of living could influence iron-related parameters in the retina [9]. The iron level also varies during retinal development and aging. Moos et al. have shown that in rats, iron entry is very high during retinal development and maturation, then decreases in adulthood, and increases again with aging [10]. In rodents, there are gender and strain-specific influences on iron regulation in the neural retina [11]. Human sex-associated differences in iron levels have also been reported, women having more retinal iron than men at all ages [12]. With aging, iron deposits are found in the RPE/choroid complex in rats and in the stroma of the choroid in non-human primate regardless of serum iron concentration [13]. Increased iron levels in the retina have also been reported in human eyes with age [12]. In rodent eyes, both neural retina and RPE/choroid present an increase of iron concentration which is associated with modifications of iron-related proteins mRNA and protein levels [14,15].

3.2. Proteins Involved in Retinal Iron Homeostasis

3.2.1. General Iron Homeostasis

Under physiological conditions, almost all non-heme iron (Fe^{3+}) in the circulation is transported bound to TF (transferrin-bound iron: TBI) with high affinity (for review on cellular iron metabolism [16]). At cellular level, the TF with two Fe^{3+} (holo-TF) is bound by its receptor (TFR1), and the complex is internalized. The Fe^{3+} is released from TF in the endosome under the effect of acidification through the action of an ATP-dependent proton pump. Iron is then reduced into the ferrous form, Fe^{2+}, by endosomal ferrireductase six transmembrane epithelial antigen of the prostate 3 (STEAP3) and exported by divalent metal transporter 1 (DMT1) in the cytosol where it contributes to the labile iron pool (LIP). In case of iron overload, TF is saturated with iron, and the non-transferrin-bound ferrous iron (NTBI) could be up-taken by iron importers such as the ZRT/IRT-like proteins (ZIPs) or DMT1 and joined intracellular LIP. The LIP consists of a transitory pool of iron species associated with a variety of ligands with low affinity (citrate, phosphate, inorganics irons) and easily oxidized, in transit to be distributed to the organelles (in particularly in mitochondria or nucleus) for cell metabolism in iron requiring proteins, stored or released.

In non-erythroid cells, the majority of iron is stored in ferritin (FT). Composed of 24 subunits of both heavy (HFT) and light (LFT) chains, FT forms a tissue-specific heterocomplex which can store up to 4500 Fe^{3+}. Fe^{2+} from LIP is transported to FT by Poly(rC)-binding proteins (PCBP1 and PCBP2) and is oxidized by ferroxidase activity of HFT in an oxygen-dependent manner. Then Fe^{3+} is stored in the cavity formed by LFT. Iron is released from FT in a controlled manner by autophagy involving a cargo receptor, the nuclear receptor coactivator 4 (NCOA4).

The only known mammalian iron exporter is ferroportin (FPN), a transmembrane protein which requires a multicopper ferroxidase to convert Fe^{2+} to Fe^{3+}, allowing binding to TF. Hephaestin (HEPC), ceruloplasmin (CP), amyloid-beta precursor protein (APP), and the newly identified zyloklopen (ZP) are co-localized with FPN at the surface membrane or secreted.

3.2.2. Iron Flux in Retina

A local retinal homeostasis of iron, independent from the systemic regulation, is suspected by the fact that main proteins involved in iron homeostasis, previously confined to systemic expression, are locally synthesized in the retina (Table 1). In addition, the outer and inner BRB prevents the entry of large quantities of iron into the eye in case of systemic iron overload. The study of mouse models invalidated for iron homeostasis proteins (Table 1) led to a hypothetical model in which iron entry and homeostasis in the retina is divided into two compartments, carried by the RPE and MGC, delimited by the external limiting membrane, and having limited exchanges in physiological condition.

Table 1. Proteins involved in iron homeostasis of the retina.

	Proteins	Expression	Functions	Knock-Out Rodent Models	Human Pathologies
Iron uptake/export	Transferrin (TF)	RPE, PR, MGC [8]	Extracellular transporter binding two ferric iron ions (Fe^{3+}) [holoTF]. Kd = 10^{22} M^{-1}	$Hpx^{-/-}$: Decrease of the electroretinogram. Decrease TF, CP, TFR1 [17]	Congenital atransferrinemia
	Transferrin receptor 1 (TFR1)	RPE, IS, OPL, INL, GCL, endothelial cells [8]	Transmembrane receptor of holoTF	ND	ND
	Lactoferrin (LF)	RPE [18]	Extracellular transporter binding two Fe^{3+}	$Lf^{-/-}$: Higher susceptibility for laser induced choroidal neovascularization [19]	ND
	Lipocalin 2 (LCN2) or (neutrophil gelatinase-associated lipocalin (NGAL) or 24p3	RPE, MGC, neural retina, microglia [20]	Extracellular transporter which binds Fe^{3+} by sequestering bacterial and mammalian siderophores (2,5-dihydroxybenzoic acid).	$Lcn2^{-/-}$: Expression of LFT, TF et TFR1 unchanged (personal data)	ND
	24p3R or (the solute carrier family 22 member 17 (SLC22A17)	RPE [21]	Transmembrane receptor of LCN2 under holo- and apo-forms		
	Megalin or (low density lipoprotein receptor-related protein 2 (LRP2)	RPE [22]	Transmembrane multiligands receptor (such lipocalin 2, lactoferrin, transferrin), co-receptor Cubulin	$Lrp2^{F/F}$ (FoxG1^{Cre+}): myopia, hypertrophic RPE and retinal degeneration [22]. Increase FT and decrease TFR1 (personal data)	Donnai-Barrow syndrome: high myopia, retinal detachment
	Ferroportin (FPN) or (SLC40A1)	RPE, IS, OPL, IPL, MGC, REC [23]	Transmembrane transporter which exports ferrous iron (Fe^{2+}) outside the cell in cooperation with ferroxidases	Fpn^{C326S}: HEPC-resistant FPN mice. Increase FT, iron deposits in RPE and choroid [24]	Hemochromatosis type 4
	Ceruloplasmin (CP)	RPE, MGC [25]	Extracellular ferroxidase that oxidizes Fe^{2+} in Fe^{3+}. Exists a glycosylphosphatidylinositol-anchored form	$Cp^{-/-}Heph^{sla/sla}$: Neovessels, deposits under RPE, loss of RPE and PR. Iron accumulation in RPE and PR. Increase FT and decrease TFR1. $Cp^{-/-}Heph^{F/F}$ (Bestrophin1^{Cre+}): no iron deposits and no retinal dystrophy [26]	Aceruloplasminemia: iron deposits in drusen and RPE. Dry-AMD like phenotype [27]
	Hephaestin (HEPH)	RPE, PR, MGC [25]	Extracellular ferroxidase. 50% of homology with CP		ND
	Amyloid-beta precursor protein (APP)	RPE, IS and OS, MGC, GCL [26]	Membrane ferroxidase	$App^{-/-}$: Disturbances of synaptic development of secondary neurons [28].	Associated with Alzheimer disease and cerebral amyloid angiopathy
	Zyklopen (ZP)	RPE, GCL [26,29]	Membrane ferroxidase	ND	ND
	DMT1 (*Divalent Metal Transporter 1*) or Natural resistance-associated macrophage protein (NRAM2) or SLC11A2	IS, horizontal and rod bipolar cells [30]	Transmembrane import of Fe^2. Iron exit from endosomal vesicle or cytosol under acidic pH (5.5).	ND	Microcytic hypochromic anemia with iron overload
	ZIP14 (*Zinc transporter 14*) or SLC39A14	CEC, RPE, PR, MGC, GCL, REC [31]	Transmembrane zinc transporter which uptakes unbound Fe^{2+} in cytosol. Optimal at physiological pH (7.4).	ND	Hypermanganesemia with dystonia 2; Hyperostosis cranialis interna.
	ZIP8 (*Zinc transporter 8*) or SLC39A8				Congenital disorder of glycosylation 2N

Table 1. *Cont.*

	Proteins	Expression	Functions	Knock-Out Rodent Models	Human Pathologies
Storage	Ferritin (FT)	Ubiquitous and highly express in RPE, IS, bipolar cells [8]	Cytosolic complex of 24 subunits of heavy (H) and light (L) chains, which can store 4,500 Fe^{3+}. The H subunits have ferroxidase activity. FT has also a nuclear localization	$Hft^{-/-}$: Higher sensibility for stress [32]	HFT: Hemochromatosis type 5LFT: Hyperferritinemia with or without cataract; Neuroferritinopathy; L-ferritin deficiency.
	Mitochondrial ferritin (FtMt)	All retina layers, with higher expression in RPE and ellipsoids of IS [30]	Mitochondria iron transporter. Share 79% of homology with HFT and has ferroxidase activity	ND	ND
	Transferrin receptor 2 (TFR2)	RPE, IS, OPL, IPL [33]	Transmembrane receptor of holo-TF which regulates transcription of HEPC in cooperation with HFE under TF iron-saturation	ND	Hemochromatosis type 3
	Hereditary hemochromatosis protein (HHE)	RPE [33]	Membrane protein which bind β2M to TFR1 or TFR2 in function of TF iron-saturation	$Hfe^{-/-}$: Hypertrophy/Hyperplasia of RPE, PR degeneration. Increase FT [34]	Hemochromatosis type 1: Dysmorphism of RPE, drusen and alteration of vision [30]. Variegate porphyria. Microvascular complications of diabetes 7
	β-2-Microglobulin (β2M)	RPE, OS, IS, OPL, INL, IPL [33]	Membrane protein involved in HFE·TFR1/2 interaction	ND	Immunodeficiency 43; Amyloidosis 8.
	Bone Morphogenetic protein 6 (BMP6)	RPE, IS, OPL, IPL, GCL	Extracellular protein which regulates HEPC transcription. Bind Activin A receptor (Acvr1A) and BMP receptor type II (BMPR2) and HJV as coreceptor, all expressed in retina	$Bmp6^{-/-}$: Iron accumulation in RPE and retina. RPE hypertrophy and PR degeneration. Decrease TFR1 and increase LFT [35]	ND
Regulation	Hemojuvelin (HJV)	RPE, PR, MGC, GCL [36]	Regulation of HEPC transcription	$Hjv^{-/-}$: Neovessels in retina, gliosis, inner BRB leakage, PR degeneration. Increase LFT [37]	Hemochromatosis type 2A
	Transmembrane serine protease 6. (TMPRSS6) or Serine protease matriptase-2	RPE, MGC GCL [38]	Membrane protein with serine protease activity which cleave HJV	$Tmprss6^{msk/msk}$: No visual alteration [38]. Increase HEPC, HJV, TFR1	Iron-refractory iron deficiency anemia
	Hepcidin (HEPC)	RPE, IS, MGC, OPL [36]	Peptide hormone which transcription is activated by TF saturation or inflammation. Induces the degradation of FPN reducing iron export	$Hamp^{-/-}$: Iron accumulation in RPE/choroid and in retina. Decrease TFR1 and increase FPN [39]	Hemochromatosis type 2B and juvenile
	Iron regulatory protein (IRP1) or cytoplasmic aconitase hydratase (ACO1)	Ubiquitous	Iron sensor protein with cluster iron-sulfur. Bind Iron responsive element (IRE) in target mRNA when intracellular iron levels are low. Under high iron condition, IRP1 is converted into an aconitase whereas IRP2 is degraded in proteasome	$Ireb1^{+/-} Ireb2^{-/-}$: No retinal alteration. Increase FPN and LFT [30]	ND
	IRP2 or Iron-responsive element-binding protein 2 (IREB2)				ND
	Hypoxia Inducible Factor (HIF)	RPE, PR ONL, INL, GCL [40,41]	Transcriptional regulator. Oxygen sensor sensitive to iron level. Bind Hypoxia responsive element (HRE) in target mRNA under hypoxia or when intracellular iron levels are low	ND	Familial erythrocytosis (HIF2α)

Legend Table 1: Proteins localization were obtained from immunostaining on sections of mouse/rat retinas. The mouse models presented are limited to those with retinal changes in iron homeostasis and retinal abnormalities, if any. The corresponding human diseases were obtained by searching the UniProt site. ND: Not determined. Legends: β2M: β-2-Microglobulin; CP: ceruloplasmin; CEC: choroidal endothelial cell; FT: ferritin; GCL: ganglion cells layer; HFE: hereditary hemochromatosis protein, HFT: ferritin heavy chain; IPL: inner plexiform layer; IRE: iron responsive element; IS: inner segments; LFT: ferritin light chain; MGC: Müller's glial cell; OPL: outer plexiform layer; OS: outer segments; PR: photoreceptor; REC: retinal endothelial cell; RPE: retinal pigment epithelium; TFR1: transferrin receptor 1.

Transferrin-Bound Iron Transport in the Retina

The RPE imports iron bound to TF from the choriocapillaries through the transcytosis of TFR1 present at the basal membrane of the RPE (Figure 2). The transcytosis of the TF/TFR1 complex along microtubules via galectin 4 and Rab11a [42] has been described in vitro. The presence of TFR1 on the apical side of RPE is ambiguous and suggests that TF/TFR1 transcytosis or a potential iron-TF uptake by RPE could egress iron from the outer retina to choriocapillaries. Six hours after an intravitreal injection of holoTF tagged with a fluorochrome, TF is localized in RPE and choroid, which favors the later hypothesis [43]. Another iron entry in RPE is the phagocytosis of PR outer segments which contains high quantities of iron [8]. Once in RPE cytosol, iron is stored in FT and in melanosomes [44]. The release of iron from cell is possible through FPN present at the basal membrane of RPE and a multicopper ferroxidase. HEPH, CP, and APP but not ZP are expressed in RPE [26].

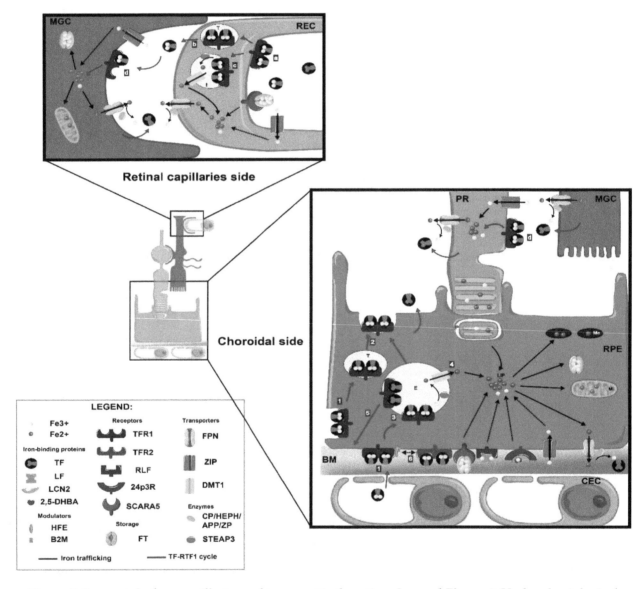

Figure 2. Iron uptake from capillaries and transport in the retina. **Legend Figure 2:** Under physiological condition, non-heme iron (Fe^{3+}) in the circulation is transported bound to transferrin (TF). A. At the

choroidal side, Fe^{3+} linked to TF is captured by its receptor 1 (TFR1) (1) at the basolateral level of the retinal pigment epithelium (RPE) (blue arrows). The internalized TF/TFR complex is transported to the apical pole by transcytosis (T) (2) or to the endosome (E) (3). In this case, Fe^{3+} is released from TF and reduced by the metaloreductase six transmembrane epithelial antigen of the prostate 3 (STEAP3) to ferrous iron (Fe^{2+}) and then exported to the cytosol by the transporter divalent metal transporter 1 (DMT1) where it constitutes the free iron pool (LIP) (4). TF and TRF1 are recycled to membrane (5). Iron is then transported from LIP to the organelles as needed, either stored in ferritin (FT) and melanosomes (Me), or exported by ferroportin (FPN) coupled to ferroxidases such as ceruloplasmin (CP) or hephaestin (HEPH), amyloid-beta precursor protein (APP) or zyloklopen (ZP) (black arrows). Hemochromatosis protein (HFE) and beta-2 microglobulin (B2M) associated to TFR1, shift to TFR2 in case of iron overload (saturation of TF) and activate hepcidin (HEPC) transcription (6). B. At retinal capillaries side, Fe^{3+} bound to TF is up-taken by TFR1 at the luminal side of retinal endothelial cells (REC) (a), and TF/TFR1 pass directly through transcytosis into the retina (b) or endocytosed then exported by FPN (c). TF synthetized by RPE, Müller glial cells (MGC) or photoreceptors (PR) up-taken retinal iron (d) and distributed it throughout the retina, especially to PR. Phototransduction performed on the outer segments of PR is a highly iron-dependent process. PR uptake Fe^{3+} bound to TF by TFR1 presents in inner segments and export it by FPN or by phagocytosis (P) of the outer segments of PR by RPE. TF-independent iron delivery to the retina can occur, especially in case of systemic iron dysregulation (black dotted lines). Serum FT has a specific receptor, the scavenger receptor class A, member 5 (SCARA5) localizes at the basal membrane of RPE, luminal side of REC, PR and MGC. Lactoferrin (LF), a member of TF superfamily and its receptors (LFR) are present in RPE. Fe^{3+} captured by a siderophore (2,5-dihydroxybenzoic acid (2,5-DHBA)) is bound by lipocalin 2 (LCN2) and its receptors (24p3R) in RPE. The non-TF-bound iron (NTBI) is up-taken by MGC, REC, PR and RPE by DMT1 or ZRT/IRT-like proteins (ZIP) importers. BM: Bruch's membrane; CEC: choroidal endothelial cell; E: endosome; Me: melanosome; MGC: Müller's glial cell; MI: mitochondria; P: phagosome; PR: photoreceptor; REC: retinal endothelial cell; RPE: retinal pigment epithelium; T: transcytosis.

In the inner retinal layers, iron is imported through retinal endothelial cells (REC) which express TFR1 at their luminal side [45]. Two mechanisms of iron transfer across the abluminal membrane of REC into the retina are evoked: TF/TFR1 transcytosis or/and TF/TFR1 endocytosis following by iron released from endosome and iron export by FPN. The abluminal membrane of REC expresses FPN colocalized with HEPC, CP, and APP [24,31]. Iron is bound by TF and distributed to the retina or the vitreous. With its unique position extending from the vitreous to PRs and its capacity to synthetize TF [46] and to express FPN [24], MGC plays a crucial role in the distribution of iron from the inner retina to the inner segment of the PR.

Iron presents in the non-vascularized subretinal space, between the apical side of RPE and the PR, is mainly bound to TF, secreted by PRs and RPE, and up-taken by PRs for their highly metabolism activities, by TFR1 express at inner segments. The PR inner segment is the iron storage compartment for PR segments, where both FT chains and mitochondrial FT are highly concentrated [30]. Iron export from the PR is ensured mostly by FPN also present in inner segments, CP and HEPH being poorly involved in favor of APP [26].

Non-Transferrin-Bound Iron Transport in the Retina

Whereas iron-bound TF is the main transport system to cross the BRB, transferrin-independent iron delivery to the retina can occur (Figure 1). Serum FT, exclusively composed of LFT has specific receptor, the scavenger receptor class A, member 5 (SCARA5) expressed in cytoplasm and nucleus in retinal endothelial cells, ganglion cells, astrocytes, the inner nuclear layer, MGC, microglia, outer nuclear layer, cones segments and RPE. After intravenous injection, serum FT remained confined in retinal endothelial cells in the inner retina [47]. Another protein possibly involved in iron transport is lactoferrin (LF), a multifunctional protein which shares 65% of homology with TF. It is synthesized in various human ocular tissues mainly in the RPE but not in the neural retina [18]. LF receptors have not been studied in the eye but are present in the brain [48]. Lipocalin 2 (LCN2) does not bind to iron directly, but through interaction with siderophores (catecholate and carboxylate) as cofactors [49] could also be implicated in iron transport in the retina [20]. β-hydroxybutyrate dehydrogenase-2 (Bdh2), an enzyme that is critical for the synthesis of 2,5-dihydroxybenzoic acid (2,5-DHBA), the mammalian siderophore, is found throughout the retina in all cell layers, including ganglion cells, MGC, and RPE cells [50]. Two major membrane-bound receptors for LCN2, megalin and 24p3R, have been identified in RPE [21,22]. Although LCN2 is being recognized as an important factor in retinal diseases [21], its exact contribution in iron retinal transport in health and diseases remain to be determined.

In case of iron overload, the NTBI could be up taken by iron importer ZIP or DMT1. This could explain why in retinal iron overload models, iron continues to accumulate despite the reduced expression of TFR1 in retina and RPE [31]. The specific localization of DMT1 in PRs and bipolar and horizontal cells suggests that it could be involved in providing iron to these cells, for phototransduction or neurotransmitter synthesis [30] ZIP8 and ZIP14 are expressed in RPE, choroid, REC, choroidal endothelial cells (CEC), ganglion cells, PRs, and MGC. At a high degree of TF saturation in the retina, there is a decreased ZIP14 expression whereas ZIP8 expression remains stable [31].

3.2.3. Iron Regulation in Retina

Cellular iron uptake and release and the intracellular LIP size are tightly controlled. Transcriptional, post-transcriptional, and post-translational processes regulate iron homeostatic proteins (for a review, see [51]). The main mechanisms of intra- and extra-cellular regulation of iron levels are limited to two extremely controlled systems.

The first system includes iron regulatory proteins (IRP) 1 and 2—intracellular iron regulatory proteins which, depending on the amount of iron, bind iron responsive element (IRE) sequences present on the mRNAs of iron homeostasis proteins such as FPN, TFR1, FT, and DMT1. Depending on the position of the IRE site, IRP controls their translation or degradation. Under conditions of increased cellular iron, IRP1 loses its IRE-binding activity by acquiring an iron in the 4Fe–4S cluster, whereas IRP2, is degraded by proteasome. In this condition, *tfr1* and *dmt1* mRNA are degraded, whereas *ft*, *fpn*, and *hif-2α* mRNA are translated. The localization of IRP1 and IRP2 has not yet been identified in the retina but their expressions are ubiquitous in mammalian cells. Mice with $Irp1^{+/-}$ $Irp2^{-/-}$ genotype show more severe neurodegenerative disease than $Irp2^{-/-}$ animals [30]. These IRP deficient retinas have increased FPN and FT in the inner segments, MGC endfeet, and inner retina compared to age and strain matched wild type retinas, suggesting that FPN and FT levels are regulated by IRPs in the retina [23]. In a model of light induced retinal degeneration, 2 h after light exposure, *Irp2* but not *Irp1* mRNA increased in the retina [32].

The second system focuses on hepcidin (HEPC), a peptide hormone principally synthetized by the liver. However, HEPC is also synthesized by PR, RPE, and MGC [39]. It is activated by two cellular signaling pathways induced by excess of iron, the transferrin receptor 2 (TFR2)/Human homeostatic iron regulator protein (HFE) pathway and the Bone Morphogenetic protein (BMP6)/Mothers against decapentaplegic homolog 1 (SMAD) pathway. When the TF saturation is high at the basolateral level of the RPE, the HFE is released from TFR1 and binds to TFR2, which activates the transcription of HEPC. BMP6 secreted by the retina and the RPE, binds to its receptors coupled to hemojuvelin (HJV) protein at the apical level of RPE in order to activate the synthesis of HEPC [35]. HEPC binds to the extracellular domain of FPN on the cell surface, leading to its internalization and degradation, effectively preventing cellular iron export and limiting the amount of iron that gets into the extracellular fluid. The specific deletion of HEPC in the retina does not lead to age-associated retinal iron accumulation, whereas liver-specific HEPC silencing leads to early serum, RPE, and retina iron accumulation followed by retinal degeneration [52].

Finally, the hypoxia inducible factor (HIF) acts as a transcription factor for certain iron homeostasis genes such as the *Tf*, *tfr1*, *Dmt1*, *Fpn*, and *Cp* genes by binding to a specific hypoxia-responsive element (HRE) site present on their mRNAs. Expression and degradation of HIF are also dependent on iron. In fact, Fe^{2+} is the cofactor of prolyl hydroxylase involved in the degradation of HIF-1α, and at the same time HIF-2α has an IRE sequence in the 5'UTR of its mRNA, which in the condition of iron deficiency, inhibits its translation. Nuclear staining of HIF-1α was observed in the GCL, the inner nuclear layer and the outer nuclear layer in human and rat [41]. Under retinal hypoxia, both HIF-1α and HIF-2α are activated but have cell specific expression within the inner retina. Specifically HIF-2α activation seems to play a key role in regulating the response of MGC to hypoxia [53].

4. Physiopathological Role of Iron in the Retina

4.1. Iron in Cellular Metabolism/Functions

4.1.1. Iron as a Fe-S Structural Motif Involved in Various Cellular Machinery Proteins

Iron sulfur (Fe-S) proteins are characterized by the presence of Fe-S clusters localized in different cell compartments (for review [54]). IRP1 is a Fe-S cluster that participates in sensing and regulating iron homeostasis in the retina. Frataxin is a nuclear-encoded mitochondrial protein involved in Fe-S cluster assembly, heme synthesis, and intracellular iron homeostasis. Frataxin is an allosteric activator which binds to this assembly complex [55]. It is present in the retina [56] and in the RPE [57] and could be responsible for retinal neurodegeneration induced by defective mitochondrial function [58]. In addition, Fe-S clusters may act as biological sensors by their binding properties to molecular oxygen and nitric oxide [59] both critical for the retinal physiology and pathology.

4.1.2. Iron in Nucleic Acids Machinery, Cell Proliferation, and DNA Repair

A recent review has reported the multiple implications of iron in DNA synthesis and repair, as well as in RNA metabolism [60]. Cytosolic and nuclear Fe-S proteins intervene in the genome stability [61]. Iron has been implicated in DNA synthesis and repair as a cofactor of sirtuin 2, an histone deacetylase, involved in iron homeostasis [62]. Sirtuin 2 maintains cellular iron levels by binding the nuclear factor erythroid-2-related factor 2 (NRF2) leading to a reduction in total and nuclear NRF2 levels. NRF2 is a transcription factor that plays key roles in retinal antioxidant and detoxification responses and has been linked with the development of age-related macular degeneration (AMD) [63].

Mitochondria are a major source of ROS and mitochondrial DNA is very susceptible to oxidative damage [64]. In RPE cells, mitochondrial DNA is damaged by hydrogen peroxide [65]. Deletions in mitochondrial DNA occurred in function of age in human neural retina [66], and the accumulation of age-related mitochondrial mutations in the eye has been correlated with a decrease in ATP production and increase ROS output, leading to oxidative stress, inflammation, and degradation [67].

4.1.3. Iron in Oxygen Transport and Regulation

Hemoglobin is synthetized in the retina [68]. It is one of the main protein synthesized in primary cultures of human RPE and secreted in vivo through the basolateral membrane [69].

Under physiological condition, free hemoglobin is bound by haptoglobin, but in case of massive hemolysis, hemoglobin releases free heme which binds hemopexin. Both hemopexin and haptoglobin have been described in the human retina [70,71]. The mRNAs for both haptoglobin and hemopexin were detected in the neural retina and PR as well as ganglion cells but not in RPE cells.

Neuroglobin is a highly conserved oxygen-binding protein reviewed in [72] and highly expressed in the retina. Its role is to facilitate oxygen metabolism, being localized in mitochondria. Hemin, the ferric chloride salt of heme enhances neuroglobin expression and protects animal model of N-methyl-N-nitrosourea-induced retinal degeneration [73]. In this model, hemin protects also cones from apoptosis. Neuroglobin has also been associated with retinal damage induced by light [74] which may reflect the changes in iron metabolism first described with light on retina [32]. It has also been associated with VEGF expression and thus could participate in retinal angiogenesis [75].

Heme, Fe^{2+} protoporphyrin IX, the prosthetic group of hemoproteins including hemoglobin, neuroglobin, oxidases/peroxidases, or cytochromes can be released after auto-oxidation. Heme transporter proteins also intervene in iron metabolism in the retina, and their dysregulation could potentially cause oxidative cell damage. All three heme transporters feline leukemia virus subgroup C receptor (FLVCR), breast cancer resistance protein (BCRP), and proton-coupled folate transporter (PCFT/HCP-1) are expressed in the retina and RPE. In the RPE, the expression of FLVCR is restricted to the apical membrane and the expression of BCRP and PCFT to the basolateral membrane. In cases of iron overload, the expression of FLVCR and PCFT is upregulated and BCRP is downregulated, suggesting an important role of heme transporter proteins in retinal iron regulation [76].

4.1.4. Iron and Visual Function

The involvement of iron in the vision cycle was discovered with the characterization of the enzyme RPE65, as an iron-dependent isomerohydrolase [77]. RPE65, abundant in the RPE [78], ensures the isomerization and hydrolysis of all-*trans* retinyl ester to 11-*cis* retinol. RPE65 is essential for vision, and mutations in *rpe65* genes induce Leber congenital amaurosis, a form of retinitis pigmentosa that leads to blindness [79]. Recently, RPE65 was also shown to intervene in the production of meso-zeaxantin, an ocular specific carotenoid which protects the fovea from oxidative stress [80].

An alternate pathway for 11-*cis* retinol recycling has been described in MGC by isomerases 1 or 2 that also appear to be iron dependent [81]. Few studies have analyzed the iron flux in the retina with the diurnal cycle conversely to what has been performed in brain in mice [82,83]. Among the sensory guanylate cyclase proteins and signaling network, guanylyl cyclase activating protein 5 is the only protein that binds strongly Fe^{2+} in zebrafish [84]. It is proposed as redox sensor in visual transduction.

Phototransduction depends on the phagocytosis of outer segments from PR by the RPE. The constant release of the outer segments from PR and their digestion during phagocytosis by RPE implies membrane biogenesis, a process which needs iron as a cofactor of fatty acid desaturase [85]. Royal College Surgeon (RCS) rats invalided for the phagocytosis protein Myeloid-epithelial-reproductive tyrosine kinase (MERTK) have increased iron in retina and particularly in RPE phagosomes and also increased retinal FT and TF expression [86].

Iron is also involved in neurotransmitters secretion as it regulates glutamate secretion by RPE cells via the cytosolic aconitase pathway [87]. Dopamine biosynthesis in specialized amacrine cells results from the conversion of the amino acid L-tyrosine in L-3,4-dihydroxyphenylalanine (L-DOPA) using oxygen and Fe^{2+} [88]. Synaptosomal nerve-associated protein 25 (SNAP-25) is a Fe-S protein involved in synapse vesicle fusion with plasma membranes highly present in retina [89].

A significant number of ATP binding cassette (ABC) transporters, involved in lipid trafficking in retinal cells, have been linked to severe genetic ocular diseases [90]. ABCA4 is present in the PR and transports 11-*cis* and all-*trans* isomers of N-retinylidene-phosphatidylethanolamine across disc membranes, preventing the accumulation of toxic bisretinoid lipofuscin compounds in PR and RPE cells. In *Abca4* null mutant mouse which presents accumulation of N-retinylidineN-ethanolamine (A2E) bisretinoids and lipofuscin in the RPE, intracellular iron accumulation is also observed which contributes to enhancing oxidative cell death [91]. The intracellular accumulation of iron in cells of the RPE in culture decreases the expression of the transporters of cholesterol ABCA1/ABCG1, increasing the level of pro-inflammatory cholesterol in retina [50].

4.2. The Dark Side of Iron

4.2.1. The Crucial Role of Iron in Oxidative Stress-Mediated Damages in the Retina

The ability of iron to change easily its valence and switch between the Fe^{2+} and Fe^{3+} forms, providing or accepting electrons, respectively, ensures a privileged position in living matter as mediator of key biochemical reactions. However, the presence of free labile iron in cell or NTBI in circulation is prone to generate highly ROS in the Fenton/Haber–Weiss reaction.

$$Fe^{2+} + H_2O_2 \rightarrow Fe^{3+} + OH^- + HO^{\cdot} : \text{Fenton reaction}$$
$$O_2^{\cdot-} + Fe^{3+} \rightarrow O_2 + Fe^{2+} : \text{Haber–Weiss reaction}$$
$$O_2^{\cdot-} + H_2O_2 \xrightarrow{Fe^{2+}; Fe^{3+}} O_2 + OH^- + HO^{\cdot} : \text{Fenton/Haber–Weiss reaction}$$

The toxicity of free iron has been extensively studied on neuronal and retinal cells, and they are not sensitive to the same doses of iron [46,92,93], the cones being the most sensitive to iron [94]. In RPE cells, the interaction of iron with bisretinoids and lipofuscin induces cell damage and retinal degeneration [91]. Conversely, melanin can bind large amounts of iron to preserve the RPE and the choroid from a pro-oxidant environment, intensified by light exposure. However, with age, the accumulation of iron in melanosomes associated with a reduction in the amount of melanin in RPE promotes the formation of free radicals [95]. Exposure of RPE cells to high non-lethal doses of iron leads to a decrease in phagocytic and lysosomal activity [15], favoring the accumulation of breakdown products of Vitamin A (lipofuscin) leading to the formation of glycation end products (AGE) present in drusen, RPE, and Bruch's membrane of AMD patients [91]. In addition, phagocytosis of PR discs, peroxidized by ferrous ions, damage the membranes of phagosomes and lysosomes in RPE cells in culture [15,96].

In hypoxic conditions, an efflux of iron from RPE to the basolateral direction [97] could explain, at least in part, that PRs tolerate better hypoxia than hyperoxia [98]. Fe^{2+} contributes also to light-induced PR cell death through the production of hydroxyl radicals [99]. The ascorbate-Fe^{2+} complex induce lipid peroxidation in rod outer segment membranes and subsequently damage proteins such as rhodopsin by carbonylation or loss of thiol groups [100]. Finally, free heme can be also a source of redox-active iron and therefore highly toxic for the retina and for RPE cells [101].

In optic neuropathy, such as glaucoma, several mechanisms involved in ganglion cell death seem to be enhanced by iron-dependent oxidative stress [102,103].

Iron is thus a key component of oxidative-induced damages in the retina and in the RPE and involved in major cell death mechanisms.

4.2.2. Retinal Cells Death Mechanisms in Iron Overload

Iron overload, induced experimentally by the implantation of iron particles in rat vitreous cavity caused apoptosis (TUNEL-positive nuclei) in the outer nuclear layer after only 2 days [104]. Rat retinal explant exposed to iron showed an early increase of necrotic markers, such as lactate deshydrogenase, receptor-interacting serine/threonine-protein (RIP) kinase, and incorporation of propidium iodide, even before intraretinal iron accumulation was detected. Using retinal organo-culture, it was observed that iron deposits in retinal explants induced a shift from necrosis to apoptosis with activation of caspase 3 and TUNEL-positive nuclei [105]. Increased intraocular iron levels following intravitreal $FeSO_4$ injection caused oxidative damage of PR, as shown by the increase of superoxide radicals; hydroxynonenal, a marker of lipid peroxidation; and increased expression of heme oxygenase 1 [94]. Retinal iron overload also activates the NOD-like receptor family, pyrin domain containing 3 (NLRP3) inflammasome signaling pathway. In fact, the expression levels of NLRP3, activated caspase-1, a downstream target of NLRP3, and interleukin (IL) 1ß were higher in the retinas of HFE KO mice, a model of genetic iron overload [106]. Ferroptosis, a newly characterized form of necrosis, is induced by the accumulation of iron in degenerative diseases and has been described in RPE cells in culture subjected to oxidative stress [107]. Glutathione depletion also induced ferroptosis, autophagy, and premature senescence in RPE cells [108].

4.2.3. Inflammation

The general implication of iron in inflammation has been recently reviewed, and it will not be detailed here [109]. In RPE cells, the intracellular accumulation of iron activated the NRLP3 inflammasome pathway via the repression of the degradation of aluRNA by double-stranded RNA-specific endoribonuclease (DICER1). This mechanism involved the sequestration of the cofactor

PCBP2 [110] and has been advocated in AMD. It has been also reported that iron induces the synthesis of complement C3 by activation of the Extracellular signal-regulated kinases (ERK)/SMAD3/CCAAT Enhancer Binding Protein Delta (CEBPD) 48 pathway [111]. The complement factor C5 carries between 13 and 15 iron atoms necessary for its conversion into an active form C5b by C5 convertase, a complex formed from the cleavage products of C3 [112], which shows the importance of iron in complement pathways activation, a recognized risk factor for AMD [113].

The prion protein (PrP^C), the principal protein implicated in the pathogenesis of human and animal prion disorders, is also implied in retinal degeneration due to iron metabolism dysfunction. This neuronal protein is expressed in many tissues of the eye, such as the retina and the cornea trabeculum. PrP^C is also expressed on the basolateral membrane of RPE, where it facilitates uptake of iron from choriocapillaries to neuroretina by functioning as a ferrireductase partner for divalent metal transporters. PrP-scrapie (PrP(Sc)), a misfolded isoform of this PrP^C accumulates in the neuroretina resulting in iron accumulation [114].

In the brain, IL6 produced by microglia in response to lipopolysaccharide, induced the production of HEPC by astrocytes [115]. HEPC prevented the iron overload-activated neuronal apoptosis [115]. LPS induced also an HFE-independent expression of HEPC in MGC and in the RPE, both in vitro and in vivo. The increase in HEPC levels in retinal cells, occurring with a decrease in FPN levels, led to oxidative stress and apoptosis within the retina in vivo [116]. On the other hand, in both in vitro and in vivo models of amyloid β-induced pathology, HEPC downregulates the inflammatory and pro-oxidant processes in astrocytes and microglia and protected neurons from cell death [117]. Microglia and MGC activation associated with reactive gliosis has been observed in HJV knockout mice ($Hjv^{-/-}$ mice) with aging and subsequent retinal iron accumulation [37].

The role of LCN2 has been suspected in AMD where its expression is increased in aqueous humor and in the infiltrating cells present in the retina and choroid [118]. An age-related increase in LCN2 was described in RPE cells of Beta-crystallin A3 (Cryba1) conditional knockout mouse, a model of AMD associated with chronic inflammation response [49], but the exact implication of LCN2 in iron metabolism in these models remains to be studied.

4.2.4. Angiogenesis

Increased iron levels in the retina could also have a role in the development of new vessels by inhibiting the anti-angiogenic effect of cleaved high molecular weight kininogen (Hka) [119], promoting the expression of succinate receptor 1 (SUCNR1 or GPR91) [120] which stimulates production of pro-angiogenic factors VEGF and angiopoietin [121]. In $Hjv^{-/-}$ mice, that leads to abnormal retinal iron overload. Proliferation of new leaky blood vessels in the vitreous was associated with reactive gliosis involving MGC and microglia [37]. In addition to proliferation by migratory cells, intravitreal hemoglobin also stimulates a transient proliferation in cells of the RPE and possibly in some supportive cells of the neural retina, such as MGC and astrocytes [122]. Iron also plays a role in HIF transcriptional regulation of pro-angiogenic genes [51]

5. Role of Iron in Retinal Diseases

5.1. Siderosis and Retinal Hemorrhages

Eye siderosis is probably the first known manifestation of iron toxicity for the eye. The presence of a foreign body containing iron inside the eyeball leads to various clinical complications including heterochromia of the iris, mydriasis, cataract, and retinal and RPE atrophy. Electroretinography analysis shows a decrease in a and b wave amplitudes, due to the progressive degeneration of the cones and rods (for a review, see [123]). The increase in iron can be observed histologically as a granular structure with FT or hemosiderin into cells. The level of vitreous iron also increases [124].

Retinal hemorrhages are present in several retinal pathologies, such as exudative AMD, diabetic retinopathy, or myopic degeneration, and they are particularly deleterious for vision when located in the subretinal space. Vision loss is dependent on the size of the hemorrhage and the ability of the tissue to shed blood [125,126]. During sub-macular hemorrhage early PR damage has been reported within 24 h [127]. In rabbits, the injection of their own blood into the subretinal space leads to a progressive degeneration of the PRs from one day after injection until a total destruction at 7 days, with an accumulation of iron in the outer segments of PR and in RPE [128]. The increased release of iron from hemoglobin induces peroxidation of unsaturated phospholipids, which are extensively present in the retina and affects particularly retinal neurons compared to the retinal glial cells [129].

5.2. Retinal Manifestations of Inherited Iron Disorders

Iron can accumulate in the retina of patients with inherited diseases involving mutations in genes encoding proteins of iron homeostasis, which can cause an imbalance in the metabolism of retinal iron. The most common hereditary hemochromatosis is related to a mutation in the *Hfe* gene resulting in excessive absorption of iron by the intestine and its accumulation in the organs. Mutations in the *Tfr2*, *Fpn*, *Hjv*, and *Hepc* genes are also involved in the development of hemochromatosis. The clinical findings associated to the retinal iron accumulation in these patients, as well as the impact on visual function, are quite rarely reported due to the variability of penetrance and the existence of a treatment reducing systemic iron overload. However, iron deposits and other changes in the RPE as well as visual acuity loss have been already reported [130].

Aceruloplasminemia is an autosomal recessive disorder caused by mutations in the Cp gene, resulting in a defect in the export of iron from cells. The retina, brain, and pancreas are overloaded with iron, leading to the clinical consequences as retinal degeneration, dementia, and diabetes. Several cases associating yellow discoloration of the fundus, atrophy of the RPE, and drusen-like deposits in the macula have been described. In post-mortem sections, an accumulation of iron associated with an enlarged RPE and loss of pigment of the RPE was observed (for a review, see [27]).

In animal models invalidated for the genes coding for iron-related proteins, an accumulation of iron in the RPE and PR is systematically observed as well as abnormalities in the RPE and PR degeneration [25,35,39,52,131].

Studies carried out in aging rodents have shown that the increase in iron intakes in food or by intravenous injection leads to local iron deposits in the choroid, the RPE, and the segments of PR, as well as deposits of complement C3 in the Bruch's membrane, hypertrophy, and vacuolation of RPE and changes in the choriocapillaries [132,133].

5.3. Age-Related Macular Degeneration

AMD is a leading cause of worldwide blindness in the elderly population, affecting 200 million individuals by 2020 and nearly 300 million by 2040 [134]. The pathological aging of the macula can cause dry or non-neovascular and wet or neovascular AMD. At the early stage, accumulation of extracellular material forms drusen between the basal lamina of the RPE and the inner layer of Bruch's membrane in the eye. At the late stages, degeneration of the PR overlying the drusen can cause severe central vision loss in the dry form, whilst formation of new abnormal blood vessels from the choroid growing into the retina can cause subretinal fluid accumulation and bleeding. The wet form progresses rapidly and is responsible for 90% of severe vision loss associated with AMD. The pathogenesis of AMD is multifactorial, with genetic and environmental factors such as smoking. It is associated with dysregulations in the angiogenic, oxidative stress, lipid, inflammatory, and complement pathways [135]. Patients with early AMD have more iron in the macula than healthy patients. Iron deposits are found in the melanosomes of the choroid and the RPE, in the central layer of the calcified Bruch's membrane, in the drusen, and at the level of the PR [136]. Part of this iron, found in the pathological retina of AMD patients, is in the toxic free form [137]. Patients with dry AMD have more than twice the concentration of iron in their aqueous humor than in patients with cataract surgery [138]. The macular region of AMD patients with geographic atrophy showed an increase in the expression of proteins involved in iron homeostasis such as TF, FT, and FPN in the PR layer and feet MGC [139]. TF and CP mRNAs are increased in the two advanced forms of AMD [140]. In the serum of patients with the different forms of AMD, a significant increase in TF and TFR1 and a significant decrease in the concentration of soluble FT were observed while iron levels were unchanged [141]. Several polymorphisms of the iron homeostasis genes have been associated with risk factors for AMD: *Tfr1*, *Tfr2* (obesity, tobacco) [142], *Dmt1* [143], *Irp1* and *Irp2* [143], and *heme oxygenases 1* and *2* (HO1/2) [144]. A recent study has shown that the expression of several miRNA, small non-coding RNA molecules binding in 3'UTR genes, was modified in the serum of AMD patients, especially those controlling the translation of the TFR1 and DMT1 proteins [145].

5.4. Diabetic Retinopathy

Diabetic retinopathy is a vision-threatening complication of diabetes affecting approximately 93 million in the middle-aged and elderly populations [146]. Chronic hyperglycemia causes progressive damage to retinal cells and to the retinal capillaries, leading to ischemia, VEGF-mediated retinal vascular abnormalization, and neovascular vessels that leak and bleed into the retina. Macular edema is also a major cause of vision loss in diabetic retinopathy [1]. Clinical reports have shown the link between iron levels in the vitreous and proliferative diabetic retinopathy [124,147]. A strong iron label was observed in the RPE and outer plexiform layer of patients with diabetic retinopathy [148]. In a mouse model of diabetic retinopathy, higher iron concentrations in the retina led to an increased expression of renin by a mechanism dependent on the GPR91 receptor [106].

5.5. Glaucoma Neuropathy

Glaucoma is increasingly a cause of irreversible blindness in the world. Its global prevalence is expected to be 76 million by 2020 and 112 million by 2040. Progressive damage to the optic nerve, leading to severe vision loss results from increased ocular pressure and other multiple favoring factors [149,150]. Although the link between iron and glaucoma is not yet fully understood, there is a change in iron homeostasis in glaucomatous eyes. TF concentration is increased in the aqueous humor [151], and mRNA of TF are increased in retina [152]. Whilst no differences were found in iron levels in aqueous humor of patients with primary open-angle glaucoma [153], serum levels of iron and FT were significantly increased [154,155], and serum CP level was lower [156]. A glaucomatous mice model had lower retinal iron concentrations than pre-glaucomatous DBA/2J and age-matched C57Bl/6J mice [157]. The expression of FT, CP, and TF was increased in monkey and rat glaucoma models [152,158]. In addition, the role of glutamate excitotoxicity in the pathogenesis of glaucoma is well documented; yet, there seems to be a link between the toxicity of glutamate and the increase in the entry of iron into neurons [159], and iron chelation seems to protect neurons against excitotoxicity and intraocular pressure-induced toxicity [160,161]. A mutation in the autophagy receptor optineurin is associated with the pathogenesis of glaucoma. It induces the degradation of the TFR1 and the Rab12-dependent autophagy mechanism leading to retinal ganglion cell death. The addition of iron in this model reduces cell death [162]. It seems that iron metabolism is dysregulated in glaucoma, but the exact role of iron is optic nerve damage and remains to be studied in the pathogenesis of glaucoma.

5.6. Inherited Retinal Dystrophies and Associated Diseases

Retinitis pigmentosa affects approximately 1.8 to 2.4 million people around the world. The disease is characterized by degeneration of the PR and progressive complete blindness [163]. Although iron has been shown to accumulate in several models of retinal degeneration, as in rd10 mouse or RCS rat [86,164], the direct link between iron and retinitis pigmentosa has not been established in human disease.

Macular telangiectasia type 2 (MacTel 2) is a complex macular disease, characterized by abnormal perifoveal vessels (telangiectasia), loss of retinal organization, and ultimately loss of macula function. MacTel2 is the only human disease recognized as primarily associated with MGC cells loss. It has been shown that iron accumulates in the retina of patients with MacTel 2. In a murine model of MGC ablation that mimics part of MacTel 2 phenotype, there is also an accumulation of iron in retina and in the RPE [148]. Knowing the importance of MGC cells in the regulation of iron levels in the retina, it could be hypothesized that iron accumulates in MacTel 2 as a consequence of MGC loss in the fovea [165].

6. Iron Neutralization as a Therapeutic Strategy for Retinal Diseases

6.1. Chemical Chelators

Whether iron dysmetabolism in the retina is a cause or a consequence of various retinal diseases, iron accumulation is pathogenic, and its neutralization was shown to protect the retina from oxidative damage and retinal cell death in various models using different neutralizing strategies [133] (Table 2). As early as in the 1970s, an iron chelator, Deferroxamine, was used in humans to reduce the amount of "rust" deposited on the eye with satisfactory results. Used in many other models of retinal degeneration (retinitis pigmentosa [166] or light-induced retinal damage models [167]), this chelator reduces the iron load and preserves the retina. Other chelators, such as Deferriprone, have shown significant protection of the retina in mice with impaired mechanisms of iron homeostasis [168–171]. These chemical chelators are mainly used clinically to treat hemosiderosis induced by frequent transfusions. Administered orally, subcutaneously or intramuscularly, they could led to several eye side effects, including vision loss [172,173]. These side effects could be explained because chemical iron chelators also bind the iron necessary for RPE and PR function [133,174].

As highlighted in a recent review [175], the clinical use of chemical chelators is complex because they should (1) target only the organ or tissue which is affected by the iron excess; (2) have a sufficient half-life; (3) cross the different barriers that surround the tissue; and (4) have a rapid elimination route.

Table 2. Comparison between chemical iron chelators and transferrin in clinical use.

	Deferoxamine	Deferiprone	Deferasirox	Transferrin
Iron Binding	1:1	3:1	2:1	2:1
Route of administration	Sub-cutaneous (every 8–12h) Intravenous (IV) (5 days/week)	Oral (t.i.d)	Oral (q.d)	Intravenous [176]
Half-Life(after IV administration)	20–30 min	3–4 h	8–16 h	4–8 d [176]
Excretion	Urinary/fecal	Urinary	Fecal	Unknown
Usual Doses (mg/Kg/d)	25–60 [177]	75–100 [177]	20–40 [177]	100 [176]
Clinical Use	Acute iron intoxicationChronic iron overload	Chronic iron overload	Chronic iron overload	Atransferrinemia [178] Haematological stem cell transplant [176]
Ocular Side effects	Pigmentary retinopathy [173], visual loss [179], impaired night vision [180], optic neuritis [173] and cataract [172].	Diplopia [181], cataract [182] and possible retinal toxicity [183].	Lens opacities [184] and retinal disorders [185]	No adverse effects observed

Legend Table 2: Tid: 3 times a day; q.d: once a day.

6.2. Natural Chelators

Other natural molecules generally coming from plants, such as curcumin, polyphenols, and flavonoids, are iron chelators and have shown effectiveness in mouse models of retinal degeneration (for a review, see [186,187]).

6.3. Transferrin

TF is part of the TF superfamily, which also includes lactoferrin, melanotransferrin, and ovotransferrin, which are found in many species of both mammals and invertebrates. It consists in two lobes, each binding a Fe^{3+} atom with a very high affinity ($10^{22}M^{-1}$). Its primary role is to maintain an environment devoid of free iron. TF synthesized by RPE, PR, and neuronal cells is found in the aqueous and vitreous humors [8,105]. By single-cell RNA sequencing of human neural retina, mRNA for TF was enriched in peripheral retina compared to fovea [188]. Its expression is amplified during inflammation or immunity to increase the buffering capacity of iron. In light-induced retinal degeneration, TF and TFR1 mRNA increased in retina immediately after light exposure and then decreased at basal level. One day after light exposure, TF was increased, whereas TFR1 was reduced compared to not illuminated mice [32]. TF has long been of therapeutic interest due to its antimicrobial capacity and the ubiquitous presence of TFR1 allowing penetration of the blood-brain barrier [189]. TF has also been used successfully in humans in iron metabolism pathologies and for its cytoprotective capacity [190].

Our laboratory is interested in the potential of TF for the treatment of retinal pathologies (Table 3). Our work has shown that administration of the iron-free form (apoTF) by intraperitoneal injections in rd10 mice, a model of retinitis pigmentosa, preserves PRs better compared to the use of other chelators or antioxidants [46,164]. Injected into the vitreous, TF is present throughout the neural retina (MGC) and is eliminated via its receptors by RPE and the choroid without any immunogenic or toxic effect on the retina [46,105]. Thus, TF administered in a model of light-induced degeneration, allows the restoration of iron homeostasis, decreases iron accumulation, reduces inflammation and apoptosis, and preserves PRs and visual function [43]. In an ex vivo model of retinal detachment, TF inhibits the degenerative processes activated by the iron excess by reducing necrosis, apoptosis, gliosis, and oxidative stress. In vivo, human TF constitutively expressed in transgenic mice (TG) reduces loss of cones, cleavage of caspase 3, an apoptosis effector, DNA breaks, and necrosis (Figure 3). In rats, TF injected at the time of the detachment, reduces retinal edema, cell death and preserves PRs. In addition to its ability to reduce the accumulation of iron in the retina following detachment, TF also acts on other cellular pathways, no doubt through its interaction with molecular partners which remain to be discovered [105].

Table 3. Transferrin as a therapeutic drug in retinal diseases models.

Model Experiment	Physiopathology	Administration Mode	Therapeutic Action of Transferrin	References
Primary culture of Müller glial cells.	Iron exposure	Cell isolation from transgenic mice carrying the human transferrin gene (TghTF)	Cell number preservation. Lower necrosis revealed by lactate dehydrogenase release. Inhibition of mRNA TF diminution.	[46]
Primary culture of Müller glial cells	Iron exposure	Addition of apo- or holo-human TF	Dose-dependent cell number preservation by apo- but not holo-human TF	[46]
rd10 mice	Model of retinitis pigmentosa presenting iron accumulation in photoreceptors (PR)	Crossing rd10 mice with TghTF mice	Preservation of retinal histology (outer and inner nuclear layers thickness). Less apoptotic-positive retinal cells. Conservation of rods and cones morphology	[164]
rd10 mice	Model of retinitis pigmentosa presenting iron accumulation in PR	Daily intraperitoneal injections of apo-human TF	Dose-dependent preservation of retinal histology (outer and inner nuclear layers thickness). Less apoptotic-positive retinal cells. Conservation of rods and cones morphology	[164]
Light-induced degeneration	Model of acute degenerative retina	Intravitreal injection of apo-human TF before and after light-induced degeneration	Preservation of retinal histology and functions. Preservation of ONL thickness and PR morphology. Lower ONL apoptotic-positive cells. Regulation of iron homeostasis balance. Lower retinal iron accumulation and oxidative stress. Regulation of retina inflammation and diminution of microglial cells activation in outer retina.	[43]
Light-induced degeneration	Model of acute degenerative retina	Electrotransfer of cDNA of human TF for *in oculo* production	Preservation of retinal histology and ONL layer thickness.	[43]
P23H rats	Model of retinitis pigmentosa	Electrotransfer of cDNA of human TF for *in oculo* production	Preservation of retinal histology and ONL layer thickness.	[43]
Bone morphogenetic protein 6 mice	Model of hemochromatosis with retinal iron accumulation	Intraperitoneal and intravitreal injections of apo-human TF	Diminution of iron accumulation in retina pigment epithelium	[43]

Table 3. *Cont.*

Model Experiment	Physiopathology	Administration Mode	Therapeutic Action of Transferrin	References
Retinal explant of mice	Retinal detachment with iron exposure	Retinas from TghTF	Preservation of cones number and rod outer segments length. Lower necrosis Prevention of iron retinal accumulation	[105]
Retinal explant of rats	Retinal detachment with iron exposure	Addition of apo-human TF after iron exposure	Preservation of rhodopsin expression level and cones number Lower necrosis and apoptosis Prevention of retinal iron accumulation	[105]
Subretinal injection of hyaluronic acid in mice	Retinal detachment presenting iron accumulation in subretinal space	TghTF mice	Preservation of retinal histology, rods outer segments length and number of cones Diminution of retinal oedema and Müller glial cells activation Lower apoptosis and necrosis Regulation of pathways involved in biological functions	[105]
Subretinal injection of hyaluronic acid in rats	Retinal detachment presenting iron accumulation in subretinal space	Intravitreal injection of apo-hTF	Preservation of retinal histology, rods outer segments length Diminution of retinal oedema	[105]

Legend Table 3: ApoTF: transferrin without iron; HoloTF: transferrin binding iron; INL: inner nuclear layer; ONL: outer nuclear layer; PR: photoreceptors; TF: transferrin; TghTf: transgenic mice carrying the complete human transferrin gene.

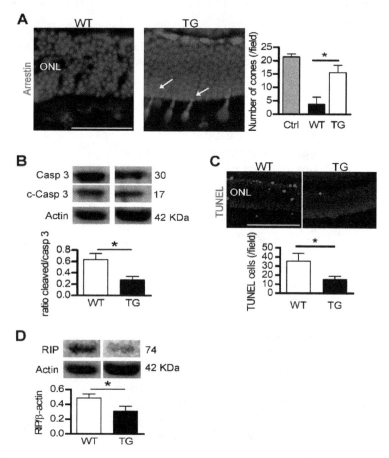

Figure 3. Transferrin expression preserves the detached retina. **Legend Figure 3:** After retinal detachment (RD), photoreceptors died by apoptosis and necrosis. Transgenic mice (TG) expressing human transferrin (TF) were used to demonstrate the protective effects of TF. (**A**) Arrestin staining revealed cones in retinal sections of TG mice (arrows) after RD. Cone number was higher in TG compared with WT mice. (**B**) The ratio of cleaved/pro–caspase 3 protein level was lower in TG mice compared to WT mice after RD. (**C**) The number of nuclei positive apoptotic-DNA breaks, stained by TUNEL, was reduced in TG mice compared to WT mice. (**D**) Necrotic RIP kinase protein level was reduced in TG mice compared with WT mice. All values are represented as the mean ± SEM. Mann–Whitney test (n = 3–6), * $p \leq 0.025$. ONL: Outer nuclear layer. Scale bar, 100 μm. From [105]. Reprinted with permission from AAAS.

7. Conclusions

Iron is one of the most common elements on Earth. Two-hundred years ago, it was discovered that, after desiccation, the residual ashes of an aged human retina could be mobilized by a magnet (as quoted in [191]). Nowadays the chemical study of iron structure and its outer electrons has been revealed by the discovery of quantum effects of iron electron in biology. The best illustrations have been described by Cedric Weber who demonstrated that very specific quantum effects are involved to explain the energy in the binding of iron to oxygen and CO to hemoglobin [192]. This transition metal plays a main role in retinal physiology, but overload leads to retinal degeneration and loss of function. Iron chelation is a potential therapeutic target to prevent retinal degeneration. TF, as an endogenous iron binding protein, avoids toxic effects of iron depletion and activates additional neuroprotective pathways.

Author Contributions: Conceptualization: E.P., Y.C., F.B.-C.; literature search: E.P., A.D.; J.Y., Y.C., F.B.-C.; figure and tables: E.P., J.Y.; writing—original draft preparation E.P., A.D.; Y.C., F.B.-C.; writing—review and editing: E.P., A.D.; Y.C., F.B.-C. All authors have read and agreed to the published version of the manuscript.

Acknowledgments: We sincerely thank Jean-Claude Jeanny and Marina Yefimova for their significant contribution in the initial description of iron and iron-related proteins in retina.

Abbreviations

ABC	ATP binding cassette
AMD	Age-Related Macular Degeneration
APP	amyloid-beta precursor protein
BMP	Bone Morphogenetic Protein
BRB	Blood Retinal Barrier
CEC	Choroidal Endothelial Cell
CP	Ceruloplasmin
DFO	Deferroxamine
DMT1	divalent metal transporter 1
Fe-S	Cluster Iron-Sulfur
FPN	Ferroportin
FT	Ferritin
HEPC	Hepcidin
HEPH	Hephaestin
HFE	Hemochromatosis protein
HFT	Heavy Ferritin chin
HIF	Hypoxia Inducible Factor
HJV	Hemojuveline
HRE	Hypoxia Responsive Element
IL	Interleukin
IRE	Iron Responsive Element
IRP	Iron Regulatory Protein
LCN2	Lipocalin 2
LF	Lactoferrin
LFT	Light Ferritin chain
LIP	Labile Iron Pool
MacTel 2	Macular telangiectasia type 2
MGC	Muller Glial cell
NTBI	Non-Transferrin Bound Iron

NLRP3	NOD-like receptor family, pyrin domain containing 3
PCBP	Poly(rC)-binding proteins
PrP^C	Prion protein
PR	photoreceptor
REC	Retinal Endothelial Cell
ROS	Reactive Oxygen Species
RPE	Retinal Pigment Epithelium
SCARA5	Scavenger receptor class A, member 5
SMAD	Mothers against decapentaplegic homolog 1
TBI	Transferrin Bound Iron
TF	Transferrin
TFR	Transferrin Receptor
VEGF	Vascular Endothelial Growth Factor
ZP	Zyloklopen
ZIP	ZRT/IRT-like proteins

References

1. Daruich, A.; Matet, A.; Moulin, A.; Kowalczuk, L.; Nicolas, M.; Sellam, A.; Rothschild, P.-R.; Omri, S.; Gélizé, E.; Jonet, L.; et al. Mechanisms of macular edema: Beyond the surface. *Prog. Retin. Eye Res.* **2018**, *63*, 20–68. [CrossRef] [PubMed]

2. Anderson, B.; Saltzman, H.A. RETINAL OXYGEN UTILIZATION MEASURED BY HYPERBARIC BLACKOUT. *Arch. Ophthalmol.* **1964**, *72*, 792–795. [CrossRef] [PubMed]

3. Linsenmeier, R.A.; Zhang, H.F. Retinal oxygen: From animals to humans. *Prog. Retin. Eye Res.* **2017**, *58*, 115–151. [CrossRef] [PubMed]

4. Wang, L.; Törnquist, P.; Bill, A. Glucose metabolism in pig outer retina in light and darkness. *Acta Physiol. Scand.* **1997**, *160*, 75–81. [CrossRef] [PubMed]

5. Hurley, J.B.; Lindsay, K.J.; Du, J. Glucose, lactate, and shuttling of metabolites in vertebrate retinas. *J. Neurosci. Res.* **2015**, *93*, 1079–1092. [CrossRef] [PubMed]

6. Kurihara, T. Development and pathological changes of neurovascular unit regulated by hypoxia response in the retina. *Prog. Brain Res.* **2016**, *225*, 201–211.

7. Yang, L.; Wang, D.; Wang, X.-T.; Lu, Y.-P.; Zhu, L. The roles of hypoxia-inducible Factor-1 and iron regulatory protein 1 in iron uptake induced by acute hypoxia. *Biochem. Biophys. Res. Commun.* **2018**, *507*, 128–135. [CrossRef]

8. Yefimova, M.G.; Jeanny, J.C.; Guillonneau, X.; Keller, N.; Nguyen-Legros, J.; Sergeant, C.; Guillou, F.; Courtois, Y. Iron, ferritin, transferrin, and transferrin receptor in the adult rat retina. *Investig. Ophthalmol. Vis. Sci.* **2000**, *41*, 2343–2351.

9. Garcia-Castineiras, S. Iron, the retina and the lens: A focused review. *Exp. Eye Res.* **2010**, *90*, 664–678. [CrossRef]

10. Moos, T.; Bernth, N.; Courtois, Y.; Morgan, E.H. Developmental iron uptake and axonal transport in the retina of the rat. *Mol. Cell. Neurosci.* **2011**, *46*, 607–613. [CrossRef]

11. Hahn, P.; Song, Y.; Ying, G.S.; He, X.; Beard, J.; Dunaief, J.L. Age-dependent and gender-specific changes in mouse tissue iron by strain. *Exp. Gerontol.* **2009**, *44*, 594–600. [CrossRef] [PubMed]

12. Hahn, P.; Ying, G.S.; Beard, J.; Dunaief, J.L. Iron levels in human retina: Sex difference and increase with age. *Neuroreport* **2006**, *17*, 1803–1806. [CrossRef] [PubMed]

13. Ugarte, M.; Osborne, N.N.; Brown, L.A.; Bishop, P.N. Iron, zinc, and copper in retinal physiology and disease. *Surv. Ophthalmol.* **2013**, *58*, 585–609. [CrossRef] [PubMed]

14. Chen, H.; Liu, B.; Lukas, T.J.; Suyeoka, G.; Wu, G.; Neufeld, A.H. Changes in iron-regulatory proteins in the aged rodent neural retina. *Neurobiol. Aging* **2009**, *30*, 1865–1876. [CrossRef] [PubMed]

15. Chen, H.; Lukas, T.J.; Du, N.; Suyeoka, G.; Neufeld, A.H. Dysfunction of the retinal pigment epithelium with age: Increased iron decreases phagocytosis and lysosomal activity. *Investig. Ophthalmol. Vis. Sci.* **2009**, *50*, 1895–1902. [CrossRef] [PubMed]

16. Lane, D.J.R.; Merlot, A.M.; Huang, M.L.-H.; Bae, D.-H.; Jansson, P.J.; Sahni, S.; Kalinowski, D.S.; Richardson, D.R. Cellular iron uptake, trafficking and metabolism: Key molecules and mechanisms and their roles in disease. *Biochim. Biophys. Acta (BBA) - Mol. Cell Res.* **2015**, *1853*, 1130–1144. [CrossRef]

17. Lederman, M.; Obolensky, A.; Grunin, M.; Banin, E.; Chowers, I. Retinal Function and Structure in the Hypotransferrinemic Mouse. *Investig. Opthalmol. Vis. Sci.* **2012**, *53*, 605. [CrossRef]

18. Rageh, A.A.; Ferrington, D.A.; Roehrich, H.; Yuan, C.; Terluk, M.R.; Nelson, E.F.; Montezuma, S.R. Lactoferrin Expression in Human and Murine Ocular Tissue. *Curr. Eye Res.* **2016**, *41*, 883–889. [CrossRef]

19. Montezuma, S.R.; Dolezal, L.D.; Rageh, A.A.; Mar, K.; Jordan, M.; Ferrington, D.A. Lactoferrin Reduces Chorioretinal Damage in the Murine Laser Model of Choroidal Neovascularization. *Curr. Eye Res.* **2015**, *40*, 946–953. [CrossRef]

20. Parmar, T.; Parmar, V.M.; Arai, E.; Sahu, B.; Perusek, L.; Maeda, A. Acute Stress Responses Are Early Molecular Events of Retinal Degeneration in Abca4−/−Rdh8−/− Mice After Light Exposure. *Investig. Ophthalmol. Vis. Sci.* **2016**, *57*, 3257–3267. [CrossRef]

21. Parmar, T.; Parmar, V.M.; Perusek, L.; Georges, A.; Takahashi, M.; Crabb, J.W.; Maeda, A. Lipocalin 2 Plays an Important Role in Regulating Inflammation in Retinal Degeneration. *J. Immunol.* **2018**, *200*, 3128–3141. [CrossRef] [PubMed]

22. Cases, O.; Obry, A.; Ben-Yacoub, S.; Augustin, S.; Joseph, A.; Toutirais, G.; Simonutti, M.; Christ, A.; Cosette, P.; Kozyraki, R. Impaired vitreous composition and retinal pigment epithelium function in the FoxG1::LRP2 myopic mice. *Biochim. Biophys. Acta* **2017**, *1863*, 1242–1254. [CrossRef] [PubMed]

23. Hahn, P.; Dentchev, T.; Qian, Y.; Rouault, T.; Harris, Z.L.; Dunaief, J.L. Immunolocalization and regulation of iron handling proteins ferritin and ferroportin in the retina. *Mol. Vis.* **2004**, *10*, 598–607. [PubMed]

24. Theurl, M.; Song, D.; Clark, E.; Sterling, J.; Grieco, S.; Altamura, S.; Galy, B.; Hentze, M.; Muckenthaler, M.U.; Dunaief, J.L. Mice with hepcidin-resistant ferroportin accumulate iron in the retina. *FASEB J.* **2016**, *30*, 813–823. [CrossRef] [PubMed]

25. Hahn, P.; Qian, Y.; Dentchev, T.; Chen, L.; Beard, J.; Harris, Z.L.; Dunaief, J.L. Disruption of ceruloplasmin and hephaestin in mice causes retinal iron overload and retinal degeneration with features of age-related macular degeneration. *Proc. Natl. Acad. Sci. USA* **2004**, *101*, 13850–13855. [CrossRef]

26. Wolkow, N.; Song, D.; Song, Y.; Chu, S.; Hadziahmetovic, M.; Lee, J.C.; Iacovelli, J.; Grieco, S.; Dunaief, J.L. Ferroxidase hephaestin's cell-autonomous role in the retinal pigment epithelium. *Am. J. Pathol.* **2012**, *180*, 1614–1624. [CrossRef]

27. Wolkow, N.; Song, Y.; Wu, T.-D.; Qian, J.; Guerquin-Kern, J.-L.; Dunaief, J.L. Aceruloplasminemia: Retinal histopathologic manifestations and iron-mediated melanosome degradation. *Arch. Ophthalmol.* **2011**, *129*, 1466–1474. [CrossRef]

28. Dinet, V.; An, N.; Ciccotosto, G.D.; Bruban, J.; Maoui, A.; Bellingham, S.A.; Hill, A.F.; Andersen, O.M.; Nykjaer, A.; Jonet, L.; et al. APP involvement in retinogenesis of mice. *Acta Neuropathol.* **2011**, *121*, 351–363. [CrossRef]

29. Chen, H.; Attieh, Z.K.; Syed, B.A.; Kuo, Y.; Stevens, V.; Fuqua, B.K.; Andersen, H.S.; Naylor, C.E.; Evans, R.W.; Gambling, L.; et al. Identification of Zyklopen, a New Member of the Vertebrate Multicopper Ferroxidase Family, and Characterization in Rodents and Human Cells123. *J. Nutr.* **2010**, *140*, 1728–1735. [CrossRef]

30. He, X.; Hahn, P.; Iacovelli, J.; Wong, R.; King, C.; Bhisitkul, R.; Massaro-Giordano, M.; Dunaief, J.L. Iron homeostasis and toxicity in retinal degeneration. *Prog. Retin. Eye Res.* **2007**, *26*, 649–673. [CrossRef]

31. Sterling, J.; Guttha, S.; Song, Y.; Song, D.; Hadziahmetovic, M.; Dunaief, J.L. Iron importers Zip8 and Zip14 are expressed in retina and regulated by retinal iron levels. *Exp. Eye Res.* **2017**, *155*, 15–23. [CrossRef] [PubMed]

32. Picard, E.; Ranchon-Cole, I.; Jonet, L.; Beaumont, C.; Behar-Cohen, F.; Courtois, Y.; Jeanny, J.-C. Light-induced retinal degeneration correlates with changes in iron metabolism gene expression, ferritin level, and aging. *Investig. Ophthalmol. Vis. Sci.* **2011**, *52*, 1261–1274. [CrossRef] [PubMed]

33. Martin, P.M.; Gnana-Prakasam, J.P.; Roon, P.; Smith, R.G.; Smith, S.B.; Ganapathy, V. Expression and polarized localization of the hemochromatosis gene product HFE in retinal pigment epithelium. *Investig. Ophthalmol. Vis. Sci.* **2006**, *47*, 4238–4244. [CrossRef] [PubMed]

34. Gnana-Prakasam, J.P.; Thangaraju, M.; Liu, K.; Ha, Y.; Martin, P.M.; Smith, S.B.; Ganapathy, V. Absence of iron-regulatory protein Hfe results in hyperproliferation of retinal pigment epithelium: Role of cystine/glutamate exchanger. *Biochem. J.* **2009**, *424*, 243–252. [CrossRef] [PubMed]

35. Hadziahmetovic, M.; Song, Y.; Wolkow, N.; Iacovelli, J.; Kautz, L.; Roth, M.P.; Dunaief, J.L. Bmp6 regulates retinal iron homeostasis and has altered expression in age-related macular degeneration. *Am. J. Pathol.* **2011**, *179*, 335–348. [CrossRef] [PubMed]

36. Gnana-Prakasam, J.P.; Zhang, M.; Martin, P.M.; Atherton, S.S.; Smith, S.B.; Ganapathy, V. Expression of the iron-regulatory protein haemojuvelin in retina and its regulation during cytomegalovirus infection. *Biochem. J.* **2009**, *419*, 533–543. [CrossRef] [PubMed]

37. Tawfik, A.; Gnana-Prakasam, J.P.; Smith, S.B.; Ganapathy, V. Deletion of hemojuvelin, an iron-regulatory protein, in mice results in abnormal angiogenesis and vasculogenesis in retina along with reactive gliosis. *Investig. Ophthalmol. Vis. Sci.* **2014**, *55*, 3616–3625. [CrossRef] [PubMed]

38. Gnana-Prakasam, J.P.; Baldowski, R.B.; Ananth, S.; Martin, P.M.; Smith, S.B.; Ganapathy, V. Retinal expression of the serine protease matriptase-2 (Tmprss6) and its role in retinal iron homeostasis. *Mol. Vis.* **2014**, *20*, 561–574. [PubMed]

39. Hadziahmetovic, M.; Song, Y.; Ponnuru, P.; Iacovelli, J.; Hunter, A.; Haddad, N.; Beard, J.; Connor, J.R.; Vaulont, S.; Dunaief, J.L. Age-Dependent Retinal Iron Accumulation and Degeneration in Hepcidin Knockout Mice. *Investig. Ophthalmol. Vis. Sci.* **2011**, *52*, 109–118. [CrossRef] [PubMed]

40. Kast, B.; Schori, C.; Grimm, C. Hypoxic preconditioning protects photoreceptors against light damage independently of hypoxia inducible transcription factors in rods. *Exp. Eye Res.* **2016**, *146*, 60–71. [CrossRef]

41. Hughes, J.M.; Groot, A.J.; van der Groep, P.; Sersansie, R.; Vooijs, M.; van Diest, P.J.; Van Noorden, C.J.F.; Schlingemann, R.O.; Klaassen, I. Active HIF-1 in the normal human retina. *J. Histochem. Cytochem.* **2010**, *58*, 247–254. [CrossRef]

42. Perez Bay, A.E.; Schreiner, R.; Benedicto, I.; Rodriguez-Boulan, E.J. Galectin-4-mediated transcytosis of transferrin receptor. *J. Cell. Sci.* **2014**, *127*, 4457–4469. [CrossRef] [PubMed]

43. Picard, E.; Le Rouzic, Q.; Oudar, A.; Berdugo, M.; El Sanharawi, M.; Andrieu-Soler, C.; Naud, M.C.; Jonet, L.; Latour, C.; Klein, C.; et al. Targeting iron-mediated retinal degeneration by local delivery of transferrin. *Free Radic. Biol. Med.* **2015**, *89*, 1105–1121. [CrossRef] [PubMed]

44. Kaczara, P.; Zaręba, M.; Herrnreiter, A.; Skumatz, C.M.B.; Żądło, A.; Sarna, T.; Burke, J.M. Melanosome-iron interactions within retinal pigment epithelium-derived cells. *Pigment Cell Melanoma Res.* **2012**, *25*, 804–814. [CrossRef] [PubMed]

45. Baumann, B.H.; Shu, W.; Song, Y.; Simpson, E.M.; Lakhal-Littleton, S.; Dunaief, J.L. Ferroportin-mediated iron export from vascular endothelial cells in retina and brain. *Exp. Eye Res.* **2019**, *187*, 107728. [CrossRef] [PubMed]

46. Picard, E.; Fontaine, I.; Jonet, L.; Guillou, F.; Behar-Cohen, F.; Courtois, Y.; Jeanny, J.C. The protective role of transferrin in Muller glial cells after iron-induced toxicity. *Mol. Vis.* **2008**, *14*, 928–941. [PubMed]

47. Mendes-Jorge, L.; Ramos, D.; Valença, A.; López-Luppo, M.; Pires, V.M.R.; Catita, J.; Nacher, V.; Navarro, M.; Carretero, A.; Rodriguez-Baeza, A.; et al. Correction: L-Ferritin Binding to Scara5: A New Iron Traffic Pathway Potentially Implicated in Retinopathy. *PLoS ONE* **2017**, *12*, e0180288. [CrossRef]

48. Rousseau, E.; Michel, P.P.; Hirsch, E.C. The Iron-Binding Protein Lactoferrin Protects Vulnerable Dopamine Neurons from Degeneration by Preserving Mitochondrial Calcium Homeostasis. *Mol. Pharm.* **2013**, *84*, 888–898. [CrossRef]

49. Valapala, M.; Edwards, M.; Hose, S.; Grebe, R.; Bhutto, I.A.; Cano, M.; Berger, T.; Mak, T.W.; Wawrousek, E.; Handa, J.T.; et al. Increased Lipocalin-2 in the retinal pigment epithelium of *Cryba1* cKO mice is associated with a chronic inflammatory response. *Aging Cell* **2014**, *13*, 1091–1094. [CrossRef]

50. Ananth, S.; Gnana-Prakasam, J.P.; Bhutia, Y.D.; Veeranan-Karmegam, R.; Martin, P.M.; Smith, S.B.; Ganapathy, V. Regulation of the cholesterol efflux transporters ABCA1 and ABCG1 in retina in hemochromatosis and by the endogenous siderophore 2,5-dihydroxybenzoic acid. *Biochim. Biophys. Acta (BBA) - Mol. Basis Dis.* **2014**, *1842*, 603–612. [CrossRef]

51. Anderson, C.P.; Shen, M.; Eisenstein, R.S.; Leibold, E.A. Mammalian iron metabolism and its control by iron regulatory proteins. *Biochim. Biophys. Acta* **2012**, *1823*, 1468–1483. [CrossRef] [PubMed]

52. Baumann, B.H.; Shu, W.; Song, Y.; Sterling, J.; Kozmik, Z.; Lakhal-Littleton, S.; Dunaief, J.L. Liver-Specific, but Not Retina-Specific, Hepcidin Knockout Causes Retinal Iron Accumulation and Degeneration. *Am. J. Pathol.* **2019**, *189*, 1814–1830. [CrossRef] [PubMed]

53. Mowat, F.M.; Luhmann, U.F.O.; Smith, A.J.; Lange, C.; Duran, Y.; Harten, S.; Shukla, D.; Maxwell, P.H.; Ali, R.R.; Bainbridge, J.W.B. HIF-1alpha and HIF-2alpha Are Differentially Activated in Distinct Cell Populations in Retinal Ischaemia. *PLoS ONE* **2010**, *5*, e11103. [CrossRef] [PubMed]

54. Maio, N.; Rouault, T.A. Iron-sulfur cluster biogenesis in mammalian cells: New insights into the molecular mechanisms of cluster delivery. *Biochim. Biophys. Acta* **2015**, *1853*, 1493–1512. [CrossRef]

55. Das, D.; Patra, S.; Bridwell-Rabb, J.; Barondeau, D.P. Mechanism of frataxin "bypass" in human iron–sulfur cluster biosynthesis with implications for Friedreich's ataxia. *J. Biol. Chem.* **2019**, *294*, 9276–9284. [CrossRef] [PubMed]

56. Efimova, M.G.; Trottier, Y. Distribution of frataxin in eye retina of normal mice and of transgenic R7E mice with retinal degeneration. *J. Evol. Biochem. Phys.* **2010**, *46*, 414–417. [CrossRef]

57. Crombie, D.E.; Van Bergen, N.; Davidson, K.C.; Anjomani Virmouni, S.; Mckelvie, P.A.; Chrysostomou, V.; Conquest, A.; Corben, L.A.; Pook, M.A.; Kulkarni, T.; et al. Characterization of the retinal pigment epithelium in Friedreich ataxia. *Biochem. Biophys. Rep.* **2015**, *4*, 141–147. [CrossRef]

58. Rouault, T.A.; Maio, N. Biogenesis and functions of mammalian iron-sulfur proteins in the regulation of iron homeostasis and pivotal metabolic pathways. *J. Biol. Chem.* **2017**, *292*, 12744–12753. [CrossRef]

59. Crack, J.C.; Green, J.; Thomson, A.J.; Brun, N.E.L. Iron–Sulfur Clusters as Biological Sensors: The Chemistry of Reactions with Molecular Oxygen and Nitric Oxide. *Acc. Chem. Res.* **2014**, *47*, 3196–3205. [CrossRef]

60. Puig, S.; Ramos-Alonso, L.; Romero, A.M.; Martínez-Pastor, M.T. The elemental role of iron in DNA synthesis and repair. *Metallomics* **2017**, *9*, 1483–1500. [CrossRef]

61. Paul, V.D.; Lill, R. Biogenesis of cytosolic and nuclear iron-sulfur proteins and their role in genome stability. *Biochim. Biophys. Acta* **2015**, *1853*, 1528–1539. [CrossRef] [PubMed]

62. Luo, H.; Zhou, M.; Ji, K.; Zhuang, J.; Dang, W.; Fu, S.; Sun, T.; Zhang, X. Expression of Sirtuins in the Retinal Neurons of Mice, Rats, and Humans. *Front. Aging Neurosci.* **2017**, *9*, 366. [CrossRef] [PubMed]

63. Zhao, Z.; Chen, Y.; Wang, J.; Sternberg, P.; Freeman, M.L.; Grossniklaus, H.E.; Cai, J. Age-Related Retinopathy in NRF2-Deficient Mice. *PLoS ONE* **2011**, *6*, e19456. [CrossRef]

64. Alexeyev, M.; Shokolenko, I.; Wilson, G.; LeDoux, S. The Maintenance of Mitochondrial DNA Integrity–Critical Analysis and Update. *Cold Spring Harb. Perspect. Biol.* **2013**, *5*, a012641. [CrossRef] [PubMed]

65. Ballinger, S.W.; Van Houten, B.; Jin, G.F.; Conklin, C.A.; Godley, B.F. Hydrogen peroxide causes significant mitochondrial DNA damage in human RPE cells. *Exp. Eye Res.* **1999**, *68*, 765–772. [CrossRef] [PubMed]

66. Barreau, E.; Brossas, J.-Y.; Courtois, Y.; Treton, J.A. Accumulation of Mitochondrial DNA Deletions in Human Retina During Aging. *Investig. Ophthalmol. Vis. Sci.* **1996**, *37*, 384–391.

67. Gkotsi, D.; Begum, R.; Salt, T.; Lascaratos, G.; Hogg, C.; Chau, K.-Y.; Schapira, A.H.V.; Jeffery, G. Recharging mitochondrial batteries in old eyes. Near infra-red increases ATP. *Exp. Eye Res.* **2014**, *122*, 50–53. [CrossRef]

68. Tezel, T.H.; Geng, L.; Lato, E.B.; Schaal, S.; Liu, Y.; Dean, D.; Klein, J.B.; Kaplan, H.J. Synthesis and Secretion of Hemoglobin by Retinal Pigment Epithelium. *Investig. Opthalmol. Vis. Sci.* **2009**, *50*, 1911. [CrossRef]

69. Promsote, W.; Makala, L.; Li, B.; Smith, S.B.; Singh, N.; Ganapathy, V.; Pace, B.S.; Martin, P.M. Monomethylfumarate Induces γ-Globin Expression and Fetal Hemoglobin Production in Cultured Human Retinal Pigment Epithelial (RPE) and Erythroid Cells, and in Intact Retina. *Investig. Opthalmol. Vis. Sci.* **2014**, *55*, 5382. [CrossRef]

70. Hunt, R.C.; Hunt, D.M.; Gaur, N.; Smith, A. Hemopexin in the human retina: Protection of the retina against heme-mediated toxicity. *J. Cell. Physiol.* **1996**, *168*, 71–80. [CrossRef]

71. Chen, W.; Lu, H.; Dutt, K.; Smith, A.; Hunt, D.M.; Hunt, R.C. Expression of the protective proteins hemopexin and haptoglobin by cells of the neural retina. *Exp. Eye Res.* **1998**, *67*, 83–93. [CrossRef] [PubMed]

72. Ascenzi, P.; di Masi, A.; Leboffe, L.; Fiocchetti, M.; Nuzzo, M.T.; Brunori, M.; Marino, M. Neuroglobin: From structure to function in health and disease. *Mol. Asp. Med.* **2016**, *52*, 1–48. [CrossRef] [PubMed]

73. Tao, Y.; Ma, Z.; Liu, B.; Fang, W.; Qin, L.; Huang, Y.F.; Wang, L.; Gao, Y. Hemin supports the survival of photoreceptors injured by N-Methyl-N-nitrosourea: The contributory role of neuroglobin in photoreceptor degeneration. *Brain Res.* **2018**, *1678*, 47–55. [CrossRef] [PubMed]

74. Yu, Z.-L.; Qiu, S.; Chen, X.-C.; Dai, Z.-H.; Huang, Y.-C.; Li, Y.-N.; Cai, R.-H.; Lei, H.-T.; Gu, H.-Y. Neuroglobin – A potential biological marker of retinal damage induced by LED light. *Neuroscience* **2014**, *270*, 158–167. [CrossRef]

75. Jin, K.; Mao, X.; Xie, L.; Greenberg, D.A. Interactions between Vascular Endothelial Growth Factor and Neuroglobin. *Neurosci. Lett.* **2012**, *519*, 47–50. [CrossRef]

76. Gnana-Prakasam, J.P.; Reddy, S.K.; Veeranan-Karmegam, R.; Smith, S.B.; Martin, P.M.; Ganapathy, V. Polarized distribution of heme transporters in retinal pigment epithelium and their regulation in the iron-overload disease hemochromatosis. *Investig. Ophthalmol. Vis. Sci.* **2011**, *52*, 9279–9286. [CrossRef]

77. Moiseyev, G.; Takahashi, Y.; Chen, Y.; Gentleman, S.; Redmond, T.M.; Crouch, R.K.; Ma, J.-X. RPE65 is an iron(II)-dependent isomerohydrolase in the retinoid visual cycle. *J. Biol. Chem.* **2006**, *281*, 2835–2840. [CrossRef]

78. Hamel, C.P.; Tsilou, E.; Pfeffer, B.A.; Hooks, J.J.; Detrick, B.; Redmond, T.M. Molecular cloning and expression of RPE65, a novel retinal pigment epithelium-specific microsomal protein that is post-transcriptionally regulated in vitro. *J. Biol. Chem.* **1993**, *268*, 15751–15757.

79. Marlhens, F.; Bareil, C.; Griffoin, J.M.; Zrenner, E.; Amalric, P.; Eliaou, C.; Liu, S.Y.; Harris, E.; Redmond, T.M.; Arnaud, B.; et al. Mutations in RPE65 cause Leber's congenital amaurosis. *Nat. Genet.* **1997**, *17*, 139–141. [CrossRef]

80. Shyam, R.; Gorusupudi, A.; Nelson, K.; Horvath, M.P.; Bernstein, P.S. RPE65 has an additional function as the lutein to *meso* -zeaxanthin isomerase in the vertebrate eye. *Proc. Natl. Acad. Sci. USA* **2017**, *114*, 10882–10887. [CrossRef]

81. Betts-Obregon, B.S.; Gonzalez-Fernandez, F.; Tsin, A.T. Interphotoreceptor retinoid-binding protein (IRBP) promotes retinol uptake and release by rat Müller cells (rMC-1) in vitro: Implications for the cone visual cycle. *Investig. Ophthalmol. Vis. Sci.* **2014**, *55*, 6265–6271. [CrossRef]

82. Unger, E.L.; Earley, C.J.; Beard, J.L. Diurnal cycle influences peripheral and brain iron levels in mice. *J. Appl. Physiol.* **2009**, *106*, 187–193. [CrossRef] [PubMed]

83. Unger, E.L.; Jones, B.C.; Bianco, L.E.; Allen, R.P.; Earley, C.J. Diurnal variations in brain iron concentrations in BXD RI mice. *Neuroscience* **2014**, *263*, 54–59. [CrossRef] [PubMed]

84. Lim, S.; Scholten, A.; Manchala, G.; Cudia, D.; Zlomke-Sell, S.-K.; Koch, K.-W.; Ames, J.B. Structural Characterization of Ferrous Ion Binding to Retinal Guanylate Cyclase Activator Protein 5 from Zebrafish Photoreceptors. *Biochemistry* **2017**, *56*, 6652–6661. [CrossRef]

85. Shichi, H. Microsomal electron transfer system of bovine retinal pigment epithelium. *Exp. Eye Res.* **1969**, *8*, 60–68. [CrossRef]

86. Yefimova, M.G.; Jeanny, J.-C.; Keller, N.; Sergeant, C.; Guillonneau, X.; Beaumont, C.; Courtois, Y. Impaired retinal iron homeostasis associated with defective phagocytosis in Royal College of Surgeons rats. *Investig. Ophthalmol. Vis. Sci.* **2002**, *43*, 537–545.

87. McGahan, M.C.; Harned, J.; Mukunnemkeril, M.; Goralska, M.; Fleisher, L.; Ferrell, J.B. Iron alters glutamate secretion by regulating cytosolic aconitase activity. *Am. J. Physiol. Cell Physiol.* **2005**, *288*, C1117–C1124. [CrossRef]

88. Kaushik, P.; Gorin, F.; Vali, S. Dynamics of tyrosine hydroxylase mediated regulation of dopamine synthesis. *J. Comput. Neurosci.* **2007**, *22*, 147–160. [CrossRef]

89. Huang, Q.; Hong, X.; Hao, Q. SNAP-25 is also an iron-sulfur protein. *FEBS Lett.* **2008**, *582*, 1431–1436. [CrossRef]

90. Molday, R.S. Insights into the Molecular Properties of ABCA4 and Its Role in the Visual Cycle and Stargardt Disease. In *Progress in Molecular Biology and Translational Science*; Elsevier: Amsterdam, The Netherlands, 2015; Volume 134, pp. 415–431. ISBN 978-0-12-801059-4.

91. Ueda, K.; Kim, H.J.; Zhao, J.; Song, Y.; Dunaief, J.L.; Sparrow, J.R. Iron promotes oxidative cell death caused by bisretinoids of retina. *Proc. Natl. Acad. Sci. USA* **2018**, *115*, 4963–4968. [CrossRef]

92. Lucius, R.; Sievers, J. Postnatal retinal ganglion cells in vitro: Protection against reactive oxygen species (ROS)-induced axonal degeneration by cocultured astrocytes. *Brain Res.* **1996**, *743*, 56–62. [CrossRef]

93. Kurz, T.; Karlsson, M.; Brunk, U.T.; Nilsson, S.E.; Frennesson, C. ARPE-19 retinal pigment epithelial cells are highly resistant to oxidative stress and exercise strict control over their lysosomal redox-active iron. *Autophagy* **2009**, *5*, 494–501. [CrossRef] [PubMed]

94. Rogers, B.S.; Symons, R.C.A.; Komeima, K.; Shen, J.; Xiao, W.; Swaim, M.E.; Gong, Y.Y.; Kachi, S.; Campochiaro, P.A. Differential sensitivity of cones to iron-mediated oxidative damage. *Investig. Ophthalmol. Vis. Sci.* **2007**, *48*, 438–445. [CrossRef] [PubMed]

95. Różanowski, B.; Burke, J.M.; Boulton, M.E.; Sarna, T.; Różanowska, M. Human RPE Melanosomes Protect from Photosensitized and Iron-Mediated Oxidation but Become Pro-oxidant in the Presence of Iron upon Photodegradation. *Investig. Ophthalmol. Vis. Sci.* **2008**, *49*, 2838–2847. [CrossRef]

96. Akeo, K.; Hiramitsu, T.; Yorifuji, H.; Okisaka, S. Membranes of retinal pigment epithelial cells in vitro are damaged in the phagocytotic process of the photoreceptor outer segment discs peroxidized by ferrous ions. *Pigment Cell Res.* **2002**, *15*, 341–347. [CrossRef]

97. Harned, J.; Nagar, S.; McGahan, M.C. Hypoxia controls iron metabolism and glutamate secretion in retinal pigmented epithelial cells. *Biochim. Biophys. Acta* **2014**, *1840*, 3138–3144. [CrossRef]

98. Reiner, A.; Fitzgerald, M.E.C.; Del Mar, N.; Li, C. Neural control of choroidal blood flow. *Prog. Retin. Eye Res.* **2018**, *64*, 96–130. [CrossRef]

99. Imamura, T.; Hirayama, T.; Tsuruma, K.; Shimazawa, M.; Nagasawa, H.; Hara, H. Hydroxyl radicals cause fluctuation in intracellular ferrous ion levels upon light exposure during photoreceptor cell death. *Exp. Eye Res.* **2014**, *129*, 24–30. [CrossRef]

100. Guajardo, M.H.; Terrasa, A.M.; Catalá, A. Lipid-protein modifications during ascorbate-Fe2+ peroxidation of photoreceptor membranes: Protective effect of melatonin. *J. Pineal Res.* **2006**, *41*, 201–210. [CrossRef]

101. Hunt, R.C.; Handy, I.; Smith, A. Heme-mediated reactive oxygen species toxicity to retinal pigment epithelial cells is reduced by hemopexin. *J. Cell. Physiol.* **1996**, *168*, 81–86. [CrossRef]

102. Tian, Y.; He, Y.; Song, W.; Zhang, E.; Xia, X. Neuroprotective effect of deferoxamine on N-methyl-d-aspartate-induced excitotoxicity in RGC-5 cells. *Acta Biochim. Biophys. Sin. (Shanghai)* **2017**, *49*, 827–834. [CrossRef] [PubMed]

103. Thaler, S.; Fiedorowicz, M.; Rejdak, R.; Choragiewicz, T.J.; Sulejczak, D.; Stopa, P.; Zarnowski, T.; Zrenner, E.; Grieb, P.; Schuettauf, F. Neuroprotective effects of tempol on retinal ganglion cells in a partial optic nerve crush rat model with and without iron load. *Exp. Eye Res.* **2010**, *90*, 254–260. [CrossRef] [PubMed]

104. Wang, Z.J.; Lam, K.W.; Lam, T.T.; Tso, M.O. Iron-induced apoptosis in the photoreceptor cells of rats. *Investig. Ophthalmol. Vis. Sci.* **1998**, *39*, 631–633. [PubMed]

105. Daruich, A.; Le Rouzic, Q.; Jonet, L.; Naud, M.-C.; Kowalczuk, L.; Pournaras, J.-A.; Boatright, J.H.; Thomas, A.; Turck, N.; Moulin, A.; et al. Iron is neurotoxic in retinal detachment and transferrin confers neuroprotection. *Sci. Adv.* **2019**, *5*, eaau9940. [CrossRef]

106. Chaudhary, K.; Promsote, W.; Ananth, S.; Veeranan-Karmegam, R.; Tawfik, A.; Arjunan, P.; Martin, P.; Smith, S.B.; Thangaraju, M.; Kisselev, O.; et al. Iron Overload Accelerates the Progression of Diabetic Retinopathy in Association with Increased Retinal Renin Expression. *Sci. Rep.* **2018**, *8*, 3025. [CrossRef]

107. Totsuka, K.; Ueta, T.; Uchida, T.; Roggia, M.F.; Nakagawa, S.; Vavvas, D.G.; Honjo, M.; Aihara, M. Oxidative stress induces ferroptotic cell death in retinal pigment epithelial cells. *Exp. Eye Res.* **2019**, *181*, 316–324. [CrossRef]

108. Sun, Y.; Zheng, Y.; Wang, C.; Liu, Y. Glutathione depletion induces ferroptosis, autophagy, and premature cell senescence in retinal pigment epithelial cells. *Cell Death Dis.* **2018**, *9*, 753. [CrossRef]

109. Muckenthaler, M.U.; Rivella, S.; Hentze, M.W.; Galy, B. A Red Carpet for Iron Metabolism. *Cell* **2017**, *168*, 344–361. [CrossRef]

110. Gelfand, B.D.; Wright, C.B.; Kim, Y.; Yasuma, T.; Yasuma, R.; Li, S.; Fowler, B.J.; Bastos-Carvalho, A.; Kerur, N.; Uittenbogaard, A.; et al. Iron Toxicity in the Retina Requires Alu RNA and the NLRP3 Inflammasome. *Cell Rep.* **2015**, *11*, 1686–1693. [CrossRef]

111. Li, Y.; Song, D.; Song, Y.; Zhao, L.; Wolkow, N.; Tobias, J.W.; Song, W.; Dunaief, J.L. Iron-induced Local Complement Component 3 (C3) Up-regulation via Non-canonical Transforming Growth Factor (TGF)-beta Signaling in the Retinal Pigment Epithelium. *J. Biol. Chem* **2015**, *290*, 11918–11934. [CrossRef]

112. Vogt, W.; Nolte, R.; Brunahl, D. Binding of iron to the 5th component of human complement directs oxygen radical-mediated conversion to specific sites and causes nonenzymic activation. *Complement Inflamm* **1991**, *8*, 313–319.

113. Toomey, C.B.; Johnson, L.V.; Bowes Rickman, C. Complement factor H in AMD: Bridging genetic associations and pathobiology. *Prog. Retin. Eye Res.* **2018**, *62*, 38–57. [CrossRef] [PubMed]

114. Asthana, A.; Baksi, S.; Ashok, A.; Karmakar, S.; Mammadova, N.; Kokemuller, R.; Greenlee, M.H.; Kong, Q.; Singh, N. Prion protein facilitates retinal iron uptake and is cleaved at the β-site: Implications for retinal iron homeostasis in prion disorders. *Sci. Rep.* **2017**, *7*, 9600. [CrossRef] [PubMed]

115. You, L.-H.; Yan, C.-Z.; Zheng, B.-J.; Ci, Y.-Z.; Chang, S.-Y.; Yu, P.; Gao, G.-F.; Li, H.-Y.; Dong, T.-Y.; Chang, Y.-Z. Astrocyte hepcidin is a key factor in LPS-induced neuronal apoptosis. *Cell Death Dis.* **2017**, *8*, e2676. [CrossRef] [PubMed]

116. Gnana-Prakasam, J.P.; Martin, P.M.; Mysona, B.A.; Roon, P.; Smith, S.B.; Ganapathy, V. Hepcidin expression in mouse retina and its regulation via lipopolysaccharide/Toll-like receptor-4 pathway independent of Hfe. *Biochem. J.* **2008**, *411*, 79–88. [CrossRef] [PubMed]

117. Urrutia, P.J.; Hirsch, E.C.; González-Billault, C.; Núñez, M.T. Hepcidin attenuates amyloid beta-induced inflammatory and pro-oxidant responses in astrocytes and microglia. *J. Neurochem.* **2017**, *142*, 140–152. [CrossRef]

118. Ghosh, S.; Shang, P.; Yazdankhah, M.; Bhutto, I.; Hose, S.; Montezuma, S.R.; Luo, T.; Chattopadhyay, S.; Qian, J.; Lutty, G.A.; et al. Activating the AKT2-nuclear factor-κB-lipocalin-2 axis elicits an inflammatory response in age-related macular degeneration: Lipocalin-2 as an indicator of early AMD. *J. Pathol.* **2017**, *241*, 583–588. [CrossRef]

119. Coffman, L.G.; Brown, J.C.; Johnson, D.A.; Parthasarathy, N.; D'Agostino, R.B.; Lively, M.O.; Hua, X.; Tilley, S.L.; Muller-Esterl, W.; Willingham, M.C.; et al. Cleavage of high-molecular-weight kininogen by elastase and tryptase is inhibited by ferritin. *Am. J. Physiol. Lung Cell Mol. Physiol.* **2008**, *294*, L505–L515. [CrossRef]

120. Gnana-Prakasam, J.P.; Ananth, S.; Prasad, P.D.; Zhang, M.; Atherton, S.S.; Martin, P.M.; Smith, S.B.; Ganapathy, V. Expression and iron-dependent regulation of succinate receptor GPR91 in retinal pigment epithelium. *Investig. Ophthalmol. Vis. Sci.* **2011**, *52*, 3751–3758. [CrossRef]

121. Arjunan, P.; Gnanaprakasam, J.P.; Ananth, S.; Romej, M.A.; Rajalakshmi, V.-K.; Prasad, P.D.; Martin, P.M.; Gurusamy, M.; Thangaraju, M.; Bhutia, Y.D.; et al. Increased Retinal Expression of the Pro-Angiogenic Receptor GPR91 via BMP6 in a Mouse Model of Juvenile Hemochromatosis. *Investig. Ophthalmol. Vis. Sci.* **2016**, *57*, 1612–1619. [CrossRef]

122. Burke, J.M.; Smith, J.M. Retinal proliferation in response to vitreous hemoglobin or iron. *Investig. Ophthalmol. Vis. Sci.* **1981**, *20*, 582–592. [PubMed]

123. Loporchio, D.; Mukkamala, L.; Gorukanti, K.; Zarbin, M.; Langer, P.; Bhagat, N. Intraocular foreign bodies: A review. *Surv. Ophthalmol.* **2016**, *61*, 582–596. [CrossRef] [PubMed]

124. Konerirajapuram, N.S.; Coral, K.; Punitham, R.; Sharma, T.; Kasinathan, N.; Sivaramakrishnan, R. Trace elements iron, copper and zinc in vitreous of patients with various vitreoretinal diseases. *Indian J. Ophthalmol.* **2004**, *52*, 145–148. [PubMed]

125. Conart, J.-B.; Berrod, J.-P. [Non-traumatic vitreous hemorrhage]. *J. Fr. Ophtalmol.* **2016**, *39*, 219–225. [CrossRef] [PubMed]

126. Levin, A.V. Retinal hemorrhage in abusive head trauma. *Pediatrics* **2010**, *126*, 961–970. [CrossRef]

127. Casini, G.; Loiudice, P.; Menchini, M.; Sartini, F.; De Cillà, S.; Figus, M.; Nardi, M. Traumatic submacular hemorrhage: Available treatment options and synthesis of the literature. *Int. J. Retin. Vitr.* **2019**, *5*, 48. [CrossRef]

128. Bhisitkul, R.B.; Winn, B.J.; Lee, O.-T.; Wong, J.; de Souza Pereira, D.; Porco, T.C.; He, X.; Hahn, P.; Dunaief, J.L. Neuroprotective effect of intravitreal triamcinolone acetonide against photoreceptor apoptosis in a rabbit model of subretinal hemorrhage. *Investig. Ophthalmol. Vis. Sci.* **2008**, *49*, 4071–4077. [CrossRef]

129. Chen-Roetling, J.; Regan, K.A.; Regan, R.F. Protective effect of vitreous against hemoglobin neurotoxicity. *Biochem. Biophys. Res. Commun.* **2018**, *503*, 152–156. [CrossRef]

130. Zerbib, J.; Pierre-Kahn, V.; Sikorav, A.; Oubraham, H.; Sayag, D.; Lobstein, F.; Massonnet-Castel, S.; Haymann-Gawrilow, P.; Souied, E.H. Unusual retinopathy associated with hemochromatosis. *Retin Cases Brief Rep.* **2015**, *9*, 190–194. [CrossRef]

131. Gnana-Prakasam, J.P.; Tawfik, A.; Romej, M.; Ananth, S.; Martin, P.M.; Smith, S.B.; Ganapathy, V. Iron-mediated retinal degeneration in haemojuvelin-knockout mice. *Biochem. J.* **2012**, *441*, 599–608. [CrossRef]

132. Kumar, P.; Nag, T.C.; Jha, K.A.; Dey, S.K.; Kathpalia, P.; Maurya, M.; Gupta, C.L.; Bhatia, J.; Roy, T.S.; Wadhwa, S. Experimental oral iron administration: Histological investigations and expressions of iron handling proteins in rat retina with aging. *Toxicology* **2017**, *392*, 22–31. [CrossRef]

133. Shu, W.; Dunaief, J.L. Potential Treatment of Retinal Diseases with Iron Chelators. *Pharmaceuticals (Basel)* **2018**, *11*, 112. [CrossRef] [PubMed]

134. Wong, W.L.; Su, X.; Li, X.; Cheung, C.M.G.; Klein, R.; Cheng, C.-Y.; Wong, T.Y. Global prevalence of age-related macular degeneration and disease burden projection for 2020 and 2040: A systematic review and meta-analysis. *Lancet Glob. Health* **2014**, *2*, e106–e116. [CrossRef]

135. Handa, J.T.; Bowes Rickman, C.; Dick, A.D.; Gorin, M.B.; Miller, J.W.; Toth, C.A.; Ueffing, M.; Zarbin, M.; Farrer, L.A. A systems biology approach towards understanding and treating non-neovascular age-related macular degeneration. *Nat. Commun.* **2019**, *10*, 3347. [CrossRef] [PubMed]

136. Biesemeier, A.; Yoeruek, E.; Eibl, O.; Schraermeyer, U. Iron accumulation in Bruch's membrane and melanosomes of donor eyes with age-related macular degeneration. *Exp. Eye Res.* **2015**, *137*, 39–49. [CrossRef]

137. Hahn, P.; Milam, A.H.; Dunaief, J.L. Maculas Affected by Age-Related Macular Degeneration Contain Increased Chelatable Iron in the Retinal Pigment Epithelium and Bruch's Membrane. *Arch. Ophthalmol.* **2003**, *121*, 1099–1105. [CrossRef]

138. Junemann, A.G.; Stopa, P.; Michalke, B.; Chaudhri, A.; Reulbach, U.; Huchzermeyer, C.; Schlotzer-Schrehardt, U.; Kruse, F.E.; Zrenner, E.; Rejdak, R. Levels of aqueous humor trace elements in patients with non-exsudative age-related macular degeneration: A case-control study. *PLoS ONE* **2013**, *8*, e56734. [CrossRef]

139. Dentchev, T.; Hahn, P.; Dunaief, J.L. Strong labeling for iron and the iron-handling proteins ferritin and ferroportin in the photoreceptor layer in age-related macular degeneration. *Arch Ophthalmol.* **2005**, *123*, 1745–1746. [CrossRef]

140. Chowers, I.; Wong, R.; Dentchev, T.; Farkas, R.H.; Iacovelli, J.; Gunatilaka, T.L.; Medeiros, N.E.; Presley, J.B.; Campochiaro, P.A.; Curcio, C.A.; et al. The iron carrier transferrin is upregulated in retinas from patients with age-related macular degeneration. *Investig. Ophthalmol. Vis. Sci.* **2006**, *47*, 2135–2140. [CrossRef]

141. Čolak, E.; Žorić, L.; Radosavljević, A.; Ignjatović, S. The Association of Serum Iron-Binding Proteins and the Antioxidant Parameter Levels in Age-Related Macular Degeneration. *Curr. Eye Res.* **2018**, *43*, 659–665. [CrossRef]

142. Wysokinski, D.; Danisz, K.; Pawlowska, E.; Dorecka, M.; Romaniuk, D.; Robaszkiewicz, J.; Szaflik, M.; Szaflik, J.; Blasiak, J.; Szaflik, J.P. Transferrin receptor levels and polymorphism of its gene in age-related macular degeneration. *Acta Biochim. Pol.* **2015**, *62*, 177–184. [CrossRef] [PubMed]

143. Synowiec, E.; Pogorzelska, M.; Blasiak, J.; Szaflik, J.; Szaflik, J.P. Genetic polymorphism of the iron-regulatory protein-1 and -2 genes in age-related macular degeneration. *Mol. Biol. Rep.* **2012**, *39*, 7077–7087. [CrossRef] [PubMed]

144. Synowiec, E.; Szaflik, J.; Chmielewska, M.; Wozniak, K.; Sklodowska, A.; Waszczyk, M.; Dorecka, M.; Blasiak, J.; Szaflik, J.P. An association between polymorphism of the heme oxygenase-1 and -2 genes and age-related macular degeneration. *Mol. Biol. Rep.* **2012**, *39*, 2081–2087. [CrossRef] [PubMed]

145. Szemraj, M.; Oszajca, K.; Szemraj, J.; Jurowski, P. MicroRNA Expression Analysis in Serum of Patients with Congenital Hemochromatosis and Age-Related Macular Degeneration (AMD). *Med. Sci. Monit.* **2017**, *23*, 4050–4060. [CrossRef] [PubMed]

146. Ding, J.; Wong, T.Y. Current epidemiology of diabetic retinopathy and diabetic macular edema. *Curr. Diab. Rep.* **2012**, *12*, 346–354. [CrossRef] [PubMed]

147. Ciudin, A.; Hernández, C.; Simó, R. Iron overload in diabetic retinopathy: A cause or a consequence of impaired mechanisms? *Exp. Diabetes Res.* **2010**, *2010*, 714108. [CrossRef]

148. Baumann, B.; Sterling, J.; Song, Y.; Song, D.; Fruttiger, M.; Gillies, M.; Shen, W.; Dunaief, J.L. Conditional Müller Cell Ablation Leads to Retinal Iron Accumulation. *Investig. Ophthalmol. Vis. Sci.* **2017**, *58*, 4223–4234. [CrossRef]

149. Weinreb, R.N.; Aung, T.; Medeiros, F.A. The pathophysiology and treatment of glaucoma: A review. *JAMA* **2014**, *311*, 1901–1911. [CrossRef]

150. Wang, H.-W.; Sun, P.; Chen, Y.; Jiang, L.-P.; Wu, H.-P.; Zhang, W.; Gao, F. Research progress on human genes involved in the pathogenesis of glaucoma (Review). *Mol. Med. Rep.* **2018**, *18*, 656–674. [CrossRef]

151. Tripathi, R.C.; Borisuth, N.S.; Tripathi, B.J.; Gotsis, S.S. Quantitative and qualitative analyses of transferrin in aqueous humor from patients with primary and secondary glaucomas. *Investig. Ophthalmol. Vis. Sci.* **1992**, *33*, 2866–2873.

152. Farkas, R.H.; Chowers, I.; Hackam, A.S.; Kageyama, M.; Nickells, R.W.; Otteson, D.C.; Duh, E.J.; Wang, C.; Valenta, D.F.; Gunatilaka, T.L.; et al. Increased expression of iron-regulating genes in monkey and human glaucoma. *Investig. Ophthalmol. Vis. Sci.* **2004**, *45*, 1410–1417. [CrossRef] [PubMed]

153. Hohberger, B.; Chaudhri, M.A.; Michalke, B.; Lucio, M.; Nowomiejska, K.; Schlötzer-Schrehardt, U.; Grieb, P.; Rejdak, R.; Jünemann, A.G.M. Levels of aqueous humor trace elements in patients with open-angle glaucoma. *J. Trace Elem. Med. Biol.* **2018**, *45*, 150–155. [CrossRef] [PubMed]

154. Fick, A.; Jünemann, A.; Michalke, B.; Lucio, M.; Hohberger, B. Levels of serum trace elements in patients with primary open-angle glaucoma. *J. Trace Elem. Med. Biol.* **2019**, *53*, 129–134. [CrossRef] [PubMed]

155. Lin, S.-C.; Wang, S.Y.; Yoo, C.; Singh, K.; Lin, S.C. Association between serum ferritin and glaucoma in the South Korean population. *JAMA Ophthalmol.* **2014**, *132*, 1414–1420. [CrossRef] [PubMed]

156. Sarnat-Kucharczyk, M.; Rokicki, W.; Zalejska-Fiolka, J.; Pojda-Wilczek, D.; Mrukwa-Kominek, E. Determination of Serum Ceruloplasmin Concentration in Patients with Primary Open Angle Glaucoma with Cataract and Patients with Cataract Only: A Pilot Study. *Med. Sci. Monit.* **2016**, *22*, 1384–1388. [CrossRef] [PubMed]

157. DeToma, A.S.; Dengler-Crish, C.M.; Deb, A.; Braymer, J.J.; Penner-Hahn, J.E.; van der Schyf, C.J.; Lim, M.H.; Crish, S.D. Abnormal metal levels in the primary visual pathway of the DBA/2J mouse model of glaucoma. *Biometals* **2014**, *27*, 1291–1301. [CrossRef]

158. Anders, F.; Teister, J.; Funke, S.; Pfeiffer, N.; Grus, F.; Solon, T.; Prokosch, V. Proteomic profiling reveals crucial retinal protein alterations in the early phase of an experimental glaucoma model. *Graefes Arch. Clin. Exp. Ophthalmol.* **2017**, *255*, 1395–1407. [CrossRef]

159. Cheah, J.H.; Kim, S.F.; Hester, L.D.; Clancy, K.W.; Patterson, S.E.; Papadopoulos, V.; Snyder, S.H. NMDA receptor-nitric oxide transmission mediates neuronal iron homeostasis via the GTPase Dexras1. *Neuron* **2006**, *51*, 431–440. [CrossRef]

160. Liu, P.; Zhang, M.; Shoeb, M.; Hogan, D.; Tang, L.; Syed, M.F.; Wang, C.Z.; Campbell, G.A.; Ansari, N.H. Metal chelator combined with permeability enhancer ameliorates oxidative stress-associated neurodegeneration in rat eyes with elevated intraocular pressure. *Free Radic. Biol. Med.* **2014**, *69*, 289–299. [CrossRef]

161. Sakamoto, K.; Suzuki, T.; Takahashi, K.; Koguchi, T.; Hirayama, T.; Mori, A.; Nakahara, T.; Nagasawa, H.; Ishii, K. Iron-chelating agents attenuate NMDA-Induced neuronal injury via reduction of oxidative stress in the rat retina. *Exp. Eye Res.* **2018**, *171*, 30–36. [CrossRef]

162. Sirohi, K.; Chalasani, M.L.S.; Sudhakar, C.; Kumari, A.; Radha, V.; Swarup, G. M98K-OPTN induces transferrin receptor degradation and RAB12-mediated autophagic death in retinal ganglion cells. *Autophagy* **2013**, *9*, 510–527. [CrossRef] [PubMed]

163. Hamel, C. Retinitis pigmentosa. *Orphanet. J. Rare Dis.* **2006**, *1*, 40. [CrossRef] [PubMed]

164. Picard, E.; Jonet, L.; Sergeant, C.; Vesvres, M.H.; Behar-Cohen, F.; Courtois, Y.; Jeanny, J.C. Overexpressed or intraperitoneally injected human transferrin prevents photoreceptor degeneration in rd10 mice. *Mol. Vis.* **2010**, *16*, 2612–2625. [PubMed]

165. Scerri, T.S.; Quaglieri, A.; Cai, C.; Zernant, J.; Matsunami, N.; Baird, L.; Scheppke, L.; Bonelli, R.; Yannuzzi, L.A.; Friedlander, M.; et al. Genome-wide analyses identify common variants associated with macular telangiectasia type 2. *Nat. Genet.* **2017**, *49*, 559–567. [CrossRef] [PubMed]

166. Obolensky, A.; Berenshtein, E.; Lederman, M.; Bulvik, B.; Alper-Pinus, R.; Yaul, R.; Deleon, E.; Chowers, I.; Chevion, M.; Banin, E. Zinc-desferrioxamine attenuates retinal degeneration in the rd10 mouse model of retinitis pigmentosa. *Free Radic. Biol. Med.* **2011**, *51*, 1482–1491. [CrossRef]

167. Li, Z.L.; Lam, S.; Tso, M.O. Desferrioxamine ameliorates retinal photic injury in albino rats. *Curr. Eye Res.* **1991**, *10*, 133–144. [CrossRef]

168. Hadziahmetovic, M.; Song, Y.; Wolkow, N.; Iacovelli, J.; Grieco, S.; Lee, J.; Lyubarsky, A.; Pratico, D.; Connelly, J.; Spino, M.; et al. The Oral Iron Chelator Deferiprone Protects against Iron Overload–Induced Retinal Degeneration. *Investig. Ophthalmol. Vis. Sci.* **2011**, *52*, 959–968. [CrossRef]

169. Song, D.; Zhao, L.; Li, Y.; Hadziahmetovic, M.; Song, Y.; Dunaief, J.L. The oral iron chelator deferiprone protects against iron overload-induced retinal degeneration in Hepcidin knockout mice. *Investig. Ophthalmol. Vis. Sci.* **2014**, *55*, 4525–4532. [CrossRef]

170. Song, D.; Song, Y.; Hadziahmetovic, M.; Zhong, Y.; Dunaief, J.L. Systemic administration of the iron chelator deferiprone protects against light-induced photoreceptor degeneration in the mouse retina. *Free Radic. Biol. Med.* **2012**, *53*, 64–71. [CrossRef]

171. Hadziahmetovic, M.; Pajic, M.; Grieco, S.; Song, Y.; Song, D.; Li, Y.; Cwanger, A.; Iacovelli, J.; Chu, S.; Ying, G.-S.; et al. The Oral Iron Chelator Deferiprone Protects Against Retinal Degeneration Induced through Diverse Mechanisms. *Transl. Vis. Sci. Technol.* **2012**, *1*, 7. [CrossRef]

172. Arora, A.; Wren, S.; Gregory Evans, K. Desferrioxamine related maculopathy: A case report. *Am. J. Hematol.* **2004**, *76*, 386–388. [CrossRef] [PubMed]

173. Lakhanpal, V.; Schocket, S.S.; Jiji, R. Deferoxamine (Desferal)-induced toxic retinal pigmentary degeneration and presumed optic neuropathy. *Ophthalmology* **1984**, *91*, 443–451. [CrossRef]

174. Jauregui, R.; Park, K.S.; Bassuk, A.G.; Mahajan, V.B.; Tsang, S.H. Deferoxamine-induced electronegative ERG responses. *Doc. Ophthalmol.* **2018**, *137*, 15–23. [CrossRef] [PubMed]

175. Mobarra, N.; Shanaki, M.; Ehteram, H.; Nasiri, H.; Sahmani, M.; Saeidi, M.; Goudarzi, M.; Pourkarim, H.; Azad, M. A Review on Iron Chelators in Treatment of Iron Overload Syndromes. *Int. J. Hematol. Oncol. Stem Cell Res.* **2016**, *10*, 239–247. [PubMed]

176. Sahlstedt, L.; von Bonsdorff, L.; Ebeling, F.; Ruutu, T.; Parkkinen, J. Effective binding of free iron by a single intravenous dose of human apotransferrin in haematological stem cell transplant patients. *Br. J. Haematol.* **2002**, *119*, 547–553. [CrossRef]

177. Brittenham, G.M. Iron-chelating therapy for transfusional iron overload. *N. Engl. J. Med.* **2011**, *364*, 146–156. [CrossRef]

178. Goya, N.; Miyazaki, S.; Kodate, S.; Ushio, B. A family of congenital atransferrinemia. *Blood* **1972**, *40*, 239–245. [CrossRef]

179. Simon, S.; Athanasiov, P.A.; Jain, R.; Raymond, G.; Gilhotra, J.S. Desferrioxamine-related ocular toxicity: A case report. *Indian J. Ophthalmol.* **2012**, *60*, 315–317. [CrossRef]

180. Di Nicola, M.; Barteselli, G.; Dell'Arti, L.; Ratiglia, R.; Viola, F. Functional and Structural Abnormalities in Deferoxamine Retinopathy: A Review of the Literature. *Biomed. Res. Int.* **2015**, *2015*, 249617. [CrossRef]

181. Beau-Salinas, F.; Guitteny, M.A.; Donadieu, J.; Jonville-Bera, A.P.; Autret-Leca, E. High doses of deferiprone may be associated with cerebellar syndrome. *BMJ* **2009**, *338*, a2319. [CrossRef]

182. Mehdizadeh, M.; Nowroozzadeh, M.H. Posterior subcapsular opacity in two patients with thalassaemia major following deferiprone consumption. *Clin. Exp. Optom.* **2009**, *92*, 392–394. [CrossRef]

183. Taneja, R.; Malik, P.; Sharma, M.; Agarwal, M.C. Multiple transfused thalassemia major: Ocular manifestations in a hospital-based population. *Indian J. Ophthalmol.* **2010**, *58*, 125–130. [PubMed]

184. Masera, N.; Rescaldani, C.; Azzolini, M.; Vimercati, C.; Tavecchia, L.; Masera, G.; De Molfetta, V.; Arpa, P. Development of lens opacities with peculiar characteristics in patients affected by thalassemia major on chelating treatment with deferasirox (ICL670) at the Pediatric Clinic in Monza, Italy. *Haematologica* **2008**, *93*, e9–e10. [CrossRef] [PubMed]

185. Pan, Y.; Keane, P.A.; Sadun, A.A.; Fawzi, A.A. Optical coherence tomography findings in deferasirox-related maculopathy. *Retin Cases Brief Rep.* **2010**, *4*, 229–232. [CrossRef]

186. Farajipour, H.; Rahimian, S.; Taghizadeh, M. Curcumin: A new candidate for retinal disease therapy? *J. Cell. Biochem.* **2018**, *120*, 6886–6893. [CrossRef]

187. Majumdar, S.; Srirangam, R. Potential of the Bioflavonoids in the Prevention/Treatment of Ocular Disorders. *J. Pharm. Pharmacol.* **2010**, *62*, 951–965. [CrossRef] [PubMed]

188. Voigt, A.P.; Whitmore, S.S.; Flamme-Wiese, M.J.; Riker, M.J.; Wiley, L.A.; Tucker, B.A.; Stone, E.M.; Mullins, R.F.; Scheetz, T.E. Molecular characterization of foveal versus peripheral human retina by single-cell RNA sequencing. *Exp. Eye Res.* **2019**, *184*, 234–242. [CrossRef]

189. Qian, Z.M.; Li, H.; Sun, H.; Ho, K. Targeted drug delivery via the transferrin receptor-mediated endocytosis pathway. *Pharm. Rev.* **2002**, *54*, 561–587. [CrossRef]

190. Gomme, P.T.; McCann, K.B.; Bertolini, J. Transferrin: Structure, function and potential therapeutic actions. *Drug Discov. Today* **2005**, *10*, 267–273. [CrossRef]

191. de Jong, P.T.V.M. A Historical Analysis of the Quest for the Origins of Aging Macula Disorder, the Tissues Involved, and Its Terminology. *Ophthalmol. Eye. Dis.* **2016**, *8*, 5–14. [CrossRef]

192. Weber, C.; Cole, D.J.; O'Regan, D.D.; Payne, M.C. Renormalization of myoglobin–ligand binding energetics by quantum many-body effects. *PNAS* **2014**, *111*, 5790–5795. [CrossRef] [PubMed]

3

The Foundation Fighting Blindness Plays an Essential and Expansive Role in Driving Genetic Research for Inherited Retinal Diseases

Ben Shaberman * and Todd Durham *

Foundation Fighting Blindness, 7168 Columbia Gateway Drive, Suite 100, Columbia, MD 21046, USA
* Correspondence: bshaberman@fightingblindness.org (B.S.); tdurham@fightingblindness.org (T.D.);

Abstract: The Foundation Fighting Blindness leads a collaborative effort among patients and families, scientists, and the commercial sector to drive the development of preventions, treatments, and cures for inherited retinal diseases (IRDs). When the nonprofit was established in 1971, it sought the knowledge and insights of leaders in the retinal research field to guide its research funding decisions. While the Foundation's early investments focused on gaining a better understanding of the genetic causes of IRDs, its portfolio of projects would come to include some of the most innovative approaches to saving and restoring vision, including gene replacement/augmentation therapies, gene editing, RNA modulation, optogenetics, and gene-based neuroprotection. In recent years, the Foundation invested in resources such as its patient registry, natural history studies, and genetic testing program to bolster clinical development and trials for emerging genetic therapies. Though the number of clinical trials for such therapies has surged over the last decade, the Foundation remains steadfast in its commitment to funding the initiatives that hold the most potential for eradicating the entire spectrum of IRDs.

Keywords: retinitis pigmentosa; Usher syndrome; Stargardt disease; Leber congenital amaurosis; RPE65; nonprofit; patient registry; translational

1. Introduction

The founders of the Foundation Fighting Blindness had no idea how challenging the development of treatments and cures for inherited retinal diseases (IRDs) would be. Little did they know, it would take nearly two decades for Foundation-funded researchers to find the first IRD gene and more than 35 years to advance a gene therapy into a human study.

The nonprofit was established in 1971, when Eliot Berson, MD, brought together Gordon and Lulie Gund and Ben and Beverly Berman to create the first IRD research center: the Berman–Gund Laboratory for the Study of Retinal Degenerations at Massachusetts Eye and Ear Infirmary.

At the time, Dr. Berson had recently diagnosed the Berman's young daughters, Mindy and Joanne, with retinitis pigmentosa (RP). Gordon had recently lost all of his vision to RP after he and Lulie had completed an exhaustive search for something—anything—to save his vision. The Gund's quest for a cure, which included a harrowing journey to a clinic in Russia at the height of the Cold War, came up empty.

It was obvious to the Foundation's founders that virtually nothing was known about the conditions. Furthermore, they understood that no other entity—public or private—would fund research for rare retinal conditions. There was simply no commercial incentive for anyone to do so at the time. Driven by passion and a personal commitment, the small group of families took it upon themselves to get the research off the ground. Their goal was clear and singular: find preventions, treatments, and cures for everyone affected. The Berman–Gund lab was their first step forward, but little did they know how difficult the path forward would be.

"If you put your shoulder to the grindstone, we'd find an answer in five or six years," said Lulie, reflecting on her expectations for conquering RP. "It just never occurred to me it could go on so long."

Today, nearly 50 years later, the Foundation is the world's largest private funding source for research to find preventions, treatments, and cures for the entire spectrum of IRDs. The nonprofit has raised more than $750 million toward its focused mission. Throughout its history, the Foundation has been led by a board and trustees comprised of families and individuals with IRDs. Likewise, it has been largely funded by grassroots donors who are also affected. Its urgent mission has been driven by those who have the greatest stake in its success.

Excitingly, there has been a tremendous surge in human research for treatments over the past 10–15 years. Nearly three dozen clinical trials for IRD therapies are underway. The US Food and Drug Administration's (FDA's) approval of LUXTURNA™ (Voretigene neparvovec)—the first gene therapy for the eye or an inherited condition to receive regulatory marketing approval—was a historical moment for the Foundation, which funded preclinical studies that made the sight-restoring treatment possible. The Foundation's leadership and supporters were ebullient about the advent of the life-changing gene therapy. Finally, something made it across the finish line. Something worked, and it worked well.

However, the Foundation recognized it must optimally leverage the LUXTURNA™ approval and clinical research momentum to save the vision for the millions who still do not have any therapies. The Foundation's funding strategy has therefore evolved from only funding basic lab research to better understand IRDs to also getting treatments across the translational chasm known as "the valley of death"—that is, to the point where biotechnology and pharmaceutical companies would invest in their clinical and commercial development.

A little de-risking from the Foundation has gone a long way. Looking at the current IRD gene therapy and genetic treatment landscape, the Foundation's footprint is virtually everywhere. Most current and emerging genetics-based treatments were made possible by lab, translational, and/or early clinical research funded in part by the Foundation.

In 2018, the Foundation launched its venture philanthropy fund, known as the Retinal Degeneration Fund (RD Fund), with initial capital of $70 million. Its charter is not only to fund translational and early stage clinical projects, but to attract more venture capital into the IRD space and re-invest returns back into research.

"Yes, we are a nonprofit, but that doesn't mean we shouldn't realize and re-invest returns for projects we are funding", said Benjamin Yerxa, PhD, the Foundation's chief executive officer. "The IRD gene therapy business is burgeoning, and we owe it to patients and families to leverage that momentum as much as possible to accelerate and expand therapy development."

While the Foundation has traditionally emphasized research to identify treatment targets and develop therapies for these genetic retinal conditions, its project portfolio has recently expanded to include natural history studies—ProgStar, for people with Stargardt disease, and RUSH2A, for those with USH2A mutations—as well as the global patient registry at www.MyRetinaTracker.org. An ancillary study of My Retina Tracker has thus far provided diagnostic genetic testing to approximately 4,000 IRD patients, at no cost to them. The overarching goal for these new initiatives is to gain a better understanding of how these genetic diseases affect vision, share de-identified patient data for disease progression, genetically diagnose more patients, and facilitate recruitment for clinical trials.

Data from both My Retina Tracker and the natural history studies can accelerate clinical development by helping researchers identify more powerful and sensitive clinical endpoints.

2. Patient Perspectives on the Progress of Genetic Research

As mentioned, the FDA's approval of LUXTURNA™ in December 2017 created tremendous excitement and hope for patients and families with IRDs. The success of the gene therapy program provided proof that a genetic treatment could, in fact, save and restore vision and be made commercially available to the people who need it. For the thousands of constituents affiliated with the Foundation—many of whom had been part of the organization for several decades—this was the most important and encouraging advancement in their journey. Also, the advent of additional gene therapy clinical trials in recent years—for several other IRDs, including choroideremia, X-linked RP, Stargardt disease, and Usher syndrome type 1B—boosted optimism for the potential for genetic research to halt and reverse vision loss. The Foundation's constituents are also eager to learn about other genetic therapies, such as clustered regularly interspaced short palindromic repeats/CRISPR-associated protein 9 (CRISPR/Cas9) and antisense oligonucleotides, especially as these approaches begin to move into human studies.

With all the enthusiasm for the current progress in research, those affected are keenly aware that only one treatment has made it through the pipeline thus far. Furthermore, LUXTURNA™ can only help a small fraction of those affected. Much more work needs to be done to address the overall need. Ultimately, sustained hope and excitement about genetic research for each patient is often predicated on the advancement of research directed toward the mutated gene causing their (or a loved one's) IRD.

Jen Walker, a woman with moderate vision loss from RP (*PDE6A* mutations), is excited about the LUXTURNA™ milestone, but recognizes well the unmet need and the urgency to meet it. "Hearing about LUXTURNA™ was life changing. It was astounding to see so many young people with visual impairments regain sight. The feeling of putting away a white cane for good is immeasurable," she said, "but more work needs to be done. This is only one gene, when there are hundreds more. We need a cure quickly, as it's going to be harder to regain sight as we lose more and more photoreceptors. I am hopeful that doctors and researchers are noticing that gene therapy for vision is an up and coming science movement, and I hope everyone gets on board sooner than later."

John Corneille, who has advanced vision loss from RP (*PDE6B* mutations), shares Jen's urgency for answers, but maintains an overall positive outlook. He said, "There are days, for sure, when I get discouraged thinking, at age 59, a treatment will not be found in time to enable me to see the faces of my children and grandchildren again. Most days, however, I remain very optimistic, given how far we have come in the last couple of decades. It was very exciting to learn that a company in France is engaged in a clinical trial for my gene! I try not to think about the complexity of gene studies, replacement, and editing. But it is very reassuring to know that there are countless incredibly talented researchers working hard, each day, to find breakthrough treatments for us."

Though gene-specific therapies are often at the top of patients' minds, more are beginning to appreciate the potential of emerging, cross-cutting genetic treatment approaches, such as optogenetics. "Perhaps most exciting is the diversity of research approaches that seem likely to eventually address any stage of these progressive and devastating diseases," said Martha Steele, who has Usher syndrome type 2A. "As someone with advanced vision loss, I realize that not all treatments under investigation will likely work for me, but some, such as optogenetics, may well be in my future."

Thanks to the advanced power and increasing affordability of gene-sequencing panels, more people are getting genetically tested and having their IRD gene mutation(s) identified. A genetic diagnosis can have a big impact on the patient and their family. Of course, the genetic diagnosis can put people on the path toward a clinical trial or future treatment.

But for many patients, the identification of their gene mutation can also be cathartic. It's a step forward in unravelling the mystery of a disease that has been progressively robbing them of their vision. For parents, the identification of their gene mutation gives them answers about the risk of passing the IRD on to their kids. Depending on the result, the knowledge can be a relief or it can raise new questions and emotions.

For Michelle Glaze, a woman with moderate vision loss from mutations in *RP1*, getting a definitive genetic diagnosis took some time, but the result helped ease her mind about her son's risk of inheriting her IRD. "I had genetic testing done about six years ago. The initial diagnosis helped me to understand what was causing my vision loss. However, there were some missing pieces, which left some things unclear. I was not sure if my son was at risk. Thanks to additional investigation by a genetic counselor,

I learned he was not at risk. Thanks to advances in genetics, and the increased ability to identify pathogenic mutations, I am now able to rest well knowing that my son will not be affected by RP. This was always a fear, always a concern in my mind, until now. As a patient and mother, I am extremely grateful for advances in research, clinical developments, and genetic testing. I have an increased hope that I may be able to see my son's sweet face clearly one day."

Michelle's story underscores how critical a genetic counselor can be to the patient's and family's understanding and journey in managing an IRD, especially when results are inconclusive or additional testing may be advised.

3. In the Beginning: The Foundation's Early Focus on Genetics

When the Foundation began funding research in the early 1970s, one of the few clues scientists had about IRDs was that they ran in families; the conditions were clearly genetic. The nonprofit and its scientific advisors—including prominent visionaries in the retinal research community, such as John Dowling, PhD, Morton Goldberg, MD, and Alan Laties, MD—understood that identifying the genetic causes would be critical to: 1) diagnosing patients, 2) elucidating disease pathways, and 3) the development of therapies.

As a result, throughout its early years and for decades to come, the Foundation aggressively funded (and continues to fund) the leading IRD genetic research labs around the world.

Despite its early and substantial investments in genetic research, it took nearly two decades for Foundation-funded investigators to find the first gene associated with RP (or any IRD). That gene was *RHO*, which was identified in 1989 by a team at Trinity College Dublin [1].

The landmark genetic breakthrough brought momentum to the search for more IRD genes, but the magnitude of the challenge was not well understood. To date, more than 270 genes have been associated with IRDs.

"In the 1980s, we expected there would only be a handful of RP genes. We now know there are more than 80 and still counting. The effort started with a small group of scientists, across the world, working together and sharing ideas, patient samples, and lab reagents," said Stephen Daiger, PhD, a world leader in IRD genetic research at The University of Texas Health Science Center in Houston, who has been funded by the Foundation for genetic research and discovery since 1986. "With the identification of *RHO* in 1989, the field took off. As the Human Genome Project got underway, the first useful byproduct was a much better map of human chromosomes. Because of this improved map, many more RP genes were mapped by 1995."

While most IRD genes have been identified, diagnostic gaps remain. Today, about two out of every three people with an IRD will have their gene mutation(s) identified when they undergo genetic diagnostic testing using a comprehensive gene panel. To address the need to genetically diagnose more patients, the Foundation is funding a five-year, $2.5 million project to find elusive IRD genes and mutations, including those in non-coding regions. The collaborative effort is being led by Dr. Daiger, Dr. Ayyagari, and Kinga Bujakowska, PhD, at Massachusetts Eye and Ear, and will include more than 140 families and an additional 400 individuals.

4. The Trajectory for Gene Therapy Development

With the discovery of the first genes associated with IRDs in the 1990s, the idea of developing gene replacement therapies—using viral vectors to replace mutated copies of an IRD gene with healthy copies—was tantalizingly attractive to the Foundation and its scientific advisors. After all, IRDs were caused by mutations in single genes and the retina was a clear and accessible target for such an approach. So, Foundation funding for IRD gene therapy, and relevant animal models for testing, began in earnest.

However, for Jean Bennett, MD, PhD, and Albert Maguire, MD, the visionaries for what eventually became LUXTURNA™, the idea of gene therapy for a condition like RP came to them in medical school, well before the first IRD gene had been discovered.

"I remember in 1985, my husband, Albert Maguire, asked me if I thought we could do a gene therapy for retinitis pigmentosa. I said, sure. But what I didn't tell him is that we didn't know the genes, we didn't have any animal models, and we didn't know how to deliver DNA to the target cells," recalled Dr. Bennett. "But that planted a seed and I started researching the state of the art. A few years later, I applied for a career development award from what was then the Retinitis Pigmentosa Foundation, now the Foundation Fighting Blindness, and got it. And that launched my whole career developing gene therapy for retinal degenerations."

The Foundation invested approximately $10 million in *RPE65* gene therapy lab studies to enable the launch of the clinical trial in 2007 at the Children's Hospital of Philadelphia (CHOP), which brought to fruition the vision of Drs. Bennett and Maguire. It was the first clinical trial of a gene therapy for an IRD. The company Spark Therapeutics was spun out of CHOP in 2013 to raise the money needed to get the treatment across the regulatory finish line and out to the patients who needed it. In early 2019, Spark was acquired by Roche for nearly $5 billion.

"The Foundation's goal has been, and always will be, to get vision-saving treatments out to the people who need them. LUXTURNA™ was an important first step in achieving that goal, and we will be in business until all inherited retinal diseases are eradicated," said Dr. Yerxa. "We are also delighted that our projects are attracting such large commercial investments, including Roche's potential acquisition of Spark. It affirms we are on the right track with the right science, the right strategies, and the right investments."

Several other clinical trials for IRD gene therapies were made possible by earlier Foundation funding. Take, for example, Nightstar Therapeutics' Phase 3 clinical trial for its choroideremia gene therapy, which has preserved or improved vision for 90 percent of patients in a Phase 1/2 study. That study would not have been possible without earlier lab research by Miguel Seabra, PhD, who received more than $1.5 million from the Foundation for his efforts to characterize the *CHM* gene, develop a rodent model of choroideremia, and evaluate early versions of the *CHM* gene therapy in lab studies. Nightstar was recently acquired by Biogen for approximately $800 million.

Large animal models and related safety and efficacy studies have been invaluable to the advancement of IRD gene therapies, and perhaps no other Foundation-funded lab has been more productive in IRD large animal research than the University of Pennsylvania School of Veterinary Medicine. Its successful studies in canines have led to gene therapy clinical trials for: Leber congenital amaurosis (*RPE65* mutations), X-linked RP (*RPGR* mutations), and achromatopsia (*CNGA3* and *CNGB3* mutations). Human trials resulting from its Best disease and RP (*RHO* mutations) gene therapy canine studies are currently being planned.

5. Beyond Gene Replacement

While momentum for the clinical development of gene replacement therapies for IRDs is strong, the approach has its limitations.

For example, the cargo capacity of the adeno-associated viruses (AAVs) commonly (and successfully) used for gene delivery in LUXTURNA™ and most ongoing clinical trials is limited to about 4.7 kb. Several genes, including *ABCA4* (Stargardt disease), *USH2A* (RP and Usher syndrome), and *CEP290* (LCA) exceed the AAV's capacity.

Also, for autosomal dominant IRDs, such as RP caused by mutations in *RHO*, the delivery of a replacement gene will not be sufficient; a therapy will need to silence the mutated allele encoding the toxic protein or the allele acting in a dominant-negative fashion.

In recent years, the Foundation's research portfolio has expanded to include gene-editing treatment approaches such as CRISPR/Cas9 for autosomal dominant RP caused by mutations in *RHO* (Johns Hopkins and Columbia) and RP1 (Massachusetts Eye and Ear), as well as Usher syndrome type 1B caused by mutations in *MYO7A* (UCLA).

In February 2018, the Foundation Fighting Blindness, through its RD Fund, announced funding of up to $7.5 million for the development of ProQR's QR-421a, an antisense oligonucleotide (AON) designed to block mutations in RNA caused by defects in exon 13 of *USH2A*. ProQR announced in March 2019 that it had dosed the first patient in its Phase 1/2 clinical trial for QR-421a. Excitingly, the company reported vision improvements for 60 percent of participants in its Phase 1/2 targeting a recurrent mutation in *CEP290*, which causes LCA10. A Phase 2/3 trial for the LCA10 AON is now underway.

6. Cross-Cutting Gene Therapies

Even before the first gene replacement therapy clinical trial got off the ground (the RPE65 trial at CHOP) in 2007, Foundation-funded scientists were envisioning neuroprotective gene-therapy paradigms that could help people regardless of the mutated gene causing their disease. That is, delivering a gene to express proteins that would slow photoreceptor degeneration.

Neuroprotection became attractive to Foundation leadership and scientific advisors because of the technical and financial infeasibility of developing a gene replacement therapy for the hundreds of mutated genes that cause IRDs. According to RetNet (https://sph.uth.edu/retnet/) there are more than 270 genes associated with IRDs. Furthermore, approximately one third of patients will not have their mutation(s) identified when genetically tested.

In 2005, José Sahel, MD, and Thierry Léveillard, PhD, at the Institut de la Vision, received the Foundation's Board of Director's Award for identifying a protein produced and secreted by rod photoreceptors that prevented cones from degenerating in models of RP. Aptly named the rod-derived cone-viability factor (RdCVF), the protein was an intriguing approach for saving cone-mediated vision in people with RP and related conditions. Perhaps most appealing was that RdCVF had the potential to work independent of the patient's mutated gene—an approach that would be desirable for those whose gene mutation could not be identified, or those for whom gene replacement or editing wasn't technically desirable.

The newly-formed French company SparingVision plans to advance RdCVF into a clinical trial soon, thanks to the culmination of many years of lab funding from the Foundation and its recent commitment of up to €7 million.

The Foundation is also funding optogenetic therapies—the delivery of a gene to retinal ganglion or bipolar cells to express a light-sensitive protein in a retina that has lost all its photoreceptors due to an advanced IRD. In fact, the Foundation funded preclinical research for retinal optogenetic approaches currently in clinical trials—studies sponsored by Allergan and GenSight. The Foundation is also funding John Flannery, PhD, UC Berkeley, who is developing optogenetic alternatives designed to work in more natural lighting conditions.

While still in early clinical trials, optogenetic therapies hold promise for restoring meaningful vision to people who have lost all of their photoreceptors, regardless of the mutated gene causing their blindness.

7. Natural History Studies: Learning about Disease Progression and Genotype–Phenotype Correlations

The successful development of any new therapy requires a thorough understanding of the disease—in the absence of treatment—ideally from the time of diagnosis to its end stages. Understanding this natural history of disease enables clinical researchers to describe the clinical manifestations of disease (the phenotype) and its association with the genotype, estimate how quickly the disease progresses over time, identify patient characteristics that predict slower or faster disease progression, and study which clinical assessments are most appropriate to measure a treatment's benefit. Addressing these objectives is particularly important for IRDs because they are highly variable in their clinical manifestations, they may progress over decades, and because they are rare diseases about which little may be known. Ultimately, the knowledge gained from natural history studies will provide a number of key insights. This fundamental work will inform the designs of clinical trials of new treatments, the patient population most likely to benefit, the length of follow-up required to demonstrate a benefit, and the outcomes that are most sensitive to change [2].

The Foundation funds and conducts natural history studies of IRDs through its Clinical Consortium, a coordinating center and an international group of over 25 leading research centers which are experts in IRDs. The Clinical Consortium's mission is to accelerate the development of treatments for IRDs through collaborative and transparent clinical research. These objectives are met by ensuring the studies are designed, led, and reported by participating investigators and by making the study datasets publicly available for wider use. Because the studies are conducted using industry standards for quality—including good clinical practice (GCP) and site certification for retinal imaging modalities—the Foundation has designed the studies so the data will have broad utility, including, in some situations, to serve as a historical control.

Currently, the Foundation's Clinical Consortium is conducting RUSH2A, a prospective, four-year, natural history study of approximately 100 patients with an IRD associated with mutations in the *USH2A* gene, the most common mutated gene in Usher syndrome type 2 and a frequent cause of non-syndromic RP. The primary objectives of the RUSH2A study are to characterize the progression of the disease with respect to functional outcome measures (e.g., visual acuity and static perimetry) and structural outcome measures (e.g., the area of the ellipsoid zone measured by SD-OCT), to investigate the relationships between structure and function, and to assess whether there are genotypic or phenotypic predictors of progression at four years.

By the end of 2019, the Clinical Consortium plans to initiate a natural history study of retinal dystrophy associated with the *EYS* gene, PRO-EYS. The PRO-EYS study has similar objectives to RUSH2A and will follow approximately 100 patients for four years. A key feature of PRO-EYS is that the patient population will be stratified by the severity of disease at study entry. Thus, the study will provide valuable information that can be used to design trials for treatments at various stages of disease progression.

Natural history studies of IRDs and their associated pathogenic genes will continue to be a major activity of the Foundation's Clinical Consortium. These studies have broad applicability; they therefore represent an ideal partnership opportunity for industry sponsors, who can save time and effort by leveraging the network's existing research infrastructure and access to IRD patients around the world.

8. My Retina Tracker: The Foundation's Global Patient Registry

Patient data for IRDs—both genetic and phenotypic information—is rare. Furthermore, IRD patient data collected by academic research centers is usually not shared widely and often limited to the conditions studied by the institution.

However, the need for comprehensive IRD patient data has become paramount with the surge in clinical trials for emerging therapies. The success of these human studies depends greatly on a sponsor's ability to recruit enough genotypically and phenotypically well-characterized patients.

In 2014, the Foundation launched its secure global patient registry, My Retina Tracker (www.MyRetinaTracker.org), to provide pre-screened researchers and companies with de-identified patient and disease data for relevant studies, including IRD clinical trials and natural history studies.

The registry is patient controlled; the patient uploads and maintains their own record. When a company or researcher searches the registry for potential clinical trial participants, they never receive patient names or personal information. Instead, they are sent an alphanumeric identifier, which Foundation administrators use to identify and notify the patient who matched the search criteria. It is then up to the patient to contact the clinical trial coordinator about possible participation in the trial or study.

As of June 2019, more than 12,260 patients (with an informative profile of their disease) were registered in My Retina Tracker. Approximately 400 new patients register every month.

The Foundation Fighting Blindness has been conducting a genetic testing study for patients registered in My Retina Tracker. Through the study, registrants obtain genetic testing, at no cost to them.

A 266 IRD gene panel (includes copy number variation testing) is being used to screen DNA samples. No cost genetic counseling is provided for those patients who don't receive genetic counseling from their clinic or physician.

"Genetically characterizing IRD patients and making their de-identified molecular and disease information available to the research community is critical for advancing human disease and therapy studies," said Brian Mansfield, PhD, the Foundation's executive vice president research and interim chief scientific officer. "Dozens of therapy developers and investigators from around the world have used data from My Retina Tracker to advance their lab and clinical research. With approximately 200,000 IRD patients in the United States alone, we still have a lot of work to do, but we are building momentum as more patients learn about My Retina Tracker and the genetic testing study."

9. Conclusion: Filling the Gaps to Advance the Field

The Foundation's role in driving genetic research for IRDs has evolved and expanded as a result of advancement in biological sciences, the development of powerful gene sequencing technologies, the mapping of the human genome, and the growth in its own revenues and membership base. Of course, success in gene therapy development—including the regulatory approval of LUXTURNA™ and the impressive results from preclinical research that propelled the *RPE65* gene therapy toward the clinic—has also brought accelerating momentum to clinical development in the field.

However, the Foundation has always maintained (and continues to maintain) a commitment to funding projects that would fill critical gaps in research that were not addressed by commercial or government sectors, especially when doing so advanced the entire IRD field.

Today, the My Retina Tracker patient registry, genetic testing study, and Stargardt disease and *USH2A* natural history studies are all prime examples of significant Foundation investments that are having a wide-reaching impact in the advancement of research, especially when it comes to the clinical development of sight-saving and -restoring therapies. In most cases, these are major investments, each costing several millions of dollars, which other organizations haven't been able or willing to make.

The Foundation's long-standing, guiding imperative—whatever the investment—is to ensure that it is based on good science and it will get more preventions, treatments, and cures for IRDs across the finish line for everyone affected.

References

1. McWilliam, P.; Farrar, G.J.; Kenna, P.; Bradley, D.G.; Humphries, M.M.; Sharp, E.M.; McConnell, D.J.; Lawler, M.; Sheils, D.; Ryan, C.; et al. Autosomal dominant retinitis pigmentosa (ADRP): Localization of an ADRP gene to the long arm of chromosome 3. *Genomics* **1989**, *5*, 619–622. [CrossRef]
2. Food and Drug Administration Center for Drug Evaluation and Research (CDER); Center for Biologics Evaluation and Research (CBER); Office of Orphan Products Development (OOPD). Rare Diseases: Natural History Studies for Drug Development. Guidance for Industry. March 2019. Available online: https://www.fda.gov/media/122425/download (accessed on 1 March 2019).

4

Characterizing the Retinal Phenotype in the High-Fat Diet and Western Diet Mouse Models of Prediabetes

Bright Asare-Bediako [1], Sunil K. Noothi [2], Sergio Li Calzi [2], Baskaran Athmanathan [3], Cristiano P. Vieira [2], Yvonne Adu-Agyeiwaah [1], Mariana Dupont [1], Bryce A. Jones [4], Xiaoxin X. Wang [5], Dibyendu Chakraborty [2], Moshe Levi [5], Prabhakara R. Nagareddy [3] and Maria B. Grant [2],*

[1]   Vision Science Graduate Program, School of Optometry, University of Alabama at Birmingham, Birmingham, AL 35233, USA; basareb@uab.edu (B.A.-B.); yvonnad@uab.edu (Y.A.-A.); mdupont@uab.edu (M.D.)

[2]   Department of Ophthalmology and Visual Sciences, School of Medicine, The University of Alabama at Birmingham, Birmingham, AL 35294, USA; sunilnooti@uabmc.edu (S.K.N.); scalzi@uabmc.edu (S.L.C.); cvieira@uabmc.edu (C.P.V.); dchakraborty@uabmc.edu (D.C.)

[3]   Division of Cardiac Surgery, Department of Surgery, Ohio State University Wexner Medical Center, Columbus, OH 43210, USA; baskaran.athmanathan@osumc.edu (B.A.); prabhakara.nagareddy@osumc.edu (P.R.N.)

[4]   Department of Pharmacology and Physiology, Georgetown University, Washington, DC 20057, USA; baj46@georgetown.edu

[5]   Department of Biochemistry and Molecular & Cellular Biology, Georgetown University, Washington, DC 20057, USA; xiaoxin.wang@georgetown.edu (X.X.W.); moshe.levi@georgetown.edu (M.L.)

*   Correspondence: mariagrant@uabmc.edu

Abstract: We sought to delineate the retinal features associated with the high-fat diet (HFD) mouse, a widely used model of obesity. C57BL/6 mice were fed either a high-fat (60% fat; HFD) or low-fat (10% fat; LFD) diet for up to 12 months. The effect of HFD on body weight and insulin resistance were measured. The retina was assessed by electroretinogram (ERG), fundus photography, permeability studies, and trypsin digests for enumeration of acellular capillaries. The HFD cohort experienced hypercholesterolemia when compared to the LFD cohort, but not hyperglycemia. HFD mice developed a higher body weight (60.33 g vs. 30.17g, $p < 0.0001$) as well as a reduced insulin sensitivity index (9.418 vs. 62.01, $p = 0.0002$) compared to LFD controls. At 6 months, retinal functional testing demonstrated a reduction in a-wave and b-wave amplitudes. At 12 months, mice on HFD showed evidence of increased retinal nerve infarcts and vascular leakage, reduced vascular density, but no increase in number of acellular capillaries compared to LFD mice. In conclusion, the HFD mouse is a useful model for examining the effect of prediabetes and hypercholesterolemia on the retina. The HFD-induced changes appear to occur slower than those observed in type 2 diabetes (T2D) models but are consistent with other retinopathy models, showing neural damage prior to vascular changes.

Keywords: retinal phenotype; neural infarcts; vascular leakage

1. Introduction

Diabetes is now considered a worldwide epidemic [1,2]. Recent reports indicate that over 90% of diabetic individuals have type 2 diabetes (T2D) [3,4]. The most common microvascular complication of diabetes is diabetic retinopathy (DR) [2]. Despite a growing number of different approaches to arrest DR, the incidence and prevalence of DR continues to rise [5]. The understanding of the pathogenesis of DR remains incomplete [4], and this is, in part, due to the lack of readily available models that completely recapitulate the metabolic phenotype [6]. The high-fat diet (HFD) mouse model has been described as a robust model for investigating obesity-associated T2D and its related metabolic complications [7]. Studies have shown that HFD-fed mice develop obesity, impaired glucose tolerance, and reduced insulin sensitivity [8,9] with systemic manifestations involving adipose tissue [10], liver [8], and kidneys [11]. However, the ocular changes associated with the HFD model have not been fully investigated. Moreover, the typical Western diet (WD; 40% fat) has also been given to rodents to recapitulate obesity-driven pathology. However, to mimic the features of T2D, the administration of low-dose Streptozotocin (STZ) is also given to the WD mice [12–14].

The retinal response to high fat exposure would likely involve local changes in the expression of lipid transport proteins, such as the liver X receptors (LXRs). The LXRs are the key transcription factors that regulate lipid and cholesterol metabolism [15]. While liver X receptor alpha (LXRα) is expressed only in some tissues, the expression of liver X receptor beta (LXRβ) is ubiquitous [12]. Previously we showed that whole body LXRα/β deficiency resulted in the generation of increased numbers of acellular capillaries, while LXR agonists improved DR in Streptozotocin (STZ)-induced diabetes [12] and in diabetic Lepr$^{db/db}$ (db/db) mice [16]; however, it is not known if the WD modulates the expression of LXR in the retina.

Retinopathy is typically characterized by macroglia activation and gliosis identified by glial fibrillary acidic protein (GFAP) overexpression, which can be considered as a marker for retinal damage [17,18]. In the healthy mammalian retina, GFAP is expressed only in astrocytes and not in Muller cells. Following inherited or acquired retinal pathology, GFAP is expressed also in Muller cells [19,20]. GFAP expression in Muller cells has been widely used as a cellular marker for retinal pathology [21–25]. Hypoxia-inducible factor 1 alpha (HIF-1α) is known to be a key regulator of a tissue's response to hypoxia [26] and plays a role in obesity-induced metabolic syndrome. It has been shown that HFD leads to gradual increase in HIF-1α and associated pathological changes in the liver [27,28]. However, the role of HIF-1α in the retina of WD-fed mice is not known.

A better understanding of DR in obesity-driven models is needed and may facilitate the optimal choice of disease models for future investigations. Thus, in the present study, we hypothesized that HFD and WD feeding would result in a distinct retinal phenotype and a time course slower than that observed in models of T2D, such as the db/db mouse [29] or the high fructose and high fat fed mouse [30]. For this purpose, we characterized not only systemic endpoints of glucose and lipid metabolism but also the function of the retina and development of retinal pathology, including retinal vascular changes and changes in expression of the critical proteins LXRβ, HIF-1α, and GFAP.

2. Materials and Methods

2.1. Animals

All animal experiments were approved by the University of Alabama at Birmingham (IACUC-20467, approved on 06/16/2016) and Georgetown University (animal project #2017-0059, approved on 10/27/2017), and followed the Association for Research in Vision and Ophthalmology Statement for the Use of Animals. Six to eight-week-old C57BL/6J mice were fed either a low-fat diet (LFD) (10%kcal fat, 70%kcal carbohydrate, 20% protein), a Western diet (40% kcal fat, 43% kcal carbohydrate, 17%kcal protein), or a HFD (60% kcal fat, 20% kcal carbohydrate, 20% kcal protein) for up to 12 months. Diets were purchased from Research Diets, Inc, New Brunswick, NJ, USA. Full details of the composition of each diet is given in Supplementary Table S1.

2.2. Body Composition, Glucose Tolerance, and Insulin Sensitivity Testing

The fat mass, lean mass, and water content of the animals were measured by magnetic resonance imaging using EchoMRI (Echo Medical Systems, LLC, Houston, TX, USA). For glucose and insulin tolerance tests, mice were fasted for 5-6 h, injected intraperitoneally with D-glucose at 1.5 g/kg of lean mass and tail bled for glucose and insulin measurements. Blood glucose and insulin levels were measured 0, 15, 30, 45, 60, and 120 min after glucose administration. The insulin sensitivity index (ISI) was estimated using the Matsuda–Defronzo method [31].

2.3. Electroretinogram (ERG)

ERGs were performed using a LKC Bigshot ERG system. Briefly, mice were dark-adapted overnight. The animals were anesthetized with ketamine (80 mg/kg total body mass) and xylazine (15 mg/kg total body mass), then dilated with atropine/phenylephrine under dim red light. Once dilated, animals were exposed to 5 full-field white light flashes at 0.25 and 2.5 cd.s/m^2 under scotopic conditions. The animals were then light-adapted for 5 min and exposed to 10–15 full-field white light flashes at 10 and 25 cd.s/m^2 under photopic conditions. Responses were averaged and analyzed using the LKC EM software.

2.4. Fundus Photography and Fluorescein Angiography

Fundus photography and fluorescein angiography were performed using the Phoenix Micron IV retinal imaging microscope (Phoenix Technology Group, Pleasanton, CA, USA). Briefly, mice were anesthetized with ketamine and xylazine, then dilated with atropine/phenlylephrine, as described above. Once dilated, the animals were placed on the instrument and fundus photographs were taken. Animals were then given intraperitoneal injection of fluorescein (AK-FLUOR 10%, Sigma Pharmaceuticals, North Liberty, IA, USA) and the retinal vasculature was imaged with blue light illumination after 5–8 min when all the vessels were filled.

2.5. Acellular Capillaries Quantification

Trypsin digestion of the retina was performed according to a previously published protocol [32,33]. Briefly, eyeballs were enucleated and incubated in 4% paraformaldehyde overnight. Retinas were isolated, washed, and digested in elastase solution (40 Units elastase/mL; Sigma-Aldrich, St. Louis, MO, USA) to remove the non-vascular tissue. The vascular beds were mounted on glass slides followed by staining with periodic acid–Schiff's base and hematoxylin. About 5–6 fields from the central to mid-periphery were imaged and the number of acellular capillaries per square millimeter were quantified.

2.6. Immunohistochemistry

Immunohistochemical staining of mouse retinas was performed according to a previously published protocol [34]. Briefly, mice were euthanized and eyes were immediately enucleated and fixed in 4% paraformaldehyde (PFA) solution for 15 min. Cornea and lenses were carefully removed and posterior cups were incubated in 15% sucrose solution in phosphate-buffered saline (PBS) overnight at 4 °C after washing briefly in PBS. Posterior cups were transferred to 30% sucrose in PBS for 3–4 h, then embedded in optimal cutting temperature (O.C.T) medium and immediately frozen on dry ice. The frozen samples were stored at −80 °C until further processing. The sections were thawed at room temperature for 4 h, washed in PBS for 5 min, and permeabilized with 0.25% Triton-X in PBS for 5 min at room temperature. Sections were blocked with 10% horse serum in 1% bovine serum albumin (BSA) for 2 h then incubated with primary antibody diluted in blocking solution (1:100 dilution) overnight at 4 °C. The antibodies used were rabbit anti-GFAP (Abcam, MA, USA), mouse mAB HIF-1α antibody (Novus Biologicals, CO, USA), LXR-β polyclonal antibody (Invitrogen, IL, USA), rabbit anti-Vimentin (Cell Signaling Technology, MA, USA), and isolectin GS-IB4 Alexa Fluor 568 (Life Technologies, OR, USA). Sections were then washed and incubated in fluorescent-labeled secondary antibodies (goat anti-rabbit IgG Alexa Fluor 488, Life Technologies, OR, USA) for 1 h at room temperature, followed by washing and incubation with 4′,6-diamidino-2-phenylindole, dihydrochloride (DAPI) solution (Life Technologies, OR, USA) for 5 min at room temperature. Finally, sections were washed and mounted with anti-fade mounting medium (Vector Laboratories, CA, USA) for imaging. Image analysis was completed in a masked fashion using four images taken at defined positions and quantified using ImageJ software.

The analysis was performed in a masked fashion by three separate observers, then averaged. To achieve unbiased results, positive and negative controls were included alongside experimental test and control groups. Fluorescent microscopy was performed by trained masked operators. To address selection bias in immunofluorescence, the entire areas of retinal cross-sections were imaged.

2.7. Statistics

All experiments were repeated at least 3 times. All data were assessed using one-way ANOVA. When the results were significant, we determined which means differed from each other using Tukey's multiple-comparisons test. Results are expressed as mean ± standard error of the mean (SEM). Statistical analysis was performed using GraphPad Prism, with $p < 0.05$ considered statistically significant. Only significant comparisons are shown in the figures. All the examiners were blinded to the identities of the samples they were analyzing.

3. Results

3.1. HFD Mice Have Normal Glucose Levels but Are Insulin-Resistant

We first sought to validate our model by confirming in our cohort that HFD feeding led to similar degrees of body weight gain as reported in the literature [10,35]. Mice on HFD showed increased body weights by 4 weeks of feeding ($p = 0.0020$). This increase was sustained throughout the 12-month observation period (Figure 1A). At 12 months, HFD mice had moderately higher lean mass (difference of 5.580 ± 1.003g, $p < 0.0001$) and water content (difference of 4.517 ± 0.876, $p = 0.0001$) but a markedly increased fat mass (difference of 21.15 ± 2.362, $p < 0.0001$) compared to LFD controls (Figure 1B). Unexpectedly, chronic high-fat feeding did not cause hyperglycemia. Despite feeding mice with a HFD for 12 months, the HbA1c levels were not different between HFD and LFD mice (Figure 1C). At 12 months, there was no difference in fasting blood glucose levels (Figure 1D, basal) and intraperitoneal glucose tolerance test (IP-GTT) did not show any significant differences between LFD and HFD mice (Figure 1D). However, due to the very high levels of insulin in HFD mice (0.6 ng/mL for LFD and 3.5 ng/mL for HFD; Figure 1E, basal), the insulin sensitivity index demonstrated that HFD mice had much lower insulin sensitivity compared to LFD mice (Figure 1E,F). Also, plasma total cholesterol levels were higher in HFD mice compared to LFD (174.4 vs. 114.9, $p = 0.0008$) (Figure 1G)

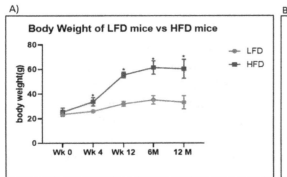
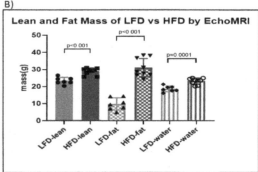

Figure 1. *Cont.*

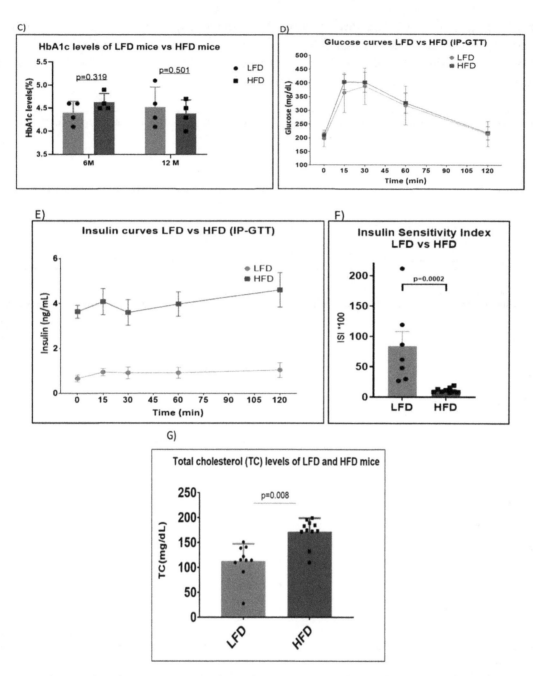

Figure 1. Body weight, glucose levels, and insulin sensitivity of high-fat diet (HFD) mice vs. low-fat diet (LFD) mice. (**A**) Body weights as measured for mice on LFD (green) and HFD (red) for 12 months. (* $p < 0.000001$; $n = 6$). (**B**) Lean mass, fat mass and water content of LFD mice vs. HFD mice. (**C**) Glycated hemoglobin (HbA1c) levels measured for the mice after 6 months and 12 months. (**D–G**) Glucose curves ($p > 0.46$ for all time points), insulin curves ($p < 0.0018$ for all time points), insulin sensitivity index, and total cholesterol levels for LFD mice vs. HFD mice, respectively, following intraperitoneal glucose tolerance test (IP-GTT) after 12 months of feeding.

3.2. HFD Mice Have Functional Deficits in Their Retinas

Full-field ERG under both scotopic and photopic conditions was performed at 6 months and 12 months of HFD feeding (Figure 2A–D). HFD mice at 6 months showed significantly reduced a- and b-wave amplitudes under scotopic conditions ($p = 0.00125$ and $p = 0.000002$ for 0.25 cd.s/m^2 and 2.5 cd.s/m^2 stimulus luminance, respectively) but not photopic conditions when compared to LFD mice. After 12 months of feeding of the respective diets, the difference was not significant ($p = 0.183$ and

$p = 0.154$ for 0.25 cd.s/m^2 and 2.5 cd.s/m^2 stimulus luminance respectively) (Figure 2C,D). Interestingly, when comparing 6 and 12 months of LFD feeding, the mice experienced marked reductions in both the a- and b- waves under both photopic and scotopic conditions at 12 months (Figure 2E,F), but no significant difference was noted in the HFD-fed mice (Figure 2G,H).

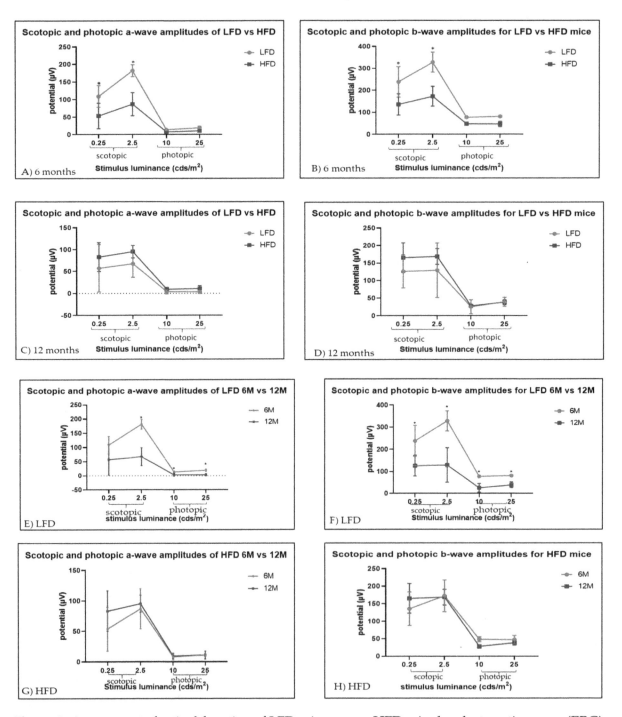

Figure 2. Assessment of retinal function of LFD mice versus HFD mice by electroretinogram (ERG). The amplitudes of a-waves and b-waves were assessed under both scotopic and photopic conditions for LFD mice and HFD mice after 6 months (**A,B**) and 12 months (**C,D**). LFD mice showed a significant reduction in retinal response between 6 months and 12 months of feeding (**E,F**), but HFD mice did not (**G,H**); (*n* = 4 for both groups).

3.3. Fundus Photography shows Neural Retinal Lesions in HFD Mice

In humans, DR is associated with retinal lesions such as hemorrhages, microaneurysms, exudates, and "cotton wool spots" [36]. Fundus photography using Micron IV demonstrated retinal pathology in the HFD mice. Though not statistically significant, HFD mice showed a trend of increased numbers of "lipid-laden-like" lesions (Figure 3A) after 6 months ($p = 0.057$). However, with 12 months of feeding, HFD mice showed significantly higher number of lesions in the retina (Figure 3B).

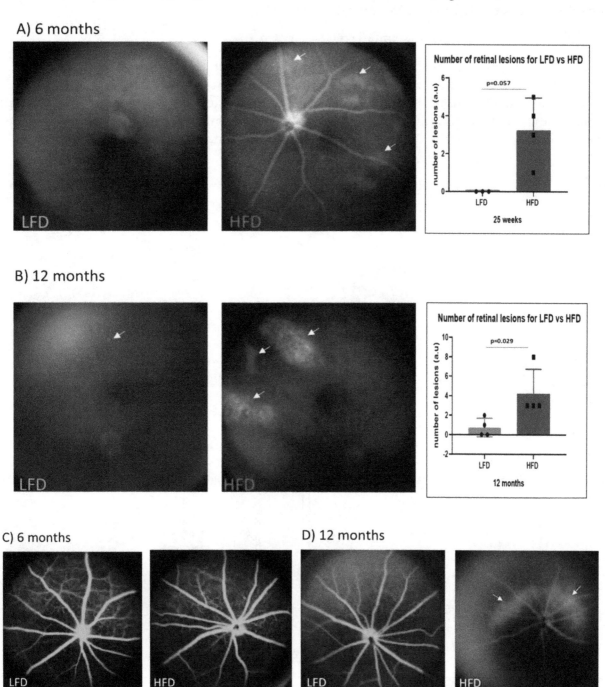

Figure 3. Assessment of retinal lesions by fundus photography (**A**,**B**) and vascular leakage by fluorescein angiography (**C**,**D**). HFD mice developed more neural infarcts ((**A**,**B**), white arrows) than LFD mice. No infarct was observed for LFD after 6 months (**A**). However, vascular leakage was observed in HFD mice after 12 months of feeding ((**D**), white arrows).

3.4. Vascular Permeability Changes in HFD Mice

A hallmark of DR in humans is increased vascular permeability, ultimately leading to diabetic macular edema in humans. To determine if HFD mice developed a breakdown in the blood–retinal barrier, we assessed vascular leakage by fluorescein angiography (FA). At 6 months of HFD feeding, FA did not show any evidence of retinal vascular leakage and were similar to FAs in LFD controls (Figure 3C). However, after 12 months of HFD feeding, increased leakage of fluorescein was observed in the retina compared to LFD control retinas (Figure 3D).

3.5. Acellular Capillary Formation in HFD Mice

A well-established feature of diabetic microvascular dysfunction is an increase in the number of acellular capillaries in the retina, defined as basal membrane tubes lacking endothelial cells and pericyte nuclei. At 12 months of HFD feeding, there was no significant increase in acellular capillary numbers in the HFD mice (Figure 4B,C) compared to the LFD mice (Figure 4A,C). However, the HFD retinas showed lower vascular densities compared to LFD retinas (Figure 4D).

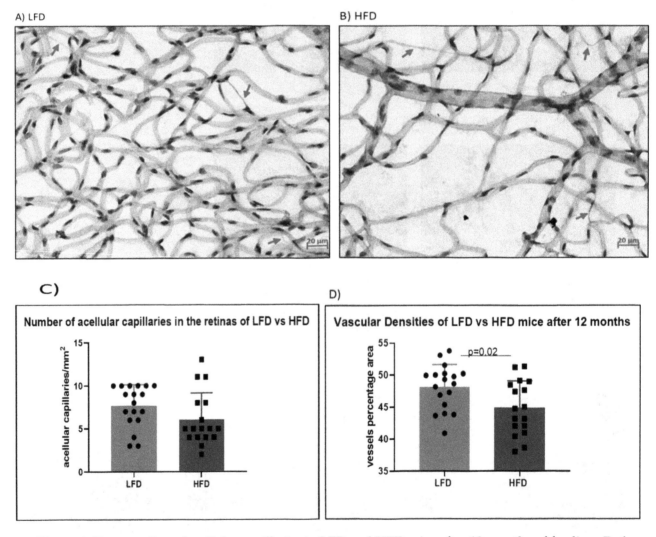

Figure 4. Enumeration of acellular capillaries in LFD and HFD mice after 12 months of feeding. Red arrows indicate acellular capillaries in the retinas of LFD (**A**) and HFD (**B**) mice. There was no significant difference in the number of acellular capillaries between both groups (**C**) ($p = 0.086$). However, HFD retinas showed lesser vascular densities compared to LFD retinas (**D**).

3.6. Retinal Damage, Hypoxia, and Lipid Transport in WD Mice

While the HFD represents a diet with 60% fat content that is used as a model of obesity and T2D, the WD with 40% fat content has garnered popularity as it represents a regimen closer to that actually ingested by humans. Since the WD diet has lower fat content and is not associated with hyperglycemia, we hypothesized that if retinal changes were present they would be subtle compared to those we observed with HFD feeding. To test the validity of our hypothesis, we performed IHC studies and first examined whether there was evidence of glial activation by examining expression of the glial marker GFAP after 6 months of WD feeding. Although there was no statistically significant difference ($p = 0.88$) in the total expression of GFAP between retinas of WD and LFD mice (Figure 5A–C), increased expression of GFAP was observed in selected Vimentin-positive Muller cells in the WD mice (Figure 5G–I) compared to LFD (Figure 5D–F). Increased expression of GFAP in Muller cells is supportive of increased oxidative stress and inflammation in these cells, and suggests that the impact of WD is not experienced uniformly across all Muller cells [37,38].

To assess whether WD feeding induced retinal hypoxia, changes in HIF-1α expression were examined by IHC. After 6 months of WD feeding, a significant increase ($p = 0.025$) in expression of HIF-1α was seen in WD mice (Figure 6D) compared to LFD mice (Figure 6C). This was not observed after 3 months of WD feeding (Figure 6A,B). Quantitation of HIF-1α expression is shown in Figure 6E, demonstrating that WD-fed mice exhibit higher levels than LFD-fed mice. Co-localization with isolectin, a known vascular endothelial cell marker, showed increased expression of HIF-1α in some endothelial cells in WD mice (I–K) but not in LFD mice (F–H). Higher magnification images from two different WD samples are shown in Figure 6L,M.

Retinal lipid content is regulated in part by liver X receptor beta (LXRβ) expression. We next examined changes in LXRβ expression in the two experimental cohorts. In control mice, LXRβ localized predominantly in the ganglion cell layer, as well as the inner nuclear layer (Figure 7A), which is the location of the bipolar cells, horizontal cells, and amacrine cells. There was a significant reduction in expression of LXRβ in WD only in the ganglion cell layer ($p = 0.0079$) after 3 months of feeding (Figure 7B). However, after 6 months of WD feeding, WD mice (Figure 7E) showed significantly reduced expression of LXRβ in the ganglion cell layer ($p = 0.0374$), inner nuclear layer ($p < 0.0001$), and outer nuclear layer, as well as in the photoreceptors of the outer nuclear layer ($p = 0.0020$). The expression of LXRβ was reduced after 6 months compared to 3 months of feeding in both LFD ($p < 0.0001$) and WD ($p < 0.0001$) in the nuclear and ganglion cell layers, suggesting an age-related loss in LXRβ.

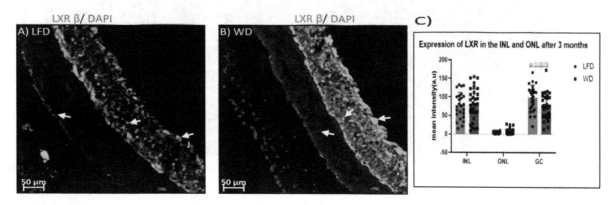

Figure 5. *Cont.*

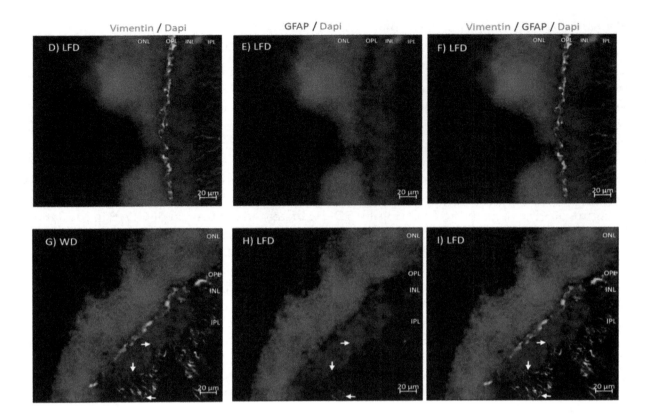

Figure 5. Retinal glial fibrillary acidic protein (GFAP) expression after 6 months of feeding. Some Muller cells in Western diet (WD) retinas express GFAP (**A,C**, white arrows), but not in LFD (**A,B**), indicating that the impact of WD is not uniform across all Muller cells. Co-localization with Vimentin, a known Mueller cell marker, showed increased expression of GFAP in some Mueller cells in WD mice (**G–I**) but not in LFD mice (**D–F**).

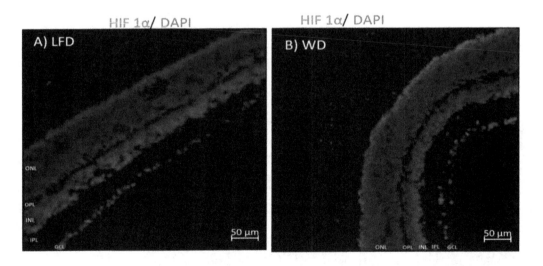

Figure 6. *Cont.*

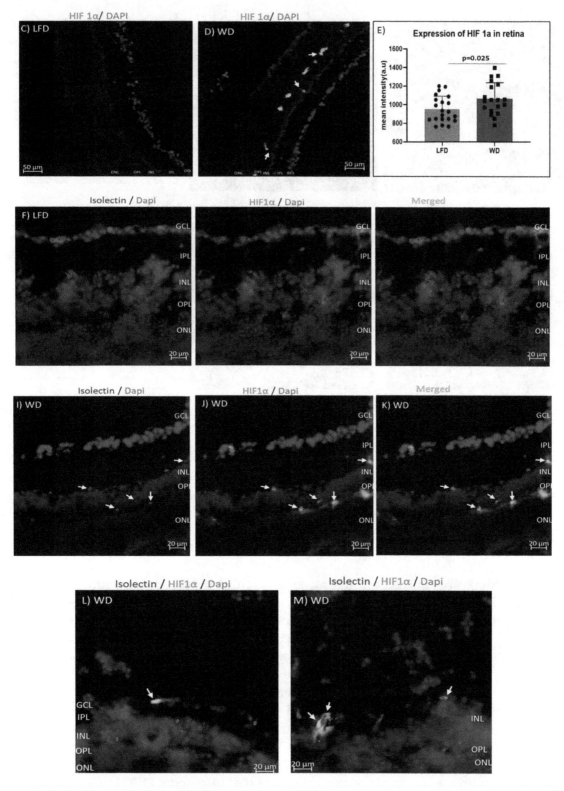

Figure 6. Retinal hypoxia-inducible factor 1 alpha (HIF-1α) expression after 3 and 6 months of WD feeding. There was increased expression of HIF-1α in WD retinas (**D**, white arrows) compared to LFD retinas (**C**), as shown by quantification (**E**). Also, there was no significant difference in expression of HIF-1α after 3 months of feeding (**A,B**). Co-localization with isolectin, a known vascular endothelial cell marker, showed increased expression of HIF-1α in some endothelial cells in WD mice (**I–K**) but not in LFD mice (**F–H**). (**L,M**) Magnified merged images from two different WD samples.

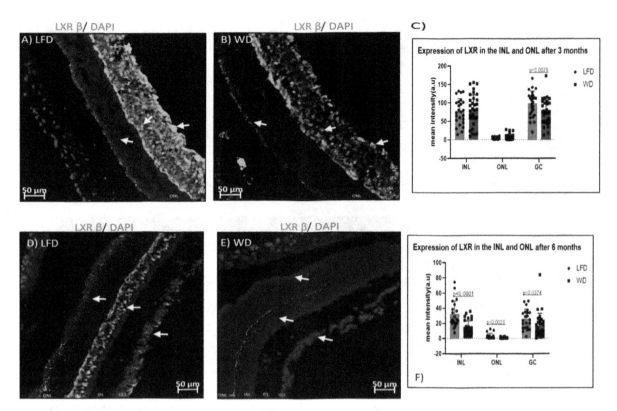

Figure 7. Retinal liver X receptor beta (LXRβ) expression after 3 and 6 months of feeding. After 3 months of either WD or LFD feeding, there was significant reduction in the expression of LXRβ in only the ganglion cell layer of WD mice (**B**) compared to LFD mice (**A**). However, after 6 months of feeding, there was reduced expression of LXRβ in the ganglion cell layer as well as inner and outer nuclear layers of WD mice (**E**, white arrows) compared to LFD mice (**D**). Quantification of LXR in the inner nuclear layer (INL) and outer nuclear layer (ONL) at 3 months shows reductions in the ganglion cell (GC) layer (**C**). At 6 months, reductions are seen in the INL, ONL, and ganglion cell (GC) layer of the WD-fed mice when compared to LFD mice.

4. Discussion

Diabetic retinopathy causes both neural and vascular defects, with neural deficits preceding vascular changes [6,39–42]. Even before the onset of clinically detectable retinopathy, diabetic patients have a reduced ERG implicit time [43] and high-frequency flicker amplitude [44]. Later, they experience decreased vascular density [45]. In this study, we have shown that HFD feeding results in a suitable model of prediabetes, with the HFD cohort exhibiting insulin resistance and hypercholesterolemia without hyperglycemia. The retinopathy that is exhibited occurs over a slower time course than in T2D models, where both hyperglycemia and hyperinsulinemia exist.

The HFD mouse has previously been described as a model for T2D [7,46], as C57BL/6J mice fed HFD develop obesity and insulin resistance [47,48], but as we show in this study, this model has a distinct timeline and different characteristics than those seen in T2D. We show that HFD mice have hypercholesterolemia and insulin resistance but the absence of hyperglycemia, which is typical of T2D models.

In agreement with the literature, our study shows that mice fed a HFD have a sustained increase in body weight [6,49,50]. As confirmed by EchoMRI, the increase in body weight is primarily due to elevated body fat mass. After 12 weeks of feeding, HFD mice showed a two-fold increase in body fat mass over control LFD mice. Despite the marked increase in fat mass, HFD mice did not develop overt hyperglycemia. Glycated hemoglobin levels measured at 6 months and 12 months showed that both groups had normal glycated hemoglobin, thus indicating a key difference between the HFD model and other T2D rodent models, many of which are genetic. However, HFD mice develop hyperinsulinemia (Figure 1E,F), and their insulin production is sufficient to maintain euglycemia, as indicated by their glycated hemoglobin levels. The marked hyperinsulinemia we observed is supported by the literature [6,51–54]. In contrast, T2D in humans is characterized by not only insulin resistance but also the presence of sustained hyperglycemia and elevated HbA1c levels. When only insulin resistance is present, individuals are described as prediabetics [55,56].

Insulin resistance is believed to play a key role in diabetic neuropathy by increasing oxidative stress and mitochondrial dysfunction [57,58], and may also drive the early neural retinal dysfunction that we observed in our HFD mice. Thus, the HFD mice secrete sufficiently elevated insulin to maintain a normal glucose level, and as such the HFD model may be better characterized as a prediabetes model. Importantly, the incidence of prediabetes is often higher than that of diabetes [59]. The prevalence of prediabetes is also increasing; it is estimated that more than 470 million people worldwide will be suffering from prediabetes by 2030 [60]. Most importantly, the three classical microvascular complications, retinopathy, neuropathy, and nephropathy, have all been documented in individuals with prediabetes [61].

While classifications of diabetes remain "glucose-centric", our study draws attention to the importance of earlier events, when glucose levels are still normal. Thus, in our model, hyperinsulinemia with hypercholesterolemia will likely lead to the retinal pathology observed. Not surprisingly, these pathologies take a longer time to develop than those typically seen when hyperglycemia is also present.

Systemic and retinal lipid abnormalities have been shown to promote retinal damage [16,62,63]. Previously, we demonstrated that diabetes-induced disruption of the LXR axis results in abnormal lipid metabolism, inadequate vascular repair, and localized and systemic inflammation [16,64]. The LXRs (LXRα and LXRβ) play important roles in cholesterol homeostasis [65]. They regulate the expression of reverse cholesterol transporters [12]. Activation of LXRs using pharmacological agents repress inflammatory genes such as TNF-α and IL-1β [66], inhibit the expression of pro-apoptotic factors [67], and prevent the development of DR [12]. We showed that use of GW3965, an LXR agonist, resulted in normalization of cholesterol homeostasis and repression of inflammatory genes, such as iNOS, IL-1β, ICAM-1, and CCL2 in the retina [16]. We found that inadequate cholesterol removal due to deficiency in LXR and reduced oxysterol production in the retina due to loss of cytochromes p450 27A1 and 46A1 resulted in widespread retinal pathology [68]. In the current study, we showed that concentrations of 40% fat in the diet were sufficient to reduce expression of LXR in the inner and outer nuclear layers.

Our study showed that HFD mice develop neural retinal deficits after 6 months of feeding, as both a-waves and b- waves were reduced under scotopic conditions. Unexpectedly, the a- and b- wave responses for LFD mice was significantly less after 12 months compared to the response after 6 months of feeding ($p < 0.01$ for both scotopic and photopic conditions), which suggests that the LFD may have detrimental effects on the neural retina. Because the composition of the diets must be isocaloric, when the amount of fat is reduced, some other dietary component needs to be increased to compensate. Inn the LFD, the amount of sucrose increases from 72 g to 354 g and 315 g of corn starch is also added so that the LFD can be isocaloric with the HFD. However, this largely occurs at the expense of making the diet high in carbohydrates. The literature supports that LFD may be detrimental [69–71]. While we were unable to find literature supporting the impact of LFD specifically on ERGs, the systemic consequences of LFD may indirectly affect the retina, for example by reduced availability of fat-soluble vitamins or changing retinal cholesterol metabolism. Moreover, the increased sucrose and cornstarch in the LFD may have direct deleterious effects [72,73]. LFDs promote insulin resistance, and while most of the research has been performed in humans, these findings may have relevance to murine studies. LFD, typically considered a high carbohydrate diet, is known to promote inflammation [74–76]. A recent study compared ERGs in HFD fed rats, Streptozotocin (STZ) rats and type 2 diabetes (T2D) rats at 6 months to controls. Kowluru found differences between the diabetic ERGs and controls, but no differences between the ERGs of the HFD rats compared to controls; however, Kowluru did not look at 12 month tests and the study was performed in rats, not in mice [77]. Thus, it is difficult to compare these findings with our results.

While neural damage was detected at 6 months, the vascular damage was not observed until much later. This is in agreement with Rajagopal et al. [6], who demonstrated that vascular damage was not observed at 6 months of HFD feeding. However, despite the absence of vascular damage after 6 months of HFD, we observed the presence of "lipid-laden like" lesions, and also neural infarcts similar to what is described in humans as "cotton-wool" spots. These lesions, which appeared to increase as the retinopathy progressed in the HFD mice, could become a useful measure of retinal damage and may be sensitive enough to use as a novel endpoint for the preclinical investigation of therapeutic agents.

GFAP is normally expressed in retinal astrocytes in rodents; however, during stress and inflammation, Muller cells [37] respond by increasing GFAP expression. In this study, we show that WD induces GFAP expression in selective Muller cells, supporting the presence of increased stress and inflammation in the retina of these mice. Kim et al. have reported increased inflammation in other tissues such as adipose tissue and intestines [78]. Lee et al. showed increased numbers of activated macrophages in the retina of HFD mice [79]. In both humans and rodents, obesity-induced diabetes is associated with hypoxia in tissues such adipose tissue, and suppression of HIF-1α mitigates tissue-specific pathological changes associated with HFD [80]. The liver, brain, kidney, and heart display tissue-specific regulation of HIF-1α under systemic hypoxia [81]. After 6 months, but not after 3 months, we observed that HIF-1α expression is increased in the WD retinas compared to LFD controls. Similar to our observation in the retina of 3-month-old mice on WD, Prasad et al. showed the absence of pimonidazole staining in the kidneys of 10–11-week old db/db mice [82], also indicating the absence of hypoxia response in the kidneys at this time point.

5. Conclusions

Our study demonstrates that HFD feeding generates a useful prediabetes model. Specifically, the combination of hypercholesterolemia and insulin resistance are sufficient to induce retinal dysfunction with a slower time course of development compared to T2D models such as the db/db mouse. In agreement with reports describing diabetes models, we show that neural functional deficits are the earliest indicator of damage in the retina of this prediabetes model before vascular changes. Key molecular targets such as HIF-1α and the LXRs provide insights into the retinal pathobiology observed in this hypercholesterolemic, hyperinsulinemic model. The appearance and frequency of neural infarcts or "lipid-laden lesions" in the retina of HFD mice could represent a novel endpoint for evaluation of therapeutic interventions.

Author Contributions: Conceptualization, M.L., P.R.N., and M.B.G.; data curation, B.A.-B. and S.K.N.; formal analysis, B.A.-B., S.K.N., B.A.J., and M.B.G.; funding acquisition, M.B.G.; investigation, B.A.-B., S.K.N., S.L.C., B.A., C.P.V., Y.A.-A., M.D., B.A.J., X.X.W., D.C., and M.B.G.; methodology, B.A.-B., S.K.N., P.R.N., and M.B.G.; project administration, P.R.N. and M.B.G.; resources, M.L., P.R.N., and M.B.G.; supervision, M.L. and P.R.N.; validation, B.A.-B. and S.L.C.; visualization, B.A.-B.; writing—original draft, B.A.-B., S.K.N., P.R.N., and M.B.G.; writing—review and editing, B.A.-B., S.K.N., S.L.C., B.A., C.P.V., Y.A.-A., B.A.J., M.L., P.R.N., and M.B.G. All authors have read and agreed to the published version of the manuscript.

References

1.   Cho, N.; Shaw, J.; Karuranga, S.; Huang, Y.; Fernandes, J.D.R.; Ohlrogge, A.; Malanda, B. IDF Diabetes Atlas: Global estimates of diabetes prevalence for 2017 and projections for 2045. *Diabetes Res. Clin. Pr.* **2018**, *138*, 271–281. [CrossRef] [PubMed]

2.   Chatterjee, S.; Khunti, K.; Davies, M.J. Type 2 diabetes. *Lancet* **2017**, *389*, 2239–2251. [CrossRef]

3.   Busik, J.V.; Tikhonenko, M.; Bhatwadekar, A.; Opreanu, M.; Yakubova, N.; Caballero, S.; Player, D.; Nakagawa, T.; Afzal, A.; Kielczewski, J.; et al. Diabetic retinopathy is associated with bone marrow neuropathy and a depressed peripheral clock. *J. Exp. Med.* **2009**, *206*, 2897–2906. [CrossRef] [PubMed]

4. Turner, R.C.; Cull, C.A.; Frighi, V.; Holman, R.R.; UK Prospective Diabetes Study (UKPDS) Group. Glycemic Control With Diet Sulfonylurea, Metformin, or Insulin in Patients with Type 2 Diabetes MellitusProgressive Requirement for Multiple Therapies (UKPDS 49). *JAMA* **1999**, *281*, 2005. [CrossRef] [PubMed]

5. Yao, Z.; Gu, Y.; Zhang, Q.; Liu, L.; Meng, G.; Wu, H.; Xia, Y.; Bao, X.; Shi, H.; Sun, S. Estimated daily quercetin intake and association with the prevalence of type 2 diabetes mellitus in chinese adults. *Eur. J. Nutr.* **2019**, *58*, 819–830. [CrossRef]

6. Rajagopal, R.; Bligard, G.W.; Zhang, S.; Yin, L.; Lukasiewicz, P.; Semenkovich, C.F. Functional Deficits Precede Structural Lesions in Mice With High-Fat Diet–Induced Diabetic Retinopathy. *Diabetes* **2016**, *65*, 1072–1084. [CrossRef]

7. Winzell, M.S.; Ahrén, B. The high-fat diet-fed mouse: A model for studying mechanisms and treatment of impaired glucose tolerance and type 2 diabetes. *Diabetes* **2004**, *53*, S215–S219. [CrossRef]

8. Liou, C.-J.; Lee, Y.-K.; Ting, N.-C.; Chen, Y.-L.; Shen, S.-C.; Wu, S.-J.; Huang, W.-C. Protective Effects of Licochalcone A Ameliorates Obesity and Non-Alcoholic Fatty Liver Disease Via Promotion of the Sirt-1/AMPK Pathway in Mice Fed a High-Fat Diet. *Cells* **2019**, *8*, 447. [CrossRef]

9. Collins, S.; Martin, T.L.; Surwit, R.S.; Robidoux, J. Genetic vulnerability to diet-induced obesity in the C57BL/6J mouse: Physiological and molecular characteristics. *Physiol. Behav.* **2004**, *81*, 243–248. [CrossRef]

10. Illesca, P.; Valenzuela, R.; Espinosa, A.; Echeverría, F.; Soto-Alarcon, S.; Ortiz, M.; Videla, L.A. Hydroxytyrosol supplementation ameliorates the metabolic disturbances in white adipose tissue from mice fed a high-fat diet through recovery of transcription factors nrf2, srebp-1c, ppar-γ and nf-κb. *Biomed. Pharmacother.* **2019**, *109*, 2472–2481. [CrossRef]

11. Declèves, A.-E.; Mathew, A.V.; Armando, A.M.; Han, X.; Dennis, E.A.; Quehenberger, O.; Sharma, K.; Decl&egraveves, A.-E. AMP-activated protein kinase activation ameliorates eicosanoid dysregulation in high-fat-induced kidney disease in mice. *J. Lipid Res.* **2019**, *60*, 937–952. [CrossRef] [PubMed]

12. Hazra, S.; Rasheed, A.; Bhatwadekar, A.; Wang, X.; Shaw, L.C.; Patel, M.; Caballero, S.; Magomedova, L.; Solis, N.; Yan, Y.; et al. Liver X Receptor Modulates Diabetic Retinopathy Outcome in a Mouse Model of Streptozotocin-Induced Diabetes. *Diabetes* **2012**, *61*, 3270–3279. [CrossRef]

13. Wang, X.X.; Jiang, T.; Shen, Y.; Caldas, Y.; Miyazaki-Anzai, S.; Santamaria, H.; Urbanek, C.; Solis, N.; Scherzer, P.; Lewis, L.; et al. Diabetic Nephropathy Is Accelerated by Farnesoid X Receptor Deficiency and Inhibited by Farnesoid X Receptor Activation in a Type 1 Diabetes Model. *Diabetes* **2010**, *59*, 2916–2927. [CrossRef] [PubMed]

14. Chen, X.; Yuan, H.; Shi, F.; Zhu, Y. Effect of garden cress in reducing blood glucose, improving blood lipids and reducing oxidative stress in a mouse model of diabetes induced by a high fat diet and streptozotocin. *J. Sci. Food Agric.* **2019**. [CrossRef] [PubMed]

15. Zheng, W.; Mast, N.; Saadane, A.; Pikuleva, I.A. Pathways of cholesterol homeostasis in mouse retina responsive to dietary and pharmacologic treatments. *J. Lipid Res.* **2015**, *56*, 81–97. [CrossRef]

16. Hammer, S.S.; Beli, E.; Kady, N.; Wang, Q.; Wood, K.; Lydic, T.A.; Malek, G.; Saban, D.R.; Wang, X.X.; Hazra, S.; et al. The Mechanism of Diabetic Retinopathy Pathogenesis Unifying Key Lipid Regulators, Sirtuin 1 and Liver X Receptor. *EBioMedicine* **2017**, *22*, 181–190. [CrossRef]

17. Li, Q.; Zemel, E.; Miller, B.; Perlman, I. Early Retinal Damage in Experimental Diabetes: Electroretinographical and Morphological Observations. *Exp. Eye Res.* **2002**, *74*, 615–625. [CrossRef]

18. Krady, J.K.; Basu, A.; Allen, C.M.; Xu, Y.; LaNoue, K.F.; Gardner, T.W.; Levison, S.W. Minocycline reduces proinflammatory cytokine expression, microglial activation, and caspase-3 activation in a rodent model of diabetic retinopathy. *Diabetes* **2005**, *54*, 1559–1565. [CrossRef]

19. Dahl, D. The radial glia of Müller in the rat retina and their response to injury. An immunofluorescence study with antibodies to the glial fibrillary acidic (GFA) protein. *Exp. Eye Res.* **1979**, *28*, 63–69. [CrossRef]

20. Osborne, N.N.; Block, F.; Sontag, K.-H. Reduction of ocular blood flow results in glial fibrillary acidic protein (GFAP) expression in rat retinal Müller cells. *Vis. Neurosci.* **1991**, *7*, 637–639. [CrossRef]

21. Penn, J.S.; Thum, A.L.; Rhem, M.N.; Dell, S.J. Effects of oxygen rearing on the electroretinogram and GFA-protein in the rat. *Investig. Ophthalmol. Vis. Sci.* **1988**, *29*, 1623–1630.

22. Tanaka, Y.; Takagi, R.; Ohta, T.; Sasase, T.; Kobayashi, M.; Toyoda, F.; Shimmura, M.; Kinoshita, N.; Takano, H.; Kakehashi, A. Pathological Features of Diabetic Retinopathy in Spontaneously Diabetic Torii Fatty Rats. *J. Diabetes Res.* **2019**, *2019*, 8724818. [CrossRef] [PubMed]

23. Fan, Y.; Lai, J.; Yuan, Y.; Wang, L.; Wang, Q.; Yuan, F. Taurine protects retinal cells and improves synaptic connections in early diabetic rats. *Curr. Eye Res.* **2020**, *45*, 52–63. [CrossRef]

24. Bahr, H.I.; Abdelghany, A.A.; Galhom, R.A.; Barakat, B.M.; Arafa, E.-S.A.; Fawzy, M.S. Duloxetine protects against experimental diabetic retinopathy in mice through retinal GFAP downregulation and modulation of neurotrophic factors. *Exp. Eye Res.* **2019**, *186*, 107742. [CrossRef]

25. Gu, L.; Xu, H.; Zhang, C.; Yang, Q.; Zhang, L.; Zhang, J. Time-dependent changes in hypoxia-and gliosis-related factors in experimental diabetic retinopathy. *Eye* **2019**, *33*, 600. [CrossRef]

26. Chen, J.; Chen, J.; Fu, H.; Li, Y.; Wang, L.; Luo, S.; Lu, H. Hypoxia exacerbates nonalcoholic fatty liver disease via the HIF-2α/PPARα pathway. *Am. J. Physiol. Metab.* **2019**, *317*, E710–E722. [CrossRef]

27. Han, J.; He, Y.; Zhao, H.; Xu, X. Hypoxia inducible factor-1 promotes liver fibrosis in nonalcoholic fatty liver disease by activating PTEN/p65 signaling pathway. *J. Cell. Biochem.* **2019**, *120*, 14735–14744. [CrossRef]

28. Carabelli, J.; Burgueño, A.L.; Rosselli, M.S.; Gianotti, T.F.; Lago, N.R.; Pirola, C.J.; Sookoian, S. High fat diet-induced liver steatosis promotes an increase in liver mitochondrial biogenesis in response to hypoxia. *J. Cell. Mol. Med.* **2011**, *15*, 1329–1338. [CrossRef]

29. Beli, E.; Yan, Y.; Moldovan, L.; Vieira, C.P.; Gao, R.; Duan, Y.; Prasad, R.; Bhatwadekar, A.; White, F.A.; Townsend, S.D.; et al. Restructuring of the Gut Microbiome by Intermittent Fasting Prevents Retinopathy and Prolongs Survival in db/db Mice. *Diabetes* **2018**, *67*, 1867–1879. [CrossRef]

30. Li, M.; Reynolds, C.M.; Gray, C.; Patel, R.; Sloboda, D.M.; Vickers, M.H. Long-term effects of a maternal high-fat: High-fructose diet on offspring growth and metabolism and impact of maternal taurine supplementation. *J. Dev. Orig. Heal. Dis.* **2019**, 1–8. [CrossRef]

31. Matsuda, M.; DeFronzo, R.A. Insulin sensitivity indices obtained from oral glucose tolerance testing: Comparison with the euglycemic insulin clamp. *Diabetes Care* **1999**, *22*, 1462–1470. [CrossRef]

32. Veenstra, A.; Liu, H.; Lee, C.A.; Du, Y.; Tang, J.; Kern, T.S. Diabetic Retinopathy: Retina-Specific Methods for Maintenance of Diabetic Rodents and Evaluation of Vascular Histopathology and Molecular Abnormalities. *Curr. Protoc. Mouse Boil.* **2015**, *5*, 247–270. [CrossRef]

33. Bhatwadekar, A.D.; Duan, Y.; Chakravarthy, H.; Korah, M.; Caballero, S.; Busik, J.V.; Grant, M.B. Ataxia telangiectasia mutated dysregulation results in diabetic retinopathy. *Stem Cells* **2016**, *34*, 405–417. [CrossRef]

34. Léger, H.; Santana, E.; Beltran, A.W.; Luca, F.C. Preparation of Mouse Retinal Cryo-sections for Immunohistochemistry. *J. Vis. Exp.* **2019**, e59683. [CrossRef]

35. Fan, S.; Zhang, Y.; Hu, N.; Sun, Q.; Ding, X.; Li, G.; Zheng, B.; Gu, M.; Huang, F.; Sun, Y.-Q.; et al. Extract of Kuding Tea Prevents High-Fat Diet-Induced Metabolic Disorders in C57BL/6 Mice via Liver X Receptor (LXR) β Antagonism. *PLoS ONE* **2012**, *7*, e51007. [CrossRef]

36. Engerman, R.L. Pathogenesis of diabetic retinopathy. *Diabetes* **1989**, *38*, 1203–1206. [CrossRef]

37. Kumar, B.; Gupta, S.K.; Nag, T.C.; Srivastava, S.; Saxena, R.; Jha, K.A.; Srinivasan, B.P. Retinal neuroprotective effects of quercetin in streptozotocin-induced diabetic rats. *Exp. Eye Res.* **2014**, *125*, 193–202. [CrossRef]

38. Eisenfeld, A.J.; Bunt-Milam, A.H.; Sarthy, P.V. Müller cell expression of glial fibrillic acidic protein after genetic and experimental photoreceptor degeneration in the rat retina. *Investig. Ophthalmol. Vis. Sci.* **1984**, *25*, 1321–1328.

39. Lieth, E.; Gardner, T.W.; Barber, A.J.; Antonetti, D.A. Retinal neurodegeneration: Early pathology in diabetes. *Clin. Exp. Ophthalmol. Viewpoint* **2000**, *28*, 3–8. [CrossRef]

40. Barber, A.J. A new view of diabetic retinopathy: A neurodegenerative disease of the eye. *Prog. Neuro-Psychopharmacol. Biol. Psychiatry* **2003**, *27*, 283–290. [CrossRef]

41. Stratton, I.M.; Kohner, E.M.; Aldington, S.J.; Turner, R.C.; Holman, R.R.; Manley, S.E.; Matthews, D.R.; UKPDS Group UKPDS 50. Risk factors for incidence and progression of retinopathy in Type II diabetes over 6 years from diagnosis. *Diabetologia* **2001**, *44*, 156–163. [CrossRef]

42. Tang, J.; Kern, T.S. Inflammation in diabetic retinopathy. *Prog. Retin. Eye Res.* **2011**, *30*, 343–358. [CrossRef]

43. Fortune, B.; Schneck, E.M.; Adams, A.J. Multifocal electroretinogram delays reveal local retinal dysfunction in early diabetic retinopathy. *Investig. Ophthalmol. Vis. Sci.* **1999**, *40*, 2638–2651.

44. McAnany, J.J.; Park, J.C.; Chau, F.Y.; Leiderman, Y.I.; Lim, J.I.; Blair, N.P. Amplitude loss of the high-frequency flicker electroretinogram in early diabetic retinopathy. *Retin.* **2019**, *39*, 2032–2039. [CrossRef] [PubMed]

45. Zeng, Y.; Cao, D.; Yu, H.; Yang, D.; Zhuang, X.; Hu, Y.; Li, J.; Yang, J.; Wu, Q.; Liu, B.; et al. Early retinal neurovascular impairment in patients with diabetes without clinically detectable retinopathy. *Br. J. Ophthalmol.* **2019**, *103*, 1747–1752. [PubMed]

46. Sone, H.; Kagawa, Y. Pancreatic beta cell senescence contributes to the pathogenesis of type 2 diabetes in high-fat diet-induced diabetic mice. *Diabetologia* **2005**, *48*, 58–67. [CrossRef]

47. Surwit, R.S.; Kuhn, C.M.; Cochrane, C.; McCubbin, A.J.; Feinglos, M.N. Diet-induced type II diabetes in C57BL/6J mice. *Diabetes* **1988**, *37*, 1163–1167. [CrossRef]

48. Surwit, R.S.; Feinglos, M.N.; Rodin, J.; Sutherland, A.; Petro, E.A.; Opara, E.C.; Kuhn, C.M.; Rebuffé-Scrive, M. Differential effects of fat and sucrose on the development of obesity and diabetes in C57BL/6J and A/J mice. *Metabolism* **1995**, *44*, 645–651. [CrossRef]

49. Cani, P.D.; Neyrinck, A.M.; Fava, F.; Knauf, C.; Burcelin, R.G.; Tuohy, K.M.; Gibson, G.R.; Delzenne, N.M. Selective increases of bifidobacteria in gut microflora improve high-fat-diet-induced diabetes in mice through a mechanism associated with endotoxaemia. *Diabetologia* **2007**, *50*, 2374–2383. [CrossRef]

50. Lin, S.; Thomas, T.; Storlien, L.; Huang, X. Development of high fat diet-induced obesity and leptin resistance in C57Bl/6J mice. *Int. J. Obes.* **2000**, *24*, 639–646. [CrossRef]

51. Membrez, M.; Blancher, F.; Jaquet, M.; Bibiloni, R.; Cani, P.D.; Burcelin, R.G.; Corthesy, I.; Chou, C.J.; Macé, K. Gut microbiota modulation with norfloxacin and ampicillin enhances glucose tolerance in mice. *FASEB J.* **2008**, *22*, 2416–2426. [CrossRef] [PubMed]

52. Rabot, S.; Membrez, M.; Bruneau, A.; Gerard, P.; Harach, T.; Moser, M.; Raymond, F.; Mansourian, R.; Chou, C.J. Germ-free C57BL/6J mice are resistant to high-fat-diet-induced insulin resistance and have altered cholesterol metabolism. *FASEB J.* **2010**, *24*, 4948–4959. [CrossRef] [PubMed]

53. Uysal, K.T.; Wiesbrock, S.M.; Marino, M.W.; Hotamisligil, G.S. Protection from obesity-induced insulin resistance in mice lacking TNF-α function. *Nature* **1997**, *389*, 610–614. [CrossRef] [PubMed]

54. Elchebly, M. Increased Insulin Sensitivity and Obesity Resistance in Mice Lacking the Protein Tyrosine Phosphatase-1B Gene. *Sci.* **1999**, *283*, 1544–1548. [CrossRef]

55. Nathan, D.M.; Buse, J.B.; Davidson, M.B.; Ferrannini, E.; Holman, R.R.; Sherwin, R.; Zinman, B. Medical management of hyperglycemia in type 2 diabetes: A consensus algorithm for the initiation and adjustment of therapy: A consensus statement of the American Diabetes Association and the European Association for the Study of Diabetes. *Diabetes Care* **2009**, *32*, 193–203. [CrossRef] [PubMed]

56. Kim, K.; Kim, E.S.; Yu, S.-Y. Longitudinal Relationship Between Retinal Diabetic Neurodegeneration and Progression of Diabetic Retinopathy in Patients With Type 2 Diabetes. *Am. J. Ophthalmol.* **2018**, *196*, 165–172. [CrossRef]

57. Kim, B.; McLean, L.L.; Philip, S.S.; Feldman, E.L. Hyperinsulinemia induces insulin resistance in dorsal root ganglion neurons. *Endocrinology* **2011**, *152*, 3638–3647. [CrossRef]

58. Kim, B.; Feldman, E.L. Insulin resistance in the nervous system. *Trends Endocrinol. Metab.* **2012**, *23*, 133–141. [CrossRef]

59. Das, A.K.; Kalra, S.; Tiwaskar, M.; Bajaj, S.; Seshadri, K.; Chowdhury, S.; Sahay, R.; Indurkar, S.; Unnikrishnan, A.G.; Phadke, U.; et al. Expert Group Consensus Opinion: Role of Anti-inflammatory Agents in the Management of Type-2 Diabetes (T2D). *J. Assoc. Physicians India* **2019**, *67*, 65–74.

60. Tabák, A.G.; Herder, C.; Rathmann, W.; Brunner, E.J.; Kivimäki, M. Prediabetes: A high-risk state for diabetes development. *Lancet* **2012**, *379*, 2279–2290. [CrossRef]

61. Lamparter, J.; Raum, P.; Pfeiffer, N.; Peto, T.; Höhn, R.; Elflein, H.; Wild, P.; Schulz, A.; Schneider, A.; Mirshahi, A. Prevalence and associations of diabetic retinopathy in a large cohort of prediabetic subjects: The Gutenberg Health Study. *J. Diabetes its Complicat.* **2014**, *28*, 482–487. [CrossRef]

62. Tikhonenko, M.; Lydic, T.A.; Opreanu, M.; Calzi, S.L.; Bozack, S.; McSorley, K.M.; Sochacki, A.L.; Faber, M.S.; Hazra, S.; Duclos, S.; et al. N-3 Polyunsaturated Fatty Acids Prevent Diabetic Retinopathy by Inhibition of Retinal Vascular Damage and Enhanced Endothelial Progenitor Cell Reparative Function. *PLoS ONE* **2013**, *8*, e55177. [CrossRef] [PubMed]

63. Busik, J.V.; Esselman, W.J.; Reid, E.G. Examining the role of lipid mediators in diabetic retinopathy. *Clin. Lipidol.* **2012**, *7*, 661–675. [CrossRef] [PubMed]

64. Hammer, S.S.; Busik, J.V. The role of dyslipidemia in diabetic retinopathy. *Vis. Res.* **2017**, *139*, 228–236. [CrossRef] [PubMed]

65. Calkin, A.C.; Tontonoz, P. Liver x receptor signaling pathways and atherosclerosis. *Arter. Thromb. Vasc. Boil.* **2010**, *30*, 1513–1518. [CrossRef] [PubMed]

66. Zelcer, N.; Tontonoz, P. Liver X receptors as integrators of metabolic and inflammatory signaling. *J. Clin. Investig.* **2006**, *116*, 607–614. [CrossRef]

67. Steffensen, K.R.; Jakobsson, T.; Gustafsson, J.-Å. Targeting liver X receptors in inflammation. *Expert Opin. Ther. Targets* **2013**, *17*, 977–990. [CrossRef]

68. Saadane, A.; Mast, N.; Trichonas, G.; Chakraborty, D.; Hammer, S.; Busik, J.V.; Grant, M.B.; Pikuleva, I.A. Retinal Vascular Abnormalities and Microglia Activation in Mice with Deficiency in Cytochrome P450 46A1–Mediated Cholesterol Removal. *Am. J. Pathol.* **2019**, *189*, 405–425. [CrossRef]

69. Sacks, F.M.; Lichtenstein, A.H.; Wu, J.H.; Appel, L.J.; Creager, M.A.; Kris-Etherton, P.M.; Miller, M.; Rimm, E.B.; Rudel, L.L.; Robinson, J.G.; et al. Dietary Fats and Cardiovascular Disease: A Presidential Advisory from the American Heart Association. *Circulation* **2017**, *136*, e1–e23. [CrossRef]

70. Andraski, A.B.; Singh, S.A.; Lee, L.H.; Higashi, H.; Smith, N.; Zhang, B.; Aikawa, M.; Sacks, F.M. Effects of Replacing Dietary Monounsaturated Fat With Carbohydrate on HDL (High-Density Lipoprotein) Protein Metabolism and Proteome Composition in Humans. *Arter. Thromb. Vasc. Boil.* **2019**, *39*, 2411–2430. [CrossRef]

71. Bolla, A.M.; Caretto, A.; Laurenzi, A.; Scavini, M.; Piemonti, L. Low-Carb and Ketogenic Diets in Type 1 and Type 2 Diabetes. *Nutrients* **2019**, *11*, 962. [CrossRef] [PubMed]

72. Gomes, J.A.; Silva, J.F.; Silva, G.C.; Gomes, G.F.; de Oliveira, A.C.; Soares, V.L.; Oliveira, M.C.; Ferreira, A.V.; Aguiar, D.C. High-refined carbohydrate diet consumption induces neuroinflammation and anxiety-like behavior in mice. *J. Nutr. Biochem.* **2019**, *77*, 108317. [CrossRef] [PubMed]

73. Tobias, D.K.; Chen, M.; Manson, J.E.; Ludwig, D.S.; Willett, W.; Hu, F.B. Effect of low-fat diet interventions versus other diet interventions on long-term weight change in adults: A systematic review and meta-analysis. *Lancet Diabetes Endocrinol.* **2015**, *3*, 968–979. [CrossRef]

74. Vega-López, S.; Venn, B.J.; Slavin, J.L. Relevance of the Glycemic Index and Glycemic Load for Body Weight, Diabetes, and Cardiovascular Disease. *Nutrients* **2018**, *10*, 1361. [CrossRef] [PubMed]

75. Livesey, G.; Taylor, R.; Livesey, H.F.; Buyken, A.E.; Jenkins, D.J.A.; Augustin, L.S.A.; Sievenpiper, J.L.; Barclay, A.W.; Liu, S.; Wolever, T.M.S.; et al. Dietary Glycemic Index and Load and the Risk of Type 2 Diabetes: Assessment of Causal Relations. *Nutrients* **2019**, *11*, 1436. [CrossRef]

76. Myette-Côté, É.; Durrer, C.; Neudorf, H.; Bammert, T.D.; Botezelli, J.D.; Johnson, J.D.; DeSouza, C.A.; Little, J.P. The effect of a short-term low-carbohydrate, high-fat diet with or without postmeal walks on glycemic control and inflammation in type 2 diabetes: A randomized trial. *Am. J. Physiol. Integr. Comp. Physiol.* **2018**, *315*, R1210–R1219.

77. Kowluru, R.A. Retinopathy in a Diet-Induced Type 2 Diabetic Rat Model, and Role of Epigenetic Modifications. *Diabetes* **2020**, db191009. [CrossRef]

78. Kim, K.-A.; Gu, W.; Lee, I.-A.; Joh, E.-H.; Kim, N.-H. High Fat Diet-Induced Gut Microbiota Exacerbates Inflammation and Obesity in Mice via the TLR4 Signaling Pathway. *PLoS ONE* **2012**, *7*, e47713. [CrossRef]

79. Lee, J.-J.; Wang, P.-W.; Yang, I.-H.; Huang, H.-M.; Chang, C.-S.; Wu, C.-L.; Chuang, J.-H. High-Fat Diet Induces Toll-Like Receptor 4-Dependent Macrophage/Microglial Cell Activation and Retinal Impairment. *Investig. Opthalmol. Vis. Sci.* **2015**, *56*, 3041. [CrossRef]

80. Krishnan, J.; Danzer, C.; Simka, T.; Ukropec, J.; Walter, K.M.; Kumpf, S.; Mirtschink, P.; Ukropcova, B.; Gasperikova, D.; Pedrazzini, T. Dietary obesity-associated hif1α activation in adipocytes restricts fatty acid oxidation and energy expenditure via suppression of the sirt2-nad+ system. *Genes Dev.* **2012**, *26*, 259–270. [CrossRef]

81. Stroka, D.M.; Burkhardt, T.; Desbaillets, I.; Wenger, R.H.; Neil, D.A.; Bauer, C.; Gassmann, M.; Candinas, D. Hif-1 is expressed in normoxic tissue and displays an organ-specific regulation under systemic hypoxia. *FASEB J.* **2001**, *15*, 2445–2453. [CrossRef] [PubMed]

82. Prasad, P.; Li, L.-P.; Halter, S.; Cabray, J.; Ye, M.; Batlle, D. Evaluation of renal hypoxia in diabetic mice by BOLD MRI. *Investig. Radiol.* **2010**, *45*, 819–822. [CrossRef] [PubMed]

Adeno-Associated Viral Vectors as a Tool for Large Gene Delivery to the Retina

Ivana Trapani [1,2]

[1]   Telethon Institute of Genetics and Medicine (TIGEM), 80078 Pozzuoli, Italy; trapani@tigem.it;

[2]   Medical Genetics, Department of Translational Medicine, Federico II University, 80131 Naples, Italy

Abstract: Gene therapy using adeno-associated viral (AAV) vectors currently represents the most promising approach for the treatment of many inherited retinal diseases (IRDs), given AAV's ability to efficiently deliver therapeutic genes to both photoreceptors and retinal pigment epithelium, and their excellent safety and efficacy profiles in humans. However, one of the main obstacles to widespread AAV application is their limited packaging capacity, which precludes their use from the treatment of IRDs which are caused by mutations in genes whose coding sequence exceeds 5 kb. Therefore, in recent years, considerable effort has been made to identify strategies to increase the transfer capacity of AAV vectors. This review will discuss these new developed strategies, highlighting the advancements as well as the limitations that the field has still to overcome to finally expand the applicability of AAV vectors to IRDs due to mutations in large genes.

Keywords: AAV; retina; gene therapy; dual AAV

1. Introduction

The eye is an ideal target for gene therapy thanks to its small and enclosed structure, relative immune privilege and easy accessibility [1,2]. This has boosted attempts at developing gene therapy approaches for the treatment of a large number of inherited retinal diseases (IRDs) over the recent decades [3,4]. Confirmation of the advancements in the retinal gene therapy field came in the last two years with the approval of the first gene therapy product for an IRD, Luxturna [5]—an adeno-associated viral (AAV) vector-based therapy for a form of Leber Congenital Amaurosis [6]—in the US, first, and then in Europe. The recombinant AAV vector on which Luxturna is based is the most widely used vector for retinal gene delivery. AAV are small (25 nm), nonenveloped, icosahedral viruses belonging to the Parvoviridae family [7]. They package a linear single-stranded DNA genome of ~4.7 kb, flanked by two 145 bp long palindromic inverted terminal repeats (ITRs) [7]. These ITRs form hairpin-loop secondary structures at the strand termini and are the only viral sequences that are retained in cis in the recombinant AAV vector genome [7]. Recombinant vectors based on AAV have fast become popular in the gene therapy field because of their excellent safety profile and low immunogenicity which allows for long-term expression of the therapeutic gene, at least in post-mitotic tissues, so that most experimental therapy studies require only a single vector administration. Additionally, dozens of different AAV variants have been identified thus far, each of them with unique transduction characteristics. This allows the user to select the most appropriate AAV serotype to transduce the retinal cell layer of interest. Indeed, following subretinal delivery, virtually all the AAV serotypes tested efficiently transduced the retinal pigment epithelium (RPE), while the levels of transduction of photoreceptors, which are the main therapeutic target cells in most IRDs, varied significantly among different serotypes [4,8]. AAV5, AAV7, AAV8 and AAV9 serotypes have all been demonstrated to efficiently transduce photoreceptors [4,8]. Additional serotypes with increased retinal transduction abilities have also been identified through either rational design or directed evolution [4,8]. This is one of the most attractive features of AAV vectors for retinal gene therapy, since alternative, both non-viral and viral, vectors tested thus far have shown more limited transduction abilities of adult photoreceptors [2,9]. For all the above described reasons, AAV have been used in many successful preclinical and clinical studies [3,4]. Clinical trial data collected over a decade have confirmed the overwhelming safety of AAV vectors delivered intraocularly and shown many instances of efficacy in treating previously incurable IRDs.

However, one of the main limitations to a broader application of AAV vectors for retinal gene therapy is their packaging capacity, which is restricted to approximately 5 kb of DNA [10]. This vector capacity is a critical issue, given the fact that approximately 6% of all human proteins have a coding sequence (CDS) that exceeds 4 kb [11] and that, in addition to the CDS of the therapeutic gene and the ITRs, a gene therapy vector needs to include, as a minimum, a promoter and a polyadenylation signal (polyA). Thus, the treatment of disorders caused by mutations in genes over 4 kb in size, including those causative of common IRDs, is currently not achievable using standard AAV vector-mediated approaches. The development of strategies to overcome AAV packaging limitation has therefore become a key area of research within the gene therapy field.

2. Strategies for Large Gene Delivery

Two types of strategies have been developed for large gene delivery via AAV: one is based on the "forced" packaging of oversized genomes (i.e., larger than 5 kb) in a single AAV vector (oversized AAV vectors); the other relies on the delivery of portions of large transgenes in two AAV vectors, which recombine through various mechanisms in the target cell, leading to the reconstitution of the full-length gene (dual AAV vectors) (Table 1).

Table 1. Adeno-associated viral (AAV) vector-based strategies for large gene delivery.

Strategy	Advantages	Limitations
Oversized AAV	No need to identify optimal splitting points/region of overlap	Genome highly heterogeneous in size
Trans-Splicing Dual AAV	Genomes with discrete nature	Non-directional concatemerization (with only one concatemer being productive) Need to identify optimal splitting points Efficiency dependent on splicing across the inverted terminal repeat (ITR) junction Potential production of shorter protein products
Overlapping Dual AAV	Genomes with discrete nature No additional foreign or artificial DNA elements required	Need to identify the optimal region of overlap for efficient homologous recombination Potential production of shorter protein products
Hybrid Dual AAV	Genomes with discrete nature Relies on two mechanisms for transgene reconstitution Transgene-independent efficacy of recombination	Need to identify optimal splitting points Efficiency dependent on splicing across the ITR junction Potential production of shorter protein products

2.1. Oversized AAV Vectors

Several research groups have tried to encapsidate large genes in a single AAV vector [12–14]. These "oversized" AAV vectors have been found to successfully express full-length proteins in vitro and in the retina of IRD models to levels which led to significant and stable improvement of the phenotype [12,15]. However, the genome contained in oversized AAV vectors was found to be not a pure population of intact large-sized genomes but rather a mixture of genomes highly heterogeneous in size [14,16–19]. Thus, it was proposed that full-length protein expression from oversized AAV vectors was achieved, following infection, through the re-assembly of truncated genomes in the target cell nucleus [14,16–19]. The efficiency of the transduction of oversized AAV vectors in the retina in comparison to alternative platforms for large gene delivery (i.e., dual AAV vectors, discussed below) has been assessed in various studies and found to be variable. Whereas some studies found considerably high levels of transgene expression from oversized AAV vectors [14,15], others showed efficient large protein reconstitution only upon dual AAV vector delivery [20,21]. Both the design and purification process of oversized AAV vectors were hypothesized to be critical for the success of the strategy, as the use of transgenes slightly above 5 kb can give rise to genomes with longer overlaps compared to the use of transgenes largely exceeding AAV cargo capacity, and this can drive more efficient re-assembly of oversized AAV vectors. Along this line, it was shown that the fractionation of oversized AAV vector preparations can be explored to promote selection of the genomes with the highest transduction properties in the final viral preparation [14]. However, despite the optimization and ability of this strategy to reconstitute large genes expression in vivo, consistently shown in various studies, the heterogenous nature of oversized AAV genomes poses major safety concerns, limiting their further application in clinical settings.

2.2. Dual AAV Vectors

An alternative strategy for AAV-mediated large gene delivery is the generation of dual AAV vectors. In this strategy, large transgenes are split into two separate AAV vectors that, upon co-infection of the same cell, reconstitute the expression of a full-length gene via intermolecular recombination between the two AAV vector genomes. This ideally doubles AAV cargo capacity, allowing delivery of transgenes up to about 9 kb. Various dual AAV vector strategies have been developed (referred to as trans-splicing [22], overlapping [23] and hybrid [24] dual AAV vector strategies), which differ in the mechanism they use to reconstitute the transgene.

2.2.1. Trans-Splicing Dual AAV Vectors

The trans-splicing approach relies on the natural ability of AAV ITRs to concatemerize in order to reconstitute full-length genomes [22,25]. In this approach, the two vectors carry two separate halves of the transgene, without regions of sequence overlap; the 5'-half vector has a splice donor (SD) signal at the 3' end of the AAV genome, while the 3'-half vector carries a splice acceptor (SA) signal at the 5' end of the AAV genome (Figure 1).

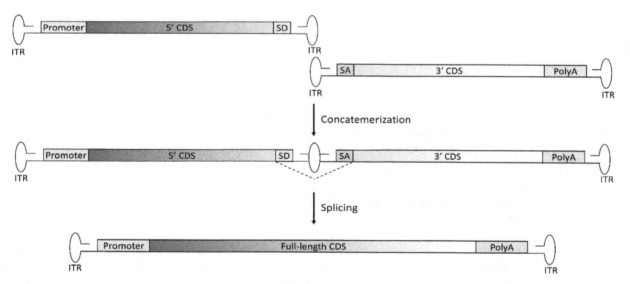

Figure 1. Schematic representation of the trans-splicing dual AAV approach for large gene reconstitution. The first vector includes the promoter, the 5'-half of the coding sequence (CDS) and the splicing donor (SD) signal; the second vector includes the splicing acceptor (SA) signal, the 3'-half of the CDS and the polyadenylation signal (PolyA). Concatemerization of the two vectors, involving the right-hand inverted terminal repeat (ITR) of the first vector and the left-hand ITR of the second vector, reconstitutes the full-length gene. After transcription, splicing leads to the removal of the ITR structure at the junction point, with restoration of the full-length, mature RNA of the transgene.

This allows splicing of the concatemerized ITR structure that forms in the middle of the therapeutic CDS following tail-to-head concatemerization of the two AAV genomes to obtain a single large mRNA molecule. This approach was first tested about 20 years ago, and historically represents the first developed approach for AAV-mediated large gene delivery. Since then, many studies have shown the efficacy of this strategy to reconstitute large genes. The major limitation of this platform, however, is that concatemerization can occur between any of the ITR of the two vectors. This may lead to the formation of both forms of circular monomers of each AAV, as well as two-vector linear concatemers in a number of orientations of which only one (i.e., tail-to-head concatemer) is productive to restore full-length gene expression [26]. Attempts at favoring the formation of concatemers in the correct orientation have been made (as discussed in the "Limitations of dual AAV vectors" paragraph). An additional limiting step of trans-splicing vectors is splicing across the ITR junction, the efficiency of which is dependent on both selection of the optimal exon–exon junction for splitting the large therapeutic gene [27] as well as the efficiency of splicing across the ITR structure [28]. To overcome the first issue, synthetic SD and SA signals have been developed, which mediate high rates of splicing independently of the gene that needs to be delivered [29]. Yet, since the sequence surrounding the splicing signals has an impact on splicing efficiency, careful selection of the splitting point is required.

2.2.2. Overlapping Dual AAV Vectors

In the overlapping approach, the transgene is split into two halves sharing homologous overlapping sequences, such that the reconstitution of the large gene expression cassette relies on homologous recombination [23] (Figure 2).

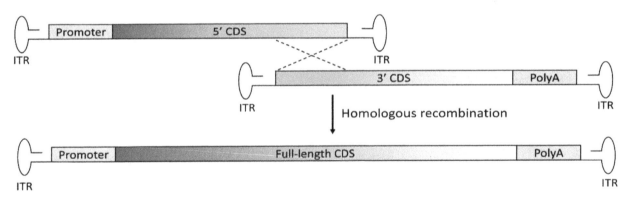

Figure 2. Schematic representation of the overlapping dual AAV approach for large gene reconstitution. The first vector includes the promoter and the 5'-half of the coding sequence (CDS) and the second vector includes the 3'-half of the CDS and the polyadenylation signal (PolyA). A portion of the sequence of the large transgene is repeated in both vectors (at the 3' end of the CDS of the first vector and at the 5' end of the CDS of the second vector). Thus, the full-length transgene expression cassette is reconstituted through homologous recombination of the overlapping regions in the two vectors. ITR: inverted terminal repeat.

As it has been designed, the overlapping approach is the simplest in design and requires less foreign or artificial DNA elements when compared to the other approaches. However, as the success of this strategy is critically dependent upon the ability of the overlapping region to mediate efficient homologous recombination, much work is needed to determine the optimal CDS overlapping region to be used for each transgene. Furthermore, data obtained so far have also highlighted that the success of this strategy is dependent on the retinal cell type being targeted, since the efficiency of the repair mechanism on which overlapping dual AAV vectors rely for large gene reconstitution is tissue dependent, as discussed below.

2.2.3. Hybrid Dual AAV Vectors

To overcome the main limitations of the previously described platforms (i.e., the lack of preference for directional tail-to-head concatemerization of the trans-splicing approach and the need for optimization of the CDS overlap for each transgene in the overlapping approach), a third transgene-independent dual AAV approach was developed: the hybrid dual AAV vectors. This approach is a combination of the trans-splicing and overlapping approaches, as it is based on the addition of a highly recombinogenic exogenous sequence to the trans-splicing vectors in order to increase recombination efficiency [24]. This recombinogenic sequence is placed downstream of the SD signal in the 5'-half vector and upstream of the SA signal in the 3'-half vector, so to be spliced out from the mRNA after recombination and transcription (Figure 3).

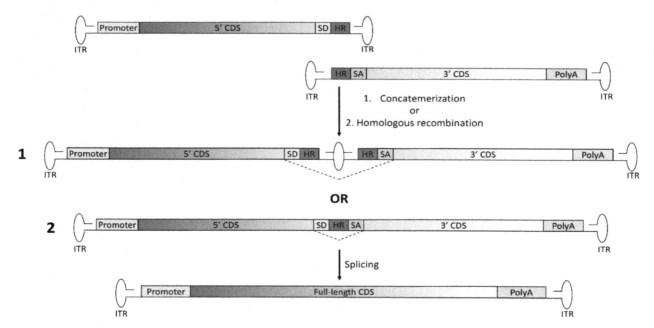

Figure 3. Schematic representation of the hybrid dual AAV approach for large gene reconstitution. The first vector includes the promoter, the 5'-half of the coding sequence (CDS), the splicing donor (SD) signal and the highly recombinogenic exogenous sequence (HR); the second vector includes the highly recombinogenic exogenous sequence, the splicing acceptor (SA) signal, the 3'-half of the CDS and the polyadenylation signal (PolyA). Joining of the two AAV vector genomes to reconstitute the full-length gene can occur through either: 1. concatemerization of the two vectors through the inverted terminal repeats (ITR), as for trans-splicing dual AAV vectors; or 2. homologous recombination mediated by the region of homology included in both vectors. In both cases, after transcription, splicing leads to the removal of the junction point, with restoration of the full-length, mature RNA of the transgene.

The hybrid dual AAV approach is potentially more effective than the other dual AAV vector approaches, since full-length gene reconstitution can occur through both homologous recombination mediated by the highly recombinogenic exogenous sequence as well as concatemerization through the ITRs [24]. The recombinogenic sequences used thus far to induce the recombination between hybrid dual AAV vectors have been derived from regions of either the alkaline phosphatase gene (AP) [24,30] or the F1 phage genome (AK) [21]. The inclusion of the exogenous sequence allows the promotion of high levels of homologous recombination between the two vector genomes, independently of the transgene to be delivered. However, similarly to the trans-splicing approach, the sequences surrounding the splicing signals still have an impact on splicing efficiency. Thus, careful selection of the splitting point is recommended to achieve maximal efficacy of large gene reconstitution.

3. The Choice of the Best Platform for Large Gene Delivery to the Retina

The efficacy of both oversized and dual AAV vectors in the retina has been evaluated in a number of studies using different reporter and therapeutic genes, such as *ABCA4* and *MYO7A* mutated in Stargardt disease (STGD1) [31] and Usher syndrome type 1B (USH1B) [32], respectively. However, literature describing these platforms is often conflicting. Initial studies in the retina reported a better performance of oversized AAV vectors compared to dual AAV strategies [14,15]. These results, however, might be due to both design and purification processes, which favor the generation of oversized vectors with high transduction properties [14], as well as to the less than optimal design of the dual AAV platform that was used as a comparison. One study, as an example, relied on the use of overlapping dual AAV vectors with a large region of overlap (1365 bases) that had not been optimized and, therefore, might potentially have a low efficiency of recombination [15]. Reconstitution from overlapping dual AAV vectors has also been found to occur at variable levels in different studies [15,20,21,26,33]. The most critical aspect of an overlapping dual AAV vector strategy is the event of recombination between the two halves of the transgene. This is influenced by both the sequence of the transgene and the cell type that is targeted, since different cell types could possibly deploy different DNA repair mechanisms. Some studies have found that long regions of overlap may lead to higher levels of transgene reconstitution [26]. However, it has recently been shown that optimization of the overlapping region is a prerequisite to achieve sustained levels of transgene expression in photoreceptors, since the efficiency of reconstitution is not directly proportional to the length of the regions of overlap [33]. It has been suggested that if the regions are too short, they might not be able to efficiently mediate interactions with the opposing viral genome, whereas longer regions of overlap may be less available for such interactions due to secondary structure formation. In line with this hypothesis, a screening of overlapping regions ranging from 23 to 1173 bp identified an overlap of 207–505 bp as the best performing for overlapping dual AAV-mediated reconstitution of *ABCA4* at therapeutic levels [33]. Thus, optimization of the overlapping region is essential to achieve sustained levels of transgene expression in photoreceptors. The targeted tissue also plays an important role in the success of the overlapping dual AAV approach since homologous recombination is typically associated with dividing cells, while low levels of homologous recombination are found in post-mitotic cells as neurons [34]. Along this line, studies have reported inefficient transduction of photoreceptors mediated by overlapping dual AAV vectors [15,21,26], whilst more efficient reconstitution was found in the RPE [21]. Other groups, however, have found efficient transduction of photoreceptors using overlapping dual AAV vectors [20,33], highlighting that the identification of highly recombinogenic regions of overlap in the transgene overcomes the limitations related to the inability of specific cell types to mediate efficient homologous recombination [33].

More consensus on the efficacy of trans-splicing and hybrid dual AAV vectors can be found in literature. A number of studies have indeed shown the ability of these strategies to reconstitute large transgenes in the retina [20,21,26,35,36] at levels which were higher compared to the other dual AAV strategies tested side by side [20,21,26], and which resulted in improvement of the retinal phenotype of animal models of IRDs [21,37]. This is possibly due to a more limited requirement of the optimization of these platforms compared to the others, since joining of the two halves of the transgene, with a discrete nature, occurs through the ITRs and/or a region of overlap known to be highly recombinogenic. Notably, the success obtained in the delivery of the large *MYO7A* gene to the retina [21] has led to the planning of a Phase I/II clinical trial, which will test the safety and efficacy of the hybrid dual AAV platform developed in the retina of USH1B patients (https://cordis.europa.eu/project/rcn/212674_it.html). Importantly, the results of this trial will definitively shed light on the efficiency of dual AAV vectors-mediated large gene delivery in the human retina.

Prompted by the success shown by dual AAV strategies, researchers have attempted at further expanding AAV cargo capacity in the retina up to 14 kb by adding a third vector to the dual system, generating triple AAV vectors [38]. This was found to be achievable, but at the expense of efficiency. Indeed, the levels of transduction achieved in the retina of a mouse model of Alstrom syndrome with triple AAV vectors have led to only a modest and transient improvement of the phenotype [38]. On the other hand, the levels of transduction mediated by triple AAV vectors in the large pig retina were found to be significantly higher than in the mouse retina, as also observed with dual AAV vectors [38]. These results bode well for further optimization of this platform.

4. Limitations of Dual AAV Vectors

Currently, all the dual AAV vector approaches have shown similar issues: variable success and expression of unwanted truncated products from single half-vectors. For all dual AAV platforms to be successful, a cell must necessarily be co-infected by at least one AAV vector including the 5′- and one including the 3′-half of the expression cassette. We and others have shown that co-transduction by two AAV vectors is quite efficient in the small subretinal space [11,21,36], which thus represents a favorable environment for developing dual AAV vector-based gene therapy approaches.

So far, however, all the studies performed have shown that none of the dual AAV approach matches the levels of expression achieved with a single AAV vector [21,26,36]. Various strategies have been explored to increase the efficiency of dual AAV vector-mediated large gene reconstitution.

One option is to increase vector dose and/or use AAV serotypes with higher tropism for the target cells in order to maximize rates of co-infection by both half vectors. A recent study has, however, suggested that an increase in vector dose does not proportionally correlate with increased levels of protein expression in the retina [26]. This suggests that, once efficient co-transduction is achieved, a further increase in vector genome amounts does not provide significant advantages [26]. Attempts at achieving higher levels of transduction by using alternative AAV serotypes have not been found consistently to result in higher transduction levels. Some studies have shown that use of capsid-engineered AAV variants with higher retinal transduction abilities, as tyrosine mutants capsids [39], led to higher levels of transgene expression from overlapping dual AAV vectors compared to naturally occurring AAV serotypes [20,33]. However, delivery of hybrid dual AAV vectors using an in-silico designed, synthetic vector (Anc80L65), which has also been shown to transduce retinal cells with a higher efficiency than AAV8 [40], led to almost identical levels of protein reconstitution compared to dual AAV8 vectors [26].

Another approach explored to increase transduction levels from dual AAV vectors has been maximizing the chances of both trans-splicing and hybrid AAV vectors to generate concatemers in the productive orientation, by forcing concatemerization of the ITRs, through the use of vectors carrying heterologous ITRs (i.e., ITR from different AAV serotypes at the opposite ends of the viral genome) [41]. Indeed, by generating trans-splicing vectors with heterologous ITR from serotypes 2 and 5 it has been shown that it is possible to reduce both the ability of each vector to form circular monomers and to increase directional tail-to-head concatemerization. This resulted in increased levels of transgene reconstitution compared to the use of vectors with homologous ITRs [41,42]. However, we have later shown that inclusion of heterologous ITRs in hybrid dual AAV vectors does not provide a significant advantage in full-length transgene reconstitution over the use of vectors with homologous ITRs [37]. This is consistent with the idea that hybrid dual AAV concatemerization is already partially driven in the correct orientation by the presence of highly recombinogenic regions. An additional strategy which has been used to direct AAV vectors concatemerization in the proper orientation is the use of a single-strand DNA oligonucleotide displaying homology to both of the distinct AAV genomes [43]. Alternatively, strategies that can improve dual AAV vector transduction efficiency by positively modulating AAV transduction steps, as the delivery of kinase inhibitors along with AAV vectors, have also been tested [44].

Another major drawback of dual AAV vectors, observed in some studies, is the production of truncated protein products from each of the single AAV vectors [20,21,33,37]. We and others have shown that, both in vitro and in the retina, truncated proteins from the 5′ half vector that contains the promoter sequence and/or from the 3′ half vector, due to the low promoter activity of the ITR, are produced. This issue can however be efficiently overcome by the use of the CL1 degron, a C-terminal destabilizing peptide that shares structural similarities with misfolded proteins and is thus recognized by the ubiquitination system [45,46]. Inclusion of this short (16 amino acids in length) degron mediates selective degradation of the truncated product from the 5′ half vector [37], without either affecting full-length protein reconstitution or significantly reducing the packaging capacity of the platform. More recently, McClements et al. have shown how the design of dual AAV vectors can also influence production of truncated proteins by the generation of unintended cryptic translation start sites and/or polyA signals [33]. Thus, the design of these platforms requires multiple considerations and adaptation, which may include codon optimizations to remove cryptic genetic signals. Furthermore, given the expression of such unwanted protein products, confirmation of the safety of dual AAV vectors is an important open question. While our preliminary data have shown no evident alterations of retinal morphology and functionality in mouse and pig eyes injected with dual AAV vectors [21,37], formal toxicity studies are required to elucidate this aspect.

5. Alternative Strategies to Allow AAV-Mediated Large Gene Delivery

Additional strategies to deliver large transgenes via AAV vectors are being actively investigated. Attempts at identifying AAV vectors with expanded cargo capacity, based on either protein libraries and directed evolution [47] or site directed mutagenesis to add positively-charged residues at lumenally exposed sites within the capsid [48], have been described. Alternatively, it has been shown that oversized AAV2 vector genomes can be effectively packaged in the capsid of human Bocavirus 1 (HBoV1) [49,50], an autonomous parvovirus relative of AAV, with a 5.5 kb genome. Testing of these vectors in the retina might lead to the identification of novel suitable vectors for large gene delivery.

The development of different short regulatory elements has also been attempted to reduce the size of the expression cassette and allow delivery of transgenes that exceed the AAV packaging capacity [51–55]. However, this often led to reduced levels of transgene expression. The combination of short synthetic enhancers and promoters was found to be useful for providing increased levels of expression of large transgenes [56]. Other studies have however shown that, despite optimization, some transgenes were more difficult than others to reconstitute from oversized AAV vectors when using short promoters [57].

The use of cDNA encoding for truncated versions of large proteins, which retain their functionality (i.e., a minigene), has also been achieved with some success [58]. However, all these approaches still cannot be easily applied to a large number of genes that exceed the AAV cargo capacity, since extensive optimization and testing would be required for each one of them.

6. Conclusions and Outlook

The growing number of clinical trials that show good safety and efficacy of the subretinal delivery of AAV vectors are contributing to the establishment of AAV as vectors of choice for retinal gene transfer. Expanding AAV cargo capacity over 5 kb is however a prerequisite to allow this platform to be used as a tool for the efficient delivery of a larger number of therapeutic genes. Recent proof-of-concept studies that used dual and triple AAV vectors to deliver large genes to the retina have shown that it is feasible to transfer genes with a CDS larger than 5 kb. Yet, these studies have highlighted that there is no one-fits-all dual AAV vector system, since dual AAV approaches have shown different relative efficiency in different studies. Clearly, the tissue being targeted, as well as the transgene that needs to be delivered, drastically influences transduction efficiency. Thus, careful design of the platform for each therapeutic application is required to achieve maximal efficacy. The planned clinical trial for USH1B will help defining whether the levels of expression achieved with dual AAV vectors are therapeutically relevant in humans. While the need of manufacturing two or more vectors to treat each disorder might represent a challenge of dual/triple AAV platforms, yet the retina is a favorable tissue for development of these approaches due to the fact that it requires delivery of only a small amount of vector. This reduces the total amount of vectors that needs to be produced.

Retinal transduction with multiple AAV vectors has been shown to reach lower levels compared to a single AAV vector. These levels were not sufficient to result in therapeutic efficacy for some diseases [38]. Consequently, alternative strategies should be explored.

Systems that rely on mechanisms different than those exploited by dual AAV vectors for large gene reconstitution might be investigated, including trans-splicing of pre-mRNAs [59] or intein-mediated protein trans-splicing [60]. Genome editing is also a rapidly expanding field of research, and could represent an interesting option for correction of mutations in genes whose delivery through AAV vectors is precluded by the large CDS size. A number of aspects for this approach however still need to be further explored. First, in the retina, where homologous recombination occurs at low rates, genome editing tools for the precise correction of a mutation will most probably need to exploit alternative repair mechanisms such as non-homologous end joining used for homology-independent targeted integration [61]. The efficiency of such approaches in the retina is still unknown. Secondly, the delivery of genome editing tools in post-mitotic tissues, such as the retina, might not be as safe as delivery in more proliferative tissues, considering the fact that their expression will persist long term after a single subretinal injection.

In conclusion, important steps forward have been made towards the treatment of IRDs due to mutations in large genes, which now seems an achievable goal. The optimization of these and the newly emerging platforms will allow expansion of the number of IRDs that are treatable using AAV-mediated gene therapy.

Acknowledgments: We thank Raffaele Castello (Scientific Office, TIGEM, Pozzuoli, Italy) for critical reading of the manuscript.

References

1. Auricchio, A.; Smith, A.J.; Ali, R.R. The Future Looks Brighter After 25 Years of Retinal Gene Therapy. *Hum. Gene Ther.* **2017**, *28*, 982–987. [CrossRef] [PubMed]

2. Trapani, I.; Auricchio, A. Seeing the Light after 25 Years of Retinal Gene Therapy. *Trends Mol. Med.* **2018**, *24*, 669–681. [CrossRef] [PubMed]

3. Moore, N.A.; Morral, N.; Ciulla, T.A.; Bracha, P. Gene therapy for inherited retinal and optic nerve degenerations. *Expert. Opin. Biol. Ther.* **2018**, *18*, 37–49. [CrossRef] [PubMed]

4. Trapani, I.; Puppo, A.; Auricchio, A. Vector platforms for gene therapy of inherited retinopathies. *Prog. Retin. Eye Res.* **2014**, *43*, 108–128. [CrossRef] [PubMed]

5. FDA approves hereditary blindness gene therapy. *Nat. Biotechnol* **2018**, *36*, 6. [CrossRef] [PubMed]

6. Pierce, E.A.; Bennett, J. The Status of RPE65 Gene Therapy Trials: Safety and Efficacy. *Cold Spring Harb. Perspect Med.* **2015**, *5*, a017285. [CrossRef]

7. Wang, D.; Tai, P.W.L.; Gao, G. Adeno-associated virus vector as a platform for gene therapy delivery. *Nat. Rev. Drug Discov.* **2019**. [CrossRef] [PubMed]

8. Day, T.P.; Byrne, L.C.; Schaffer, D.V.; Flannery, J.G. Advances in AAV vector development for gene therapy in the retina. *Adv. Exp. Med. Biol.* **2014**, *801*, 687–693.

9. Planul, A.; Dalkara, D. Vectors and Gene Delivery to the Retina. *Annu. Rev. Vis. Sci.* **2017**, *3*, 121–140. [CrossRef]

10. Salganik, M.; Hirsch, M.L.; Samulski, R.J. Adeno-associated Virus as a Mammalian DNA Vector. *Microbiol. Spectr.* **2015**, *3*. [CrossRef]

11. Palfi, A.; Chadderton, N.; McKee, A.G.; Blanco Fernandez, A.; Humphries, P.; Kenna, P.F.; Farrar, G.J. Efficacy of codelivery of dual AAV2/5 vectors in the murine retina and hippocampus. *Hum. Gene. Ther.* **2012**, *23*, 847–858. [CrossRef] [PubMed]

12. Allocca, M.; Doria, M.; Petrillo, M.; Colella, P.; Garcia-Hoyos, M.; Gibbs, D.; Kim, S.R.; Maguire, A.; Rex, T.S.; Di Vicino, U.; et al. Serotype-dependent packaging of large genes in adeno-associated viral vectors results in effective gene delivery in mice. *J. Clin. Invest.* **2008**, *118*, 1955–1964. [CrossRef] [PubMed]

13. Grieger, J.C.; Samulski, R.J. Packaging capacity of adeno-associated virus serotypes: Impact of larger genomes on infectivity and postentry steps. *J. Virol.* **2005**, *79*, 9933–9944. [CrossRef]

14. Hirsch, M.L.; Li, C.; Bellon, I.; Yin, C.; Chavala, S.; Pryadkina, M.; Richard, I.; Samulski, R.J. Oversized AAV transductifon is mediated via a DNA-PKcs-independent, Rad51C-dependent repair pathway. *Mol. Ther.* **2013**, *21*, 2205–2216. [CrossRef]

15. Lopes, V.S.; Boye, S.E.; Louie, C.M.; Boye, S.; Dyka, F.; Chiodo, V.; Fofo, H.; Hauswirth, W.W.; Williams, D.S. Retinal gene therapy with a large MYO7A cDNA using adeno-associated virus. *Gene. Ther.* **2013**, *20*, 824–833. [CrossRef] [PubMed]

16. Dong, B.; Nakai, H.; Xiao, W. Characterization of genome integrity for oversized recombinant AAV vector. *Mol. Ther.* **2010**, *18*, 87–92. [CrossRef] [PubMed]

17. Hirsch, M.L.; Agbandje-McKenna, M.; Samulski, R.J. Little vector, big gene transduction: Fragmented genome reassembly of adeno-associated virus. *Mol. Ther.* **2010**, *18*, 6–8. [CrossRef]

18. Lai, Y.; Yue, Y.; Duan, D. Evidence for the failure of adeno-associated virus serotype 5 to package a viral genome > or = 8.2 kb. *Mol. Ther.* **2010**, *18*, 75–79. [CrossRef]

19. Wu, Z.; Yang, H.; Colosi, P. Effect of genome size on AAV vector packaging. *Mol. Ther.* **2010**, *18*, 80–86. [CrossRef]

20. Dyka, F.M.; Boye, S.L.; Chiodo, V.A.; Hauswirth, W.W.; Boye, S.E. Dual adeno-associated virus vectors result in efficient in vitro and in vivo expression of an oversized gene, MYO7A. *Hum. Gene. Ther. Methods* **2014**, *25*, 166–177. [CrossRef]

21. Trapani, I.; Colella, P.; Sommella, A.; Iodice, C.; Cesi, G.; de Simone, S.; Marrocco, E.; Rossi, S.; Giunti, M.; Palfi, A.; et al. Effective delivery of large genes to the retina by dual AAV vectors. *EMBO Mol. Med.* **2014**, *6*, 194–211. [CrossRef]

22. Yan, Z.; Zhang, Y.; Duan, D.; Engelhardt, J.F. Trans-splicing vectors expand the utility of adeno-associated virus for gene therapy. *Proc. Natl. Acad. Sci. USA* **2000**, *97*, 6716–6721. [CrossRef]

23. Duan, D.; Yue, Y.; Engelhardt, J.F. Expanding AAV packaging capacity with trans-splicing or overlapping vectors: A quantitative comparison. *Mol. Ther.* **2001**, *4*, 383–391. [CrossRef]

24. Ghosh, A.; Yue, Y.; Lai, Y.; Duan, D. A hybrid vector system expands adeno-associated viral vector packaging capacity in a transgene-independent manner. *Mol. Ther.* **2008**, *16*, 124–130. [CrossRef]

25. Yang, J.; Zhou, W.; Zhang, Y.; Zidon, T.; Ritchie, T.; Engelhardt, J.F. Concatamerization of adeno-associated virus circular genomes occurs through intermolecular recombination. *J. Virol.* **1999**, *73*, 9468–9477.

26. Carvalho, L.S.; Turunen, H.T.; Wassmer, S.J.; Luna-Velez, M.V.; Xiao, R.; Bennett, J.; Vandenberghe, L.H. Evaluating Efficiencies of Dual AAV Approaches for Retinal Targeting. *Front Neurosci.* **2017**, *11*, 503. [CrossRef]

27. Lai, Y.; Yue, Y.; Liu, M.; Ghosh, A.; Engelhardt, J.F.; Chamberlain, J.S.; Duan, D. Efficient in vivo gene expression by trans-splicing adeno-associated viral vectors. *Nat. Biotechnol.* **2005**, *23*, 1435–1439. [CrossRef] [PubMed]

28. Xu, Z.; Yue, Y.; Lai, Y.; Ye, C.; Qiu, J.; Pintel, D.J.; Duan, D. Trans-splicing adeno-associated viral vector-mediated gene therapy is limited by the accumulation of spliced mRNA but not by dual vector coinfection efficiency. *Hum. Gene. Ther.* **2004**, *15*, 896–905. [CrossRef] [PubMed]

29. Lai, Y.; Yue, Y.; Liu, M.; Duan, D. Synthetic intron improves transduction efficiency of trans-splicing adeno-associated viral vectors. *Hum. Gene. Ther.* **2006**, *17*, 1036–1042. [CrossRef]

30. Ghosh, A.; Yue, Y.; Duan, D. Efficient transgene reconstitution with hybrid dual AAV vectors carrying the minimized bridging sequences. *Hum. Gene. Ther.* **2011**, *22*, 77–83. [CrossRef]

31. Tanna, P.; Strauss, R.W.; Fujinami, K.; Michaelides, M. Stargardt disease: clinical features, molecular genetics, animal models and therapeutic options. *Br. J. Ophthalmol.* **2017**, *101*, 25–30. [CrossRef]

32. Williams, D.S. Usher syndrome: Animal models, retinal function of Usher proteins, and prospects for gene therapy. *Vision Res.* **2008**, *48*, 433–441. [CrossRef]

33. McClements, M.E.; Barnard, A.R.; Singh, M.S.; Charbel Issa, P.; Jiang, Z.; Radu, R.A.; MacLaren, R.E. An AAV Dual Vector Strategy Ameliorates the Stargardt Phenotype in Adult Abca4(-/-) Mice. *Hum. Gene. Ther.* **2018**. [CrossRef]

34. Fishel, M.L.; Vasko, M.R.; Kelley, M.R. DNA repair in neurons: so if they don't divide what's to repair? *Mutat. Res.* **2007**, *614*, 24–36. [CrossRef] [PubMed]

35. Reich, S.J.; Auricchio, A.; Hildinger, M.; Glover, E.; Maguire, A.M.; Wilson, J.M.; Bennett, J. Efficient trans-splicing in the retina expands the utility of adeno-associated virus as a vector for gene therapy. *Hum. Gene. Ther.* **2003**, *14*, 37–44. [CrossRef]

36. Colella, P.; Trapani, I.; Cesi, G.; Sommella, A.; Manfredi, A.; Puppo, A.; Iodice, C.; Rossi, S.; Simonelli, F.; Giunti, M.; et al. Efficient gene delivery to the cone-enriched pig retina by dual AAV vectors. *Gene. Ther.* **2014**, *21*, 450–456. [CrossRef] [PubMed]

37. Trapani, I.; Toriello, E.; de Simone, S.; Colella, P.; Iodice, C.; Polishchuk, E.V.; Sommella, A.; Colecchi, L.; Rossi, S.; Simonelli, F.; et al. Improved dual AAV vectors with reduced expression of truncated proteins are safe and effective in the retina of a mouse model of Stargardt disease. *Hum. Mol. Genet.* **2015**, *24*, 6811–6825. [CrossRef]

38. Maddalena, A.; Tornabene, P.; Tiberi, P.; Minopoli, R.; Manfredi, A.; Mutarelli, M.; Rossi, S.; Simonelli, F.; Naggert, J.K.; Cacchiarelli, D.; et al. Triple Vectors Expand AAV Transfer Capacity in the Retina. *Mol. Ther.* **2018**, *26*, 524–541. [CrossRef]

39. Petrs-Silva, H.; Dinculescu, A.; Li, Q.; Min, S.H.; Chiodo, V.; Pang, J.J.; Zhong, L.; Zolotukhin, S.; Srivastava, A.; Lewin, A.S.; et al. High-efficiency transduction of the mouse retina by tyrosine-mutant AAV serotype vectors. *Mol. Ther.* **2009**, *17*, 463–471. [CrossRef]

40. Zinn, E.; Pacouret, S.; Khaychuk, V.; Turunen, H.T.; Carvalho, L.S.; Andres-Mateos, E.; Shah, S.; Shelke, R.; Maurer, A.C.; Plovie, E.; et al. In Silico Reconstruction of the Viral Evolutionary Lineage Yields a Potent Gene Therapy Vector. *Cell Rep.* **2015**, *12*, 1056–1068. [CrossRef]

41. Yan, Z.; Zak, R.; Zhang, Y.; Engelhardt, J.F. Inverted terminal repeat sequences are important for intermolecular recombination and circularization of adeno-associated virus genomes. *J. Virol.* **2005**, *79*, 364–379. [CrossRef] [PubMed]

42. Yan, Z.; Lei-Butters, D.C.; Zhang, Y.; Zak, R.; Engelhardt, J.F. Hybrid adeno-associated virus bearing nonhomologous inverted terminal repeats enhances dual-vector reconstruction of minigenes in vivo. *Hum. Gene. Ther.* **2007**, *18*, 81–87. [CrossRef]

43. Hirsch, M.L.; Storici, F.; Li, C.; Choi, V.W.; Samulski, R.J. AAV recombineering with single strand oligonucleotides. *PLoS ONE* **2009**, *4*, e7705. [CrossRef]

44. Maddalena, A.; Dell'Aquila, F.; Giovannelli, P.; Tiberi, P.; Wanderlingh, L.G.; Montefusco, S.; Tornabene, P.; Iodice, C.; Visconte, F.; Carissimo, A.; et al. High-Throughput Screening Identifies Kinase Inhibitors That Increase Dual Adeno-Associated Viral Vector Transduction In Vitro and in Mouse Retina. *Hum. Gene. Ther.* **2018**, *29*, 886–901. [CrossRef]

45. Bence, N.F.; Sampat, R.M.; Kopito, R.R. Impairment of the ubiquitin-proteasome system by protein aggregation. *Science* **2001**, *292*, 1552–1555. [CrossRef]

46. Gilon, T.; Chomsky, O.; Kulka, R.G. Degradation signals for ubiquitin system proteolysis in Saccharomyces cerevisiae. *EMBO J.* **1998**, *17*, 2759–2766. [CrossRef] [PubMed]

47. Turunen, H.T.; Vandenberghe, L.H. Generating Novel AAV Capsid Mutants for Large Genome Packaging Through Protein Libraries and Directed Evolution. In Proceedings of the American Society of Gene & Cell Therapy 17th Annual Meeting, Washigton, DC, USA, 21–24 May 2014; p. S118.

48. Tiffany, M.; Kay, M.A. Expanded Packaging Capacity of AAV by Lumenal Charge Alteration. In Proceedings of the American Society of Gene & Cell Therapy 19th Annual Meeting, Washigton, DC, USA, 22 April 2016; pp. S99–S100.

49. Yan, Z.; Keiser, N.W.; Song, Y.; Deng, X.; Cheng, F.; Qiu, J.; Engelhardt, J.F. A novel chimeric adenoassociated virus 2/human bocavirus 1 parvovirus vector efficiently transduces human airway epithelia. *Mol. Ther.* **2013**, *21*, 2181–2194. [CrossRef]

50. Fakhiri, J.; Schneider, M.A.; Puschhof, J.; Stanifer, M.; Schildgen, V.; Holderbach, S.; Voss, Y.; El Andari, J.; Schildgen, O.; Boulant, S.; et al. Novel Chimeric Gene Therapy Vectors Based on Adeno-Associated Virus and Four Different Mammalian Bocaviruses. *Mol. Ther. Methods Clin. Dev.* **2019**, *12*, 202–222. [CrossRef] [PubMed]

51. Ostedgaard, L.S.; Rokhlina, T.; Karp, P.H.; Lashmit, P.; Afione, S.; Schmidt, M.; Zabner, J.; Stinski, M.F.; Chiorini, J.A.; Welsh, M.J. A shortened adeno-associated virus expression cassette for CFTR gene transfer to cystic fibrosis airway epithelia. *Proc. Natl. Acad. Sci. USA* **2005**, *102*, 2952–2957. [CrossRef] [PubMed]

52. McFarland, T.J.; Zhang, Y.; Atchaneeyaskul, L.O.; Francis, P.; Stout, J.T.; Appukuttan, B. Evaluation of a novel short polyadenylation signal as an alternative to the SV40 polyadenylation signal. *Plasmid* **2006**, *56*, 62–67. [CrossRef]

53. Pellissier, L.P.; Hoek, R.M.; Vos, R.M.; Aartsen, W.M.; Klimczak, R.R.; Hoyng, S.A.; Flannery, J.G.; Wijnholds, J. Specific tools for targeting and expression in Muller glial cells. *Mol. Ther. Methods Clin. Dev.* **2014**, *1*, 14009. [CrossRef]

54. Choi, J.H.; Yu, N.K.; Baek, G.C.; Bakes, J.; Seo, D.; Nam, H.J.; Baek, S.H.; Lim, C.S.; Lee, Y.S.; Kaang, B.K. Optimization of AAV expression cassettes to improve packaging capacity and transgene expression in neurons. *Mol. Brain* **2014**, *7*, 17. [CrossRef]

55. Wang, D.; Fischer, H.; Zhang, L.; Fan, P.; Ding, R.X.; Dong, J. Efficient CFTR expression from AAV vectors packaged with promoters—The second generation. *Gene. Ther.* **1999**, *6*, 667–675. [CrossRef] [PubMed]

56. Yan, Z.; Sun, X.; Feng, Z.; Li, G.; Fisher, J.T.; Stewart, Z.A.; Engelhardt, J.F. Optimization of Recombinant Adeno-Associated Virus-Mediated Expression for Large Transgenes, Using a Synthetic Promoter and Tandem Array Enhancers. *Hum. Gene. Ther.* **2015**, *26*, 334–346. [CrossRef] [PubMed]

57. Holehonnur, R.; Lella, S.K.; Ho, A.; Luong, J.A.; Ploski, J.E. The production of viral vectors designed to express large and difficult to express transgenes within neurons. *Mol. Brain* **2015**, *8*, 12. [CrossRef]

58. Lai, Y.; Thomas, G.D.; Yue, Y.; Yang, H.T.; Li, D.; Long, C.; Judge, L.; Bostick, B.; Chamberlain, J.S.; Terjung, R.L.; et al. Dystrophins carrying spectrin-like repeats 16 and 17 anchor nNOS to the sarcolemma and enhance exercise performance in a mouse model of muscular dystrophy. *J. Clin. Invest.* **2009**, *119*, 624–635. [CrossRef]

59. Yang, Y.; Walsh, C.E. Spliceosome-mediated RNA trans-splicing. *Mol. Ther.* **2005**, *12*, 1006–1012. [CrossRef]

60. Li, Y. Split-inteins and their bioapplications. *Biotechnol. Lett.* **2015**, *37*, 2121–2137. [CrossRef] [PubMed]

61. Suzuki, K.; Tsunekawa, Y.; Hernandez-Benitez, R.; Wu, J.; Zhu, J.; Kim, E.J.; Hatanaka, F.; Yamamoto, M.; Araoka, T.; Li, Z.; et al. In vivo genome editing via CRISPR/Cas9 mediated homology-independent targeted integration. *Nature* **2016**, *540*, 144–149. [CrossRef]

6

Lack of Overt Retinal Degeneration in a K42E *Dhdds* Knock-In Mouse Model of RP59

Sriganesh Ramachandra Rao [1,2,†], Steven J. Fliesler [1,2,†], Pravallika Kotla [3], Mai N. Nguyen [3] and Steven J. Pittler [3,*]

[1]   Research Service, VA Western NY Healthcare System, Buffalo, NY 14215, USA;
      sramacha@buffalo.edu (S.R.R.); fliesler@buffalo.edu (S.J.F.)
[2]   Departments of Ophthalmology and Biochemistry and Neuroscience Graduate Program,
      The State University of New York- University at Buffalo, Buffalo, NY 14209, USA
[3]   Department of Optometry and Vision Science, Vision Science Research Center, University of Alabama at
      Birmingham, School of Optometry, Birmingham, AL 35294, USA; pkotla@uab.edu (P.K.);
      mnnguyen@uab.edu (M.N.N.)
*   Correspondence: pittler@uab.edu;
†   These authors contributed equally to this work.

Abstract: Dehydrodolichyl diphosphate synthase (DHDDS) is required for protein N-glycosylation in eukaryotic cells. A K42E point mutation in the DHDDS gene causes an autosomal recessive form of retinitis pigmentosa (RP59), which has been classified as a congenital disease of glycosylation (CDG). We generated K42E *Dhdds* knock-in mice as a potential model for RP59. Mice heterozygous for the *Dhdds* K42E mutation were generated using CRISPR/Cas9 technology and crossed to generate *Dhdds*$^{K42E/K42E}$ homozygous mice. Spectral domain-optical coherence tomography (SD-OCT) was performed to assess retinal structure, relative to age-matched wild type (WT) controls. Immunohistochemistry against glial fibrillary acidic protein (GFAP) and opsin (1D4 epitope) was performed on retinal frozen sections to monitor gliosis and opsin localization, respectively, while lectin cytochemistry, plus and minus PNGase-F treatment, was performed to assess protein glycosylation status. Retinas of *Dhdds*$^{K42E/K42E}$ mice exhibited grossly normal histological organization from 1 to 12 months of age. Anti-GFAP immunoreactivity was markedly increased in *Dhdds*$^{K42E/K42E}$ mice, relative to controls. However, opsin immunolocalization, ConA labeling and PNGase-F sensitivity were comparable in mutant and control retinas. Hence, retinas of *Dhdds*$^{K42E/K42E}$ mice exhibited no overt signs of degeneration, yet were markedly gliotic, but without evidence of compromised protein N-glycosylation. These results challenge the notion of RP59 as a DHDDS loss-of-function CDG and highlight the need to investigate unexplored RP59 disease mechanisms.

Keywords: retinitis pigmentosa; knock-in mouse model; congenital disorder of glycosylation; retina

1. Introduction

Retinitis pigmentosa (RP) represents a group of hereditary retinal degenerative disorders of diverse genetic origins that have as their common trait the progressive, irreversible dysfunction, degeneration, and demise of retinal photoreceptor cells, with rods initially undergoing these pathological changes followed eventually by cones [1,2]. Relatively recently, a K42E point mutation in the dehydrodolichyl diphosphate synthase (DHDDS) gene was shown to cause a rare, recessive form of RP (RP59; OMIM #613861) [3–5]. DHDDS catalyzes *cis*-prenyl chain elongation in the synthesis of dolichyl diphosphate (Dol-PP), which is required for protein N-glycosylation [6,7]. DHDDS catalyzes the condensation of multiple units of isopentenyl pyrophosphate (IPP, also called isopentenyl diphosphate) to farnesyl pyrophosphate (FPP, also called farnesyl diphosphate) to produce Dol-PP [8,9]. This is used as the "lipid carrier" onto which oligosaccharide chains are built that are ultimately transferred to specific asparagine (N) residues on nascent polypeptide chains in the lumen of the endoplasmic reticulum (ER) to form N-linked glycoproteins [10]. The monophosphate (Dol-P) is used as a sugar carrier, transferring sugars from their corresponding sugar-nucleotide adducts (e.g., UDP-glucose, GDP-mannose, etc.) to the growing Dol-PP-linked oligosaccharide chains in the ER. Mutations in rhodopsin that block its glycosylation have been shown to cause retinal degeneration in vertebrate animals [11,12]. In addition, pharmacological inhibition of protein N-glycosylation with tunicamycin has been shown to disrupt retinal photoreceptor outer segment (OS) disc membrane morphogenesis in vitro [13], as well as to cause retinal degeneration with progressive shortening and loss of photoreceptor OSs in vivo [14].

In the present study, we created a DHDDS K42E homozygous knock-in mouse model (hereafter called $Dhdds^{K42E/K42E}$) of RP59—since K42E is the most prevalent point mutation in the RP59 patient population [3–5]—to study its underlying pathological mechanism, with the working hypothesis that defective protein N-glycosylation underlies the retinal dysfunction and degeneration observed in human RP59. Herein, we present a description of the generation and initial characterization of the phenotypic features of the $Dhdds^{K42E/K42E}$ mouse model. Surprisingly, although we expected to observe an early onset, progressive, and potentially severe retinal degeneration, this was not the case. The retina appeared histologically intact and normal according to spectral domain optical coherence tomography (SD-OCT) analysis for up to at least one year of age. However, there was evidence of gliotic reactivity (glial fibrillary acidic protein (GFAP) immunostaining), despite the lack of obvious neuronal degeneration or cell death/loss. Also, despite the homozygous mutation in $Dhdds$, we found no evidence of compromised protein N-glycosylation in mutant mouse retinas.

2. Materials and Methods

2.1. Animals

Heterozygous (K42E/+) $Dhdds$ knock-in (KI) mice were generated on a C57Bl/6J background by Applied StemCell (Milipitas, CA, USA). Briefly, CRISPR guide RNA (5′-TCGCTATGCCAAGAAGTGTC-3′ with PAM site AGG) was generated using in vitro transcription and was used to create a double strand break in the murine $Dhdds$ locus to promote introduction of a single-stranded oligodeoxynucleotide (SSO) carrying the K42E mutation and a second silent DNA polymorphism to eliminate the PAM recognition site required for cleavage by CAS9 (5′-ATTATCTGTTCTCTTCTACAGGCTGGCCCAGTACCCAAACATATCGCGTTCATAATGGACGGC AACCGTCGCTATGCCAAGGAGTGTCAAGTGGAGCGCCAGGAGGGCCACACACAGGGCTTCA ATAAGCTTGCTGAGGTGGGTGCGGGTGACAGAGCCTAGA-3′). Mouse zygotes were injected with 100, 100, and 250 ng/µL of Cas9 enzyme, guide RNA, and SSO, respectively, which were then transferred into pseudo pregnant CD-1 females. Three potential founder (F0) pups were identified out of 13 mice tested, and an F0 founder was verified by DNA sequence analysis. Sequence-validated heterozygous ($Dhdds^{K42E/+}$) mice were crossed to generate homozygous ($Dhdds^{K42E/K42E}$) mice, as confirmed by PCR and DNA sequencing (see below). C57Bl/6J wild type (WT) mice, age- and sex-matched, were used as controls. All procedures conformed to the ARVO Statement for the Use of Animals in Ophthalmic and Vision Research, and were approved by the Institutional Animal Care and Use Committee (IACUC) of the University of Alabama at Birmingham. All animals were maintained on a standard 12/12 h light/dark cycle (20–40 lux ambient room illumination), fed standard rodent chow, provided water ad libitum, and housed in plastic cages with standard rodent bedding.

2.2. PCR Genotyping and DNA Analysis

PCR primers were designed that spanned the targeted region (forward primer, 5′-TCTAGGCTCTGTCACCCGCA-3′ and reverse primer 5′-TCTAGGCTCTGTCACCCGCA-3′) amplifying a 292 bp segment of DNA in both WT and $Dhdds^{K42E/K42E}$ mice. For initial verification of the knock-in, PCR products were sequenced in the UAB Heflin Center for Genomic Sciences. The presence of the knock-in sequence was confirmed in subsequent generations by restriction enzyme digestion with StyI, which cleaves the knock-in allele only (data not shown). Knock-in alleles were independently verified by Transnetyx, Inc. (Cordova, TN, USA) using proprietary technology. While the analysis was set up to recognize and differentiate the knock-in mutation and the PAM site polymorphism, only the knock-in mutation was maintained in all subsequent breeding.

2.3. Spectral Domain Optical Coherence Tomography (SD-OCT)

In vivo retinal imaging was performed as previously described in detail by DeRamus et al. [15], using a Bioptigen Model 840 Envisu Class-R high-resolution SD-OCT instrument (Bioptigen/Leica, Inc.; Durham, NC, USA). Data were collected from $Dhdds^{K42E/K42E}$ and WT mice at postnatal day (PN) 1 (KI, n = 5; WT, n = 9), 2 (KI, n = 4; WT, n = 8), 3 (KI, n = 5; WT, n = 3), 8 (KI, n = 4; WT n = 5), and 12 months (mos) (KI, n = 3; WT n = 3) to assess retinal structure. Layer thicknesses were determined manually using Bioptigen InVivoVue® and Bioptigen Diver® V. 3.4.4 software and the data were analyzed and graphed using Microsoft Excel software.

2.4. Immunohistochemistry (IHC)

Procedures utilized for fixation, O.C.T. embedment, and sectioning of mouse eyes were as described in detail previously by Ramachandra Rao et al. [16]. In brief, eyes were immersion fixed overnight in phosphate-buffered saline (PBS) containing freshly prepared paraformaldehyde (4% v/v), appropriately cryopreserved, embedded in O.C.T., and cryosectioning was performed on a Leica Model CM3050 S Cryostat (Leica Biosystems, Wetzlar, Germany). Retinal sections were first "blocked" with 0.1% BSA, 0.5% serum (species corresponding to secondary antibody host) in Tris-buffered saline containing 0.1% Tween-20 (TBST), then incubated for 1 h at room temperature with a rabbit polyclonal antibody against glial fibrillary acidic protein (GFAP;, DAKO/Agilent, Santa Clara, CA, USA; 1:500 dilution in TBST) and a mouse monoclonal antibody against the C-terminal epitope of opsin (1D4; Novus Biologicals, Littleton, CO, USA; 1:500 dilution in TBST), followed by incubation with fluor-conjugated secondary antibodies (AlexaFluor®-488 conjugated anti-mouse IgG, AlexaFluor®-568 conjugated anti-rabbit IgG; Thermo Fisher Scientific, Waltham, MA, USA; 1:500 dilution in TBST). Sections were then counterstained with DAPI and cover slipped with anti-fade mounting medium (Vectashield®; Vector Laboratories, Burlingame, CA, USA) and viewed with a Leica TCS SPEII DMI4000 scanning laser confocal microscope (Leica Biosystems). Images were captured using a 40X oil immersion (RI 1.518) objective under normal laser intensity (10% of laser power source), arbitrary gain (850 V) and offset (−0.5) values, to optimize signal-to-noise ratio. Digital images were captured and stored as TIFF files on a PC computer.

2.5. Lectin Cytochemistry

Paraformaldehyde-fixed eyes (as described above) were processed for paraffin embedment. Paraffin sections of mouse eyes were then incubated (45 min at room temperature) with biotinylated Concanavalin-A (ConA, B-1005; Vector Laboratories; 1:200 dilution in PBS), followed by incubation with AlexaFluor®-488 conjugated streptavidin (Thermo Fisher Scientific; 1:500 dilution in PBS) and AlexaFluor®-647-conjugated peanut agglutinin (PNA, L32460; Thermo Fisher Scientific; 1:250 dilution in PBS), with or without pre-treatment (37 °C, overnight) with peptide:N-glycosidase F (PNGase-F, 200 U, P0704S; New England Biolabs, Inc., Ipswich, MA, USA). Sections were DAPI-stained and mounted using Vectashield mounting media, and digital images obtained using scanning laser confocal microscopy as described above [16].

3. Results

3.1. Generation and Validation of K42E DHDDS Knock-In Mutation

K42E knock-in mice were generated commercially using CRISPR-Cas9 technology. The K42E knock-in mutations in both heterozygous and homozygous mice were confirmed by DNA sequence for one of the heterozygous F0 founder mice, which is shown in Figure 1. Both the A-to-G and G-to-A transitions that lead to the K42E mutation and the Q44Q silent polymorphism, respectively, are heterozygous (arrows). Intra-litter mating was done to establish at least fourth generation homozygous mice that were used for all subsequent analyses. Heterozygous mice were initially characterized by SD-OCT and histology and found not to differ from WT (not shown).

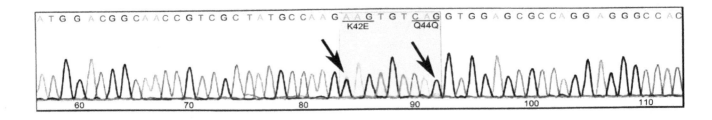

Figure 1. DNA sequence analysis of a tail DNA from a K42E/+ founder mouse. Tail DNA was amplified with primers that cover a 292 bp segment spanning the target region. The sequence analysis confirmed the presence (arrows) of the K42E (A-to-G) mutation and the Q44Q (G-to-A) polymorphism that was included to eliminate the CRISPR-related PAM site.

3.2. SD-OCT Analysis Reveals No Evidence for Retinal Degeneration in Dhdds$^{K42E/K42E}$ Mice

SD-OCT provides a non-invasive means of assessing retinal morphology *in vivo*. Qualitative SD-OCT images obtained from wild type (WT) and *Dhdds*$^{K42E/K42E}$ mice are presented in Figure 2. From these images, it is clear that the gross morphology of the retina in the homozygous knock-in animals, from PN 1 to 12 months of age, are comparable to that observed in fully mature, age-matched WT control mice. All retinal histological layers were intact and of normal appearance. Hence, there was no evidence of retinal degeneration, even up to one year of age.

We used SD-OCT to perform quantitative analysis of retinal morphology to compare ocular tissue layer thicknesses in WT and knock-in mice. Figure 3 compares data obtained at PN 1, 2, 3, 8, and 12 mos for *Dhdds*$^{K42E/K42E}$ mice, compared to age-matched WT control littermates. The data are shown both with respect to outer nuclear layer (ONL) thickness (yellow and gray lines) as well as total neural retina thickness (blue and orange lines) as a function of distance from the optic nerve head (ONH, point 4 in each graph) along the vertical meridian, for both the inferior and superior hemispheres. No differences in these quantitative metrics of retinal morphology were observed with respect to genotype, consistent with the representative OCT images shown in Figure 2.

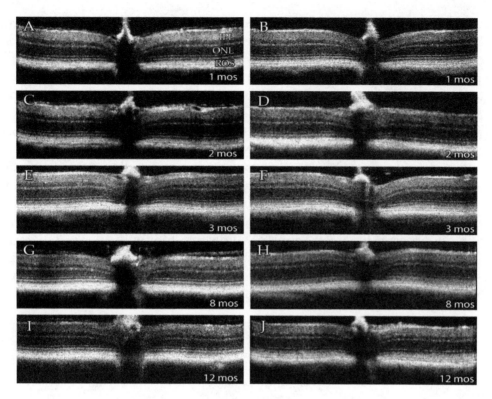

Figure 2. Representative averaged SD-OCT images of retinas from (left panels: **A,C,E,G,I**) 1-, 2-, 3-, 8- and 12-months (mos) old wild type (WT), and (right panels: **B,D,F,H,J**) 1-, 2-, 3-, 8-, and 12-months old $Dhdds^{K42E/K42E}$ mice. Abbreviations: IPL, inner plexiform layer; ONL, outer nuclear layer; ROS, rod outer segment layer. No changes were observed at any age in retinas of $Dhdds^{K42E/K42E}$ mice compared to WT mice.

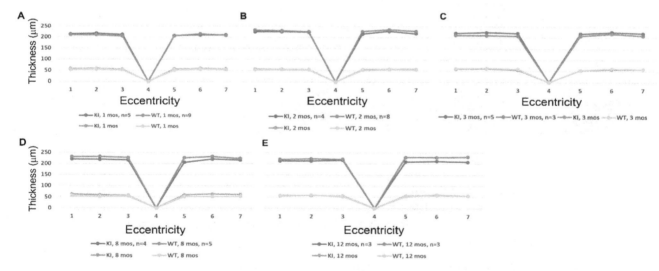

Figure 3. Analysis of the ONL thickness (yellow and gray lines) and total retinal thickness (blue and orange lines) in WT and $Dhdds^{K42E/K42E}$ mice ranging in age from PN 1 to 12 months. (**A**) 1 month, (**B**) 2 months, (**C**) 3 months, (**D**) 8 months, (**E**) 12 months. Outer nuclear layer (ONL) thickness and total retina thickness measurements (in microns), as a function of genotype and distance from the optic nerve head (ONH) along the vertical meridian in both the inferior and superior hemispheres. Genotypes: WT and $Dhdds^{K42E/K42E}$ mice. No significant differences were observed between the groups.

3.3. Gliotic Reactivity, Despite Lack of Overt Neural Retina Degeneration, in Dhdds^{K42E/K42E} Mice

We performed immunohistochemical analysis on frozen sections of fixed, O.C.T.-embedded WT and $Dhdds^{K42E/K42E}$ mouse eyes at PN 2 months of age, probing with antibodies against GFAP (polyclonal) and a C-terminal epitope of rod opsin (1D4 monoclonal). As shown in Figure 4, whereas WT control retinas only exhibited GFAP immunoreactivity (pseudocolored red) along the vitreoretinal interface, corresponding to astrocytes and Müller glia "end feet", retinas from $Dhdds^{K42E/K42E}$ mice exhibited extensive, robust anti-GFAP labeling in a radial pattern. This extended throughout the inner retinal layers to the outer plexiform layer (OPL), in addition to intense labeling along the vitreoretinal interface. The latter results are indicative of massive gliotic activation, which is remarkable considering the lack of overt retinal degeneration or loss of retinal neurons (per the SD-OCT data; see Figures 2 and 3). Gliosis in $Dhdds^{K42E/K42E}$ mouse retinas was also detected at PN one month and persisted even at PN six months of age (data not shown). Anti-opsin immunolabeling (pseudocolored green) was comparable in both WT and $Dhdds^{K42E/K42E}$ retinas. Notably, the label was confined to the OS layer; there was no mislocalization of opsin to the plasma membrane of the cell in the IS or ONL layer—unlike what is often observed in degenerating photoreceptor cells in various animal models—suggesting normal trafficking of opsin to the outer segment, and consistent with a lack of overt photoreceptor degeneration. It is worth noting that the green labeling in a few cells in the inner retina in Figure 4 is due to mouse-on-mouse binding of the monoclonal antibody to endogenous IgG in blood vessels. It does not represent true anti-opsin immunolabeling.

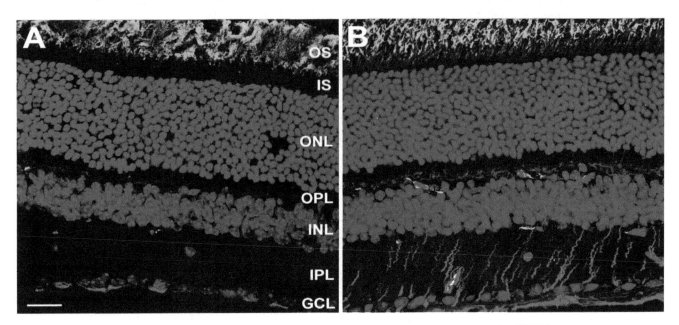

Figure 4. Laser confocal microscopy images of (**A**) WT control and (**B**) $Dhdds^{K42E/K42E}$ mouse retina frozen sections at PN 2 months of age, stained with antibodies to GFAP (pseudocolor: red) and rod opsin (pseudocolor: green), and counterstained with DAPI (blue). Scale bar (both panels) is 20 μm. Abbreviations: OS, outer segment layer; IS, inner segment layer; ONL, outer nuclear layer; OPL, outer plexiform layer; INL, inner nuclear layer; IPL, inner plexiform layer; GCL, ganglion cell layer. Scale bar (both panels) is 20 μm.

3.4. Lack of Defective Protein Glycosylation in Dhdds$^{K42E/K42E}$ Mouse Retinas

The N-linked oligo-saccharides of glycoproteins contain alpha-linked mannose residues as constituents, which are cognate ligands for the lectin concanavalin A (Con A) [17]. Hence, ConA lectin cytochemistry offers a reliable means of detecting the presence (or absence) of N-linked oligo-saccharides in tissue sections of $Dhdds^{K42E/K42E}$ mice, and a way to directly test the current hypothesis that RP59 is driven by lack of glycosylation. This is because the synthesis of oligosaccharide chains in cells and tissues obligatorily depends upon the presence of Dol-PP and Dol-P (which requires upstream DHDDS activity). Furthermore, N-linked oligosaccharide chains are selectively susceptible to hydrolysis by peptide:N-glycosidase F (PNGase-F) [18]; hence, tissue sections treated with PNGase-F should exhibit a marked loss of Con A binding (serving as a true negative control), thereby mimicking the scenario where upstream DHDDS activity may be lacking. We performed ConA lectin cytochemical analysis on retinal sections from WT control and $Dhdds^{K42E/K42E}$ mice at PN six months of age, with and without pre-treatment with PNGase-F. The results are shown in Figure 5.

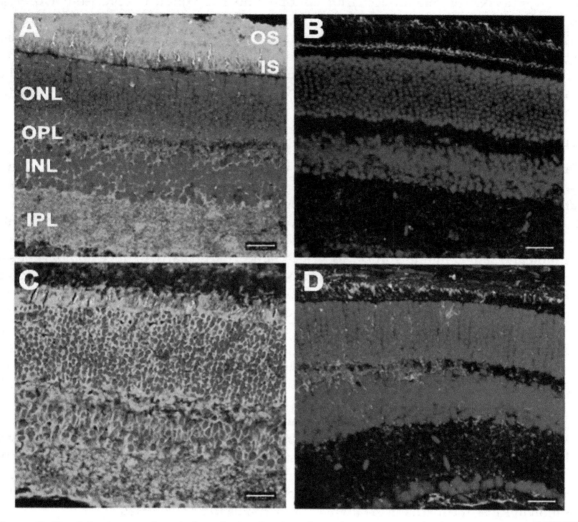

Figure 5. ConA lectin cytochemical analysis of retinas from (**A,B**) WT control and (**C,D**) $Dhdds^{K42E/K42E}$ mice at PN 6 months of age, with (**B,D**) or without (**A,C**) pretreatment with PNGase-F. ConA binding (green); PNA binding (magenta); DAPI counterstain (blue). Abbreviations are the same as in the Figure 4 legend. Scale bar (all panels): 20 μm.

Normally, N-linked glycoproteins are present throughout the retina, being notably enriched in photoreceptor cells and the synaptic endings of neurons (IPL, OPL). Hence, the inner and outer segment layers (IS and OS, respectively), including the glycoconjugate-rich interphotoreceptor matrix (IPM), as well as the inner and outer plexiform layers (IPL and OPL, respectively) were robustly labeled with fluor-tagged ConA in untreated WT retinal sections (Figure 5 A). As expected, treatment of WT retinal tissue sections with PNGase-F dramatically reduced the level of ConA binding throughout the retina (Figure 5B). Notably, retinal sections from $Dhdds^{K42E/K42E}$ mice also exhibited robust, pan-retinal ConA binding (Figure 5C), comparable to that of WT controls. Upon treatment with PNGase-F, most of the ConA staining was lost (Figure 5D). These results obviate any significant DHDDS loss-of-function in $Dhdds^{K42E/K42E}$ mice.

Peanut agglutinin (PNA) binds to the disaccharide Gal-β(1-3)-GalNAc in glycoproteins and glycolipids [17]. Oligosaccharides containing this disaccharide are highly enriched in the extracellular matrix surrounding cone photoreceptor outer segments (the "cone matrix sheath") [19,20]. Thus, PNA binding can be used to selectively label cone photoreceptors in retinal tissue sections, since rod photoreceptors and their associated "rod matrix sheath" lack such glycan chains [21]. Furthermore, oligosaccharides containing Gal-β(1-3)-GalNAc are generally O-linked (e.g., through Ser or Thr residues), rather than N-linked, and their synthesis is not dolichol-dependent in mammalian cells [22]. Furthermore, the PNA-binding disaccharide epitope is not susceptible to PNGase-F hydrolysis [17]. Hence, we expected to observe no appreciable differences in the binding of PNA to retinal tissue sections from $Dhdds^{K42E/K42E}$ retinas vs. WT controls, nor effects of PNGase-F treatment on PNA binding, either with regard to labeling intensity or distribution. These expectations were realized, as illustrated in Figure 5 (magenta staining, all four panels). Both $Dhdds^{K42E/K42E}$ and control retinas exhibited comparable distribution of PNA-positive cone matrix sheaths, suggesting persistence of viable cone photoreceptors in the K42E mutants.

4. Discussion

Here, we have presented the generation and initial characterization of a novel mouse model of RP59, where we have achieved global homozygous knock-in of the K42E Dhdds mutation specifically associated with RP59 [3–5]. Based upon the clinical presentation of RP59 in human patients [3–5], as well as the demonstrable importance of dolichol-dependent protein glycosylation in maintaining the normal structure and function of the vertebrate retina [11–14], we expected to observe retinal degeneration and retinal thinning in $Dhdds^{K42E/K42E}$ mice, particularly in mice homozygous for the K42E mutation. This expectation was also predicated on a preliminary report [23], using a similar K42E mouse knock-in model, that claimed nearly 50% loss of OS length and reduction in ONL thickness by about two-thirds at PN 3 months of age, compared to WT mouse retinas. However, we observed no evidence of retinal degeneration in $Dhdds^{K42E/K42E}$ mice up to one year of age. Furthermore, despite the confirmed mutation of Dhdds, we found no evidence for defective protein N-glycosylation in the retinas of these mice. The retinas were labeled robustly with fluor-tagged ConA lectin, irrespective of genotype. These findings are in good agreement with observations made by Sabry et al. [24] who found normal mannose incorporation into N-linked oligosaccharides using either siRNA silencing of DHDDS in a HepG2 cell line or in RP59 (severe mutation) patient fibroblasts. The ConA binding observed in our study is further consistent with observations made by Wen et al., who observed that rather than any loss in dolichols, there was an alteration in dolichol chain lengths (increased D17:D18 ratio) in RP59 patients compared to normal human subjects, but without obvious hypoglycosylation of serum transferrin [25]. These findings collectively suggest hypoglycosylation-independent retinal degeneration in RP59, the mechanism of which still remains to be elucidated.

Understanding the pathophysiological and biochemical mechanisms underlying RP59 remains limited due to the lack of a validated vertebrate animal model that faithfully mimics the key hallmarks of the disease. Heretofore, only a zebrafish model of RP59 has been documented, using global knock-down of DHDDS expression by injection of morpholino oligonucleotides at the one-cell embryo stage [26]. In that case, the fish exhibited defective photoresponses and their cone outer segments (as assessed indirectly by PNA staining) were dramatically shortened, if not nearly absent. It should be noted that zebrafish have a highly cone-rich retina, unlike humans or mice (which have highly rod-dominant retinas). Also, the reduction and loss of PNA binding in the zebrafish knock-down retinas most likely reflects degeneration and death of cone photoreceptors, with concomitant degeneration and loss of their outer segments, due to their requirement for dolichol. Unlike the zebrafish Dhdds knock-down model, the murine RP59 model generated in the present study exhibits robust PNA staining in the outer retina, suggesting persistence of viable cone photoreceptors. In a parallel study (Ramachandra Rao et al., unpublished), we have observed Dhdds transcript distribution in all retinal nuclear layers by in situ hybridization, consistent with the fact that all cells require dolichol derivatives to support protein N-glycosylation. Taken together, these findings suggest that the K42E Dhdds mutation does not affect cone photoreceptor viability. Recently (Ramachandra Rao et al., manuscript submitted for publication), we also generated a conditional Dhdds knockout mouse model, with targeted ablation of Dhdds in retinal rod photoreceptors, using a Cre-lox approach; however, unlike the K42E knock-in model, the rod-specific *Dhdds* knockout model exhibits profound, rapid retinal degeneration, with almost complete loss of photoreceptors by PN 6 weeks. Yet, there was no evidence of compromised protein *N*-glycosylation prior to the onset of photoreceptor degeneration. In addition, as reported in a companion article in this Special Issue of *Cells* [27], targeted ablation of *Dhdds* in retinal pigment epithelium, (RPE) cells in mice also results in a progressive, but somewhat slower, retinal degeneration.

As pointed out by Zelinger et al. [4], the phenotype of RP59 only involves the retina; there is no observable dysfunction or pathology in other tissues and organs in RP59 patients. Hence, those authors speculated that the K42E mutation, "alters, rather than abolishes, enzymatic function, perhaps either by reducing the level of DHDDS protein or by preventing requisite interactions between DHDDS and a photoreceptor-specific protein" [4]. They also suggested, alternatively, that mutation of DHDDS might result in, "a toxic accumulation of isoprenoid compounds," such as occurs in various forms of neuronal ceroid lipofuscinosis (e.g., Batten disease). While such speculations may turn out to be true, there is no direct empirical evidence extant to support this hypothesis. It is also entirely possible, however, that mutations (whether K42E or others) in DHDDS may affect its interactions with its enzymatic partner, Nogo-B receptor (NgBR, encoded by the *Nus1* gene) [8,9], with concomitant alterations in dolichol synthesis and protein *N*-glycosylation [28,29]. At present, nothing is known about the expression of Nogo-B receptor or its interactions with DHDDS, specifically in the retina. Our *Dhdds*$^{K42E/K42E}$ mouse line and retinal cell type-specific conditional DHDDS knockout mice offer potentially valuable model systems in which to pursue further investigations along these lines. In addition, we are currently pursuing studies employing dual, targeted ablation of DHDDS and NgBR in the retina. (See also the article by DeRamus et al., in this Special Issue of *Cells*, regarding an RPE-specific DHDDS knockout mouse model [27].)

Our findings bring into question the current concept that RP59 is a member of a large and diverse class of diseases known as "congenital disorders of glycosylation" (CDGs) [30,31]. While, in principle, it would be reasonable to consider RP59 as a CDG, due to the associated mutation(s) in DHDDS, there is no direct evidence to demonstrate a glycosylation defect in the human retinal disease or in any animal model of RP59 generated to date. The mechanism underlying the DHDDS-dependent retinal degeneration in human arRP patients remains to be elucidated, but is more complex than simply loss-of-function of DHDDS.

Author Contributions: Conceptualization, S.J.P. and S.J.F.; methodology, S.J.P., S.J.F., S.R.R., P.K.; M.N.N.; validation, S.R.R., M.N.N., P.K., S.J.P. and S.J.F.; formal analysis, M.N.N., S.J.P., S.J.F. and S.R.R.; investigation, S.J.P., S.R.R., P.K.; resources, S.J.P. and S.J.F.; data curation, S.J.P. and S.J.F.; writing—original draft preparation, S.J.F.; writing—review and editing, S.J.F., S.J.P., P.K., M.N.N. and S.R.R.; visualization, S.J.F., S.R.R. and S.J.P.; supervision, S.J.P. and S.J.F.; project administration, S.J.P. and S.J.F.; funding acquisition, S.J.P. and S.J.F. All authors have read and agreed to the published version of the manuscript.

Acknowledgments: We thank Isaac Cobb for technical assistance with OCT and genotyping. The opinions expressed herein do not reflect those of the Department of Veteran Affairs or the U.S. Government.

References

1.   Hartong, D.T.; Berson, E.L.; Dryja, T.P. Retinitis pigmentosa. *Lancet* **2006**, *368*, 1795–1809. [CrossRef]
2.   Zhang, Q. Retinitis Pigmentosa: Progress and Perspective. *Asia Pac. J. Ophthalmol. (Phila)* **2016**, *5*, 265–271. [CrossRef] [PubMed]

3. Zuchner, S.; Dallman, J.; Wen, R.; Beecham, G.; Naj, A.; Farooq, A.; Kohli, M.A.; Whitehead, P.L.; Hulme, W.; Konidari, I.; et al. Whole-exome sequencing links a variant in DHDDS to retinitis pigmentosa. *Am. J. Hum. Genet.* **2011**, *88*, 201–206. [CrossRef]

4. Zelinger, L.; Banin, E.; Obolensky, A.; Mizrahi-Meissonnier, L.; Beryozkin, A.; Bandah-Rozenfeld, D.; Frenkel, S.; Ben-Yosef, T.; Merin, S.; Schwartz, S.B.; et al. A missense mutation in DHDDS, encoding dehydrodolichyl diphosphate synthase, is associated with autosomal-recessive retinitis pigmentosa in Ashkenazi Jews. *Am. J. Hum. Genet.* **2011**, *88*, 207–215. [CrossRef] [PubMed]

5. Lam, B.L.; Zuchner, S.L.; Dallman, J.; Wen, R.; Alfonso, E.C.; Vance, J.M.; Pericak-Vance, M.A. Mutation K42E in dehydrodolichol diphosphate synthase (DHDDS) causes recessive retinitis pigmentosa. *Adv. Exp Med. Biol.* **2014**, *801*, 165–170. [CrossRef] [PubMed]

6. Parodi, A.J.; Leloir, L.F. The role of lipid intermediates in the glycosylation of proteins in the eucaryotic cell. *Biochim. Biophys. Acta* **1979**, *559*, 1–37. [CrossRef]

7. Hemming, F.W. Control and manipulation of the phosphodolichol pathway of protein N-glycosylation. *Biosci. Rep.* **1982**, *2*, 203–221. [CrossRef]

8. Giladi, M.; Edri, I.; Goldenberg, M.; Newman, H.; Strulovich, R.; Khananshvili, D.; Haitin, Y.; Loewenstein, A. Purification and characterization of human dehydrodolychil diphosphate synthase (DHDDS) overexpressed in E. coli. *Protein Expr. Purif.* **2017**, *132*, 138–142. [CrossRef]

9. Lisnyansky Bar-El, M.; Lee, S.Y.; Ki, A.Y.; Kapelushnik, N.; Loewenstein, A.; Chung, K.Y.; Schneidman-Duhovny, D.; Giladi, M.; Newman, H.; Haitin, Y. Structural Characterization of Full-Length Human Dehydrodolichyl Diphosphate Synthase Using an Integrative Computational and Experimental Approach. *Biomolecules* **2019**, *9*. [CrossRef]

10. Behrens, N.H.; Leloir, L.F. Dolichol monophosphate glucose: An intermediate in glucose transfer in liver. *Proc. Natl. Acad. Sci. USA* **1970**, *66*, 153–159. [CrossRef]

11. Tam, B.M.; Moritz, O.L. The role of rhodopsin glycosylation in protein folding, trafficking, and light-sensitive retinal degeneration. *J. Neurosci.* **2009**, *29*, 15145–15154. [CrossRef] [PubMed]

12. Murray, A.R.; Vuong, L.; Brobst, D.; Fliesler, S.J.; Peachey, N.S.; Gorbatyuk, M.S.; Naash, M.I.; Al-Ubaidi, M.R. Glycosylation of rhodopsin is necessary for its stability and incorporation into photoreceptor outer segment discs. *Hum. Mol. Genet.* **2015**, *24*, 2709–2723. [CrossRef] [PubMed]

13. Fliesler, S.J.; Rayborn, M.E.; Hollyfield, J.G. Membrane morphogenesis in retinal rod outer segments: Inhibition by tunicamycin. *J. Cell Biol.* **1985**, *100*, 574–587. [CrossRef] [PubMed]

14. Fliesler, S.J.; Rapp, L.M.; Hollyfield, J.G. Photoreceptor-specific degeneration caused by tunicamycin. *Nature* **1984**, *311*, 575–577. [CrossRef]

15. DeRamus, M.L.; Stacks, D.A.; Zhang, Y.; Huisingh, C.E.; McGwin, G.; Pittler, S.J. GARP2 accelerates retinal degeneration in rod cGMP-gated cation channel beta-subunit knockout mice. *Sci. Rep.* **2017**, *7*, 42545. [CrossRef]

16. Ramachandra Rao, S.; Pfeffer, B.A.; Mas Gomez, N.; Skelton, L.A.; Keiko, U.; Sparrow, J.R.; Rowsam, A.M.; Mitchell, C.H.; Fliesler, S.J. Compromised phagosome maturation underlies RPE pathology in cell culture and whole animal models of Smith-Lemli-Opitz Syndrome. *Autophagy* **2018**, 1–22. [CrossRef]

17. Goldstein, I.J.; Hayes, C.E. The lectins: Carbohydrate-binding proteins of plants and animals. *Adv. Carbohydr. Chem. Biochem.* **1978**, *35*, 127–340. [CrossRef]

18. Wang, T.; Voglmeir, J. PNGases as valuable tools in glycoprotein analysis. *Protein Pept. Lett.* **2014**, *21*, 976–985. [CrossRef]

19. Blanks, J.C.; Johnson, L.V. Specific binding of peanut lectin to a class of retinal photoreceptor cells. A species comparison. *Invest. Ophthalmol. Vis. Sci.* **1984**, *25*, 546–557.

20. Johnson, L.V.; Hageman, G.S.; Blanks, J.C. Interphotoreceptor matrix domains ensheath vertebrate cone photoreceptor cells. *Invest. Ophthalmol. Vis. Sci.* **1986**, *27*, 129–135.

21. Fariss, R.N.; Anderson, D.H.; Fisher, S.K. Comparison of photoreceptor-specific matrix domains in the cat and monkey retinas. *Exp. Eye Res.* **1990**, *51*, 473–485. [CrossRef]

22. Gemmill, T.R.; Trimble, R.B. Overview of N- and O-linked oligosaccharide structures found in various yeast species. *Biochim. Biophys. Acta* **1999**, *1426*, 227–237. [CrossRef]

23. Li, Y.; Lam, B.L.; Guan, Z.; Wang, Z.; Wang, N.; Chen, Y.; Wen, R. Photoreceptor degeneration in the DHDDSK42E/K42E mouse. *Invest. Ophthalmol. Vis. Sci.* **2014**, *55*, 4371.

24. Sabry, S.; Vuillaumier-Barrot, S.; Mintet, E.; Fasseu, M.; Valayannopoulos, V.; Heron, D.; Dorison, N.; Mignot, C.; Seta, N.; Chantret, I.; et al. A case of fatal Type I congenital disorders of glycosylation (CDG I) associated with low dehydrodolichol diphosphate synthase (DHDDS) activity. *Orphanet. J. Rare Dis.* **2016**, *11*, 84. [CrossRef]

25. Wen, R.; Lam, B.L.; Guan, Z. Aberrant dolichol chain lengths as biomarkers for retinitis pigmentosa caused by impaired dolichol biosynthesis. *J. Lipid Res.* **2013**, *54*, 3516–3522. [CrossRef]

26. Wen, R.; Dallman, J.E.; Li, Y.; Zuchner, S.L.; Vance, J.M.; Pericak-Vance, M.A.; Lam, B.L. Knock-down DHDDS expression induces photoreceptor degeneration in zebrafish. *Adv. Exp. Med. Biol.* **2014**, *801*, 543–550. [CrossRef]

27. DeRamus, M.L.; Davis, S.J.; Rao, S.R.; Nyankerh, C.; Stacks, D.; Kraft, T.W.; Fliesler, S.J.; Pittler, S.J. Selective Ablation of Dehydrodolichyl Diphosphate Synthase in Murine Retinal Pigment Epithelium (RPE) Causes RPE Atrophy and Retinal Degeneration. *Cells* **2020**, *9*, 771. [CrossRef]

28. Harrison, K.D.; Park, E.J.; Gao, N.; Kuo, A.; Rush, J.S.; Waechter, C.J.; Lehrman, M.A.; Sessa, W.C. Nogo-B receptor is necessary for cellular dolichol biosynthesis and protein N-glycosylation. *EMBO J.* **2011**, *30*, 2490–2500. [CrossRef]

29. Park, E.J.; Grabinska, K.A.; Guan, Z.; Stranecky, V.; Hartmannova, H.; Hodanova, K.; Baresova, V.; Sovova, J.; Jozsef, L.; Ondruskova, N.; et al. Mutation of Nogo-B receptor, a subunit of cis-prenyltransferase, causes a congenital disorder of glycosylation. *Cell Metab.* **2014**, *20*, 448–457. [CrossRef]

30. Haeuptle, M.A.; Hennet, T. Congenital disorders of glycosylation: An update on defects affecting the biosynthesis of dolichol-linked oligosaccharides. *Hum. Mutat.* **2009**, *30*, 1628–1641. [CrossRef]

31. Ng, B.G.; Freeze, H.H. Perspectives on Glycosylation and Its Congenital Disorders. *Trends Genet.* **2018**, *34*, 466–476. [CrossRef] [PubMed]

7

Molecular Therapies for Choroideremia

Jasmina Cehajic Kapetanovic [1,2,*], **Alun R. Barnard** [1,2] **and Robert E. MacLaren** [1,2]

[1]   Nuffield Laboratory of Ophthalmology, University of Oxford, Oxford OX3 9DU, UK;
      alun.barnard@eye.ox.ac.uk (A.R.B.); robert.maclaren@eye.ox.ac.uk (R.E.M.)
[2]   Oxford Eye Hospital, Oxford University Hospitals NHS Foundation Trust, Oxford OX3 9DU, UK
*   Correspondence: enquiries@eye.ox.ac.uk

Abstract: Advances in molecular research have culminated in the development of novel gene-based therapies for inherited retinal diseases. We have recently witnessed several groundbreaking clinical studies that ultimately led to approval of Luxturna, the first gene therapy for an inherited retinal disease. In parallel, international research community has been engaged in conducting gene therapy trials for another more common inherited retinal disease known as choroideremia and with phase III clinical trials now underway, approval of this therapy is poised to follow suit. This chapter discusses new insights into clinical phenotyping and molecular genetic testing in choroideremia with review of molecular mechanisms implicated in its pathogenesis. We provide an update on current gene therapy trials and discuss potential inclusion of female carries in future clinical studies. Alternative molecular therapies are discussed including suitability of *CRISPR* gene editing, small molecule nonsense suppression therapy and vision restoration strategies in late stage choroideremia.

Keywords: choroideremia; gene therapy; REP1; inherited retinal disease; treatment

1. Introduction

Choroideremia is a rare X-linked recessive inherited retinal disease caused by sequence variations or deletions in the *CHM* gene which are usually functionally null mutations, leading to deficiency in Rab escort protein 1 (REP1) [1–3]. The estimated prevalence is 1 in 50,000 males. Although REP1 is expressed ubiquitously, in humans choroideremia appears only to affect the retinal pigment epithelium (RPE) layer of the eye, leading to a characteristic clinical phenotype of progressive centripetal retinal degeneration. In Ancient Greek, the name choroid derives from χόριον (khórion, "skin") and εἶδος (eîdos, "resembling"). The suffix 'eremia' (ἐρημία) was added to describe the barren appearance (from the root word meaning wasteland or desert). Hence the literal translation of choroideremia is, in relation to the eye, 'the skin-resembling part is deserted'. Interestingly, the incorrect spelling *'choroideraemia'* has been used previously, but this may be based on misinterpretation of the suffix being derived from αἷμα (haima, blood), into which the 'ae' diphthong is still substituted in many non-US English usages. Importantly however, despite reference to the choroid in the name, the disease is now known to be driven primarily by the loss of the RPE, followed by the secondary degeneration of photoreceptors and choroidal atrophy [4]. Recent evidence has shed light on the molecular mechanisms of REP1 contribution to retinal degeneration in choroideremia, describing its essential role in post-translational modification of proteins and in intracellular trafficking of molecules [5]. The process affects primarily the RPE and pigment clumping is the first sign, long before photoreceptor loss. However, since the RPE has an essential role in retinal isomerization in the visual cycle which is more important for rod compared to cone function and hence rod function is impaired quite early in the disease process. As a result, the disease presents with early childhood nyctalopia, but the majority of patients retain excellent visual acuity until the very end stages of disease, presumably because Müller cells can still contribute to the cone visual cycle in the absence of RPE [6–8].

In this chapter we review advances in molecular therapies that have resulted in the development of adeno-associated vector (AAV) gene replacement therapy for choroideremia. The therapy is currently being explored in multiple clinical trials worldwide, having recently reached phase III in the development (Table 1). We discuss new insights into the clinical phenotyping and genotyping of choroideremia male patients and female carriers, including progress from the natural history studies, that will aid disease characterisation, monitoring of disease progression and interpretation of clinical trial endpoints. The review discusses current knowledge and progress in molecular mechanisms of choroideremia and the development of emerging potential therapies.

Table 1. Summary of interventional gene therapy clinical trials in choroideremia.

Clinical trial	Intervention	Clinical centre	References
Phase I/II NCT01461213 Start date: 2011 Completed 2018	Gene therapy involving subretinal delivery of AAV2-REP1	University of Oxford, UK	Lancet, 2014 [9] NEJM, 2016 [10] Nat Med, 2018 [11]
Phase I/II NCT02341807 Start date: 2015 Ongoing	Gene therapy involving subretinal delivery of AAV2-REP1	Philadelphia, USA Spark Therapeutics	No reports to date
Phase I/II NCT02077361 Start date: 2015 Completed 2018	Gene therapy involving subretinal delivery of AAV2-REP1	University of Alberta, Canada	Am J Ophthalmol, 2018 [12]
Phase II NCT02553135 Start date: 2015 Completed 2019	Gene therapy involving subretinal delivery of AAV2-REP1	University of Miami, USA	Am J Ophthalmol, 2019 [13]
Phase II NCT02671539 THOR TRIAL Start date: 2016 Completed 2018	Gene therapy involving subretinal delivery of AAV2-REP1	University of Tubingen, Germany	Retina, 2018 [14]
Phase II NCT02407678 REGENERATE TRIAL Start date: 2016 Ongoing	Gene therapy involving subretinal delivery of AAV2-REP1	University of Oxford and Moorfields Eye Hospital, UK	No reports to date
Phase II NCT03507686 GEMINI TRIAL Start date: 2017 Ongoing	Gene therapy involving bilateral subretinal delivery of AAV2-REP1	Nightstar Therapeutics (now Biogen) International, Multi-centre	No reports to date
Phase III NCT03496012 STAR TRIAL Start date: 2017 Ongoing	Gene therapy involving subretinal delivery of AAV2-REP1	Nightstar Therapeutics (now Biogen), International, Multi-centre	No reports to date
Observational NCT03584165 SOLSTICE TRIAL Start date: 2018 Ongoing	Long-term follow up study evaluating the safety and efficacy of AAV2-REP1 used in antecedent interventional choroideremia studies, 100 participants	Nightstar Therapeutics (now Biogen), International, Multi-centre	No reports to date

2. Choroideremia Phenotype

Choroideremia manifests with a pathognomonic fundus appearance characterised by progressive degeneration of retina and choroid (Figure 1). The degeneration starts in a ring around the mid-periphery of the retina and expands both centripetally towards the fovea and anteriorly to the pars plana [7,15,16]. The anatomical changes are accompanied by loss of functional scotopic vision and the reduction of the mid-peripheral visual field that begins during the first and second decade of life. The visual acuity is generally well preserved until late in the disease process, usually until the fifth decade of life, when the degeneration starts to encroach onto the fovea [6–8,15,16].

It remains somewhat unclear whether the RPE, the retina and the choroid are all primarily affected, or whether one or more of these tissues is secondarily affected during the pathogenesis of choroideremia [4].

There is however mounting indirect evidence that the RPE is the primary site of the disease in choroideremia, with the inner (photoreceptor) and outer (choroidal) layers degenerating through secondary mechanisms [5]. The unique pattern of preserved retina and RPE, as seen on autofluorescence imaging (Figure 1), with sharply demarcated edges is very different from many other retinal diseases where preserved regions are more circular or oval. This appearance is, however, almost identical in dominantly inherited *RPE65* retinal diseases. Since *RPE65* is only expressed in the RPE, we know that this phenotype is a feature specific to the RPE (presumably, RPE cell death), giving indirect evidence that choroideremia is a disease driven by RPE loss. The confounding variable in choroideremia is that the REP1 protein is expressed throughout the body [17] and the name 'choroideremia' gives the impression that this is primarily a choroidal degeneration. This is not the case, however, because any disease or treatments such as cryotherapy that destroys the RPE layer alone, will eventually lead to secondary atrophy of the underlying choroid, in a similar manner. In other words, choroideremia is the phenotype of complete RPE cell loss. The other relevant factor is that male patients with choroideremia can develop choroidal new vessels (Figure 2) and this clearly shows that the choroidal vasculature has the capacity to regenerate in certain cases. Finally, we know from female carriers (Figure 3) that the pattern of RPE loss is very similar to that in carriers of ocular albinism. There is no evidence of X inactivation leading to patchy loss of the choroid independently in female carriers.

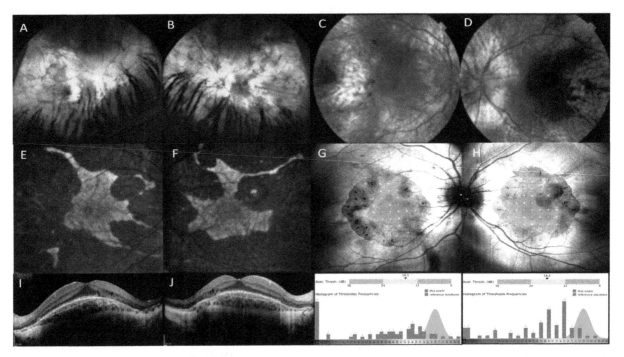

Figure 1. Retinal imaging in choroideremia. Widefield optomaps, Optos, Dumfernline, UK (**A,B**) and Heidelberg Spectralis imaging, Heidelberg, Germany (**C–F**) showing choroideremia phenotype in an affected male. Colour fundus photographs (**C,D**) show extensive retinal degeneration with choroidal atrophy and visualisation of underlying pale sclera. Fundus autofluorescence (**E,F**) shows typical patterns of sharply demarcated areas of remaining tissue (hyperfluorescent) against atrophic retina (hypofluorescent background). Mesopic microperimetry, MAIA CenterVue SpA, Padova, Italy (**G,H**) measures central retinal sensitivity that closely maps areas of residual retina as seen on autofluorescence. Sensitivity maps are shown with corresponding histograms of threshold frequencies. Spectral domain optical coherence tomography, Heidelberg, Germany (**I,J**) shows retinal structure in cross-section with distribution of ellipsoid zone (yellow line) and preserved inner retinal layers.

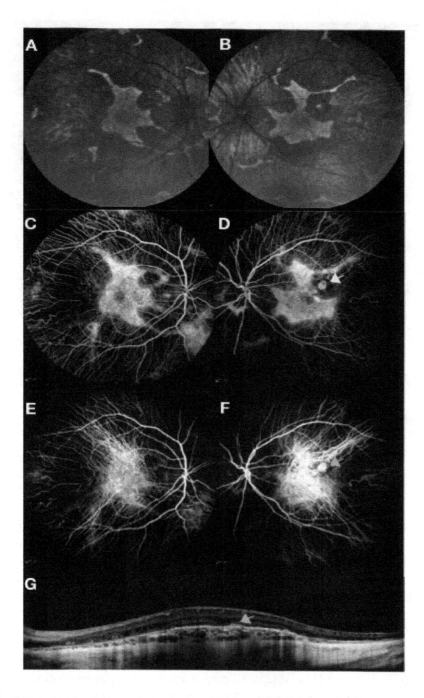

Figure 2. Retinal imaging in a choroideremia patient showing an area of scaring from an old choroidal neovascular membrane in the left eye. Fundus autofluorescence (**A,B**), fluorescein angiography (**C,D**), indocyanine green angiography (**E,F**) and spectral domain optical coherence tomography (**G**) with arrows marking the old scar. Imaging was performed with Heidelberg Spectralis, Heidelberg, Germany.

It is also possible that REP1 expression may be important for rod photoreceptor function [18]. Processing of post-mortem tissue from patients can make histological analyses difficult, and studies using advanced imaging techniques have provided somewhat equivocal results in terms of evidence of independent rod degeneration in humans in areas of the retina where the underlying RPE cells are unaffected by the disease [6,8,18–20]. Since patients with choroideremia maintain excellent visual acuity until the very late stages of the disease [6–8], it is likely that the REP1 deficiency is not a significant factor for the cone photoreceptors.

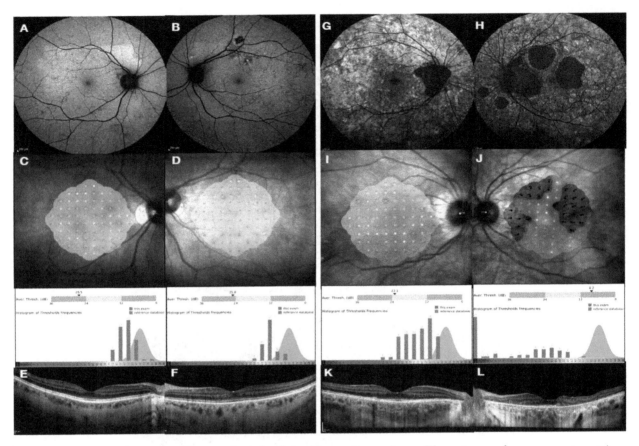

Figure 3. Retinal imaging in two female choroideremia carriers. Phenotype of an asymptomatic mild carrier with Snellen visual acuity of 6/5 in both eyes is shown from (**A–F**) and a carrier with a 'geographic-pattern' phenotype and reduced visual acuity of 6/7.5 in the right eye and 6/12 in the left eye is shown from (**G–L**). Fundus autofluorescence showing very early signs of fine 'salt and pepper' mottling (**A,B**) compared with coarse mottling and atrophic patches resembling geographic patterns (**G,H**). Mesopic microperimetry, MAIA CenterVue SpA, Padova, Italy showing sensitivity maps with corresponding histograms of threshold frequencies. Near-normal central retinal sensitivity is found in mild, asymptomatic carriers (**C,D**) compared to reduced retinal sensitivity in affected carriers especially in the left eye of the above case (**I,J**). OCT imaging is clinically insignificant in mild, asymptomatic carriers (**E,F**) whereas some disruption of retinal pigment epithelium (RPE) and ellipsoid zone is observed in the affected carrier, particularly in the left eye (**K,L**).

Elucidating the pattern of degeneration in choroideremia may help us understand the basis of the disease and how it progresses [16]. It is not known why the degeneration in choroideremia starts in the equatorial region before spreading anteriorly and posteriorly to reach the macula. The retinal pigment epithelial cell density is roughly similar at 5000 cells per mm^2 throughout the posterior eyecup. Gyrate atrophy of the choroid however may develop in a similar distribution, although this is in contrast to age-related macular degeneration, which is very much focused in the region around the fovea. In a recent study it was shown that the rate of degeneration in choroideremia followed an exponential decay function and was very similar across patients of different ages [21], but the key factor that determined the severity of the disease was the age of onset of degeneration. It may therefore be possible to predict the severity of the disease simply by measuring the residual area in a patient at a given age, because the progression is likely to be constant in the absence of treatment.

The centripetal degeneration in choroideremia has two phases by fundus autofluorescence-mottled RPE up to the edge and a more central zone of smooth RPE, both of which shrink progressively. In more advanced stages of the disease there is a total loss of smooth zone. The anatomical basis for these two zones is not immediately clear, but it may be that the slightly increased RPE cell density and much thicker choroid at the posterior pole provides some degree of protection against the metabolic stress caused by REP1 deficiency. Recent evidence suggests that there is less preserved autoflourescence area in nasal macula that may be more vulnerable to degeneration [16]. Further studies are necessary to determine whether the RPE zones can predict the health status of the overlying photoreceptors and how these might be affected following treatment.

3. Choroideremia Genotype

The choroideremia gene, *CHM* (OMIM #300390), encodes the REP1 protein, a 653 amino acid polypeptide essential for intracellular trafficking and post-translational prenylation of proteins within the human eye. Currently, there are 346 mutations registered on Leiden Open Variation Database, LOVD[3] (www.lovd.nl/CHM). Almost all of the identified sequence variations regardless of mechanism, are predicted to be null [3,22–25]. The mechanisms include insertions and deletions (minor, a few nucleotides, and major involving up to the entire gene length), splice site mutations, missense changes and point mutations that result in stop codons (premature termination codons). Novel mutations have recently been identified involving a deep-intronic region [26] and a promoter region [27] of the *CHM* gene.

Compared with other genetic diseases including inherited retinal disease, choroideremia has a surprisingly low number of disease-causing missense mutations. This would suggest that the REP1 protein, with 3 principal domains, has no catalytic domains with corresponding mutational hotspots within the gene. This is in contrast to genes that encode enzymes (such as *retinitis pigmentosa GTPase regulator* gene) that typically have such hotspot regions (e.g., ORF15 region). This supports the role of REP1 as a chaperone protein, enhancing activity of another protein, which is important in cell structure and stability.

Recent evidence shows that the majority of missense mutations are disproportionately found to be single point C to T transitions at C-phosphate-G (CpG) dinucleotides, spread across 5 of only 24 CpG dinucleotides in the entire *CHM* gene [25]. This is consistent with the evolutionary loss of CpG dinucleotides through destabilising methylation and subsequent deamination. Notably, the 5 locations were the only sites at which C to T transitions resulted in a stop codon. Future de novo mutations are likely to arise within these destabilised hotspot loci.

Molecular genetic testing offers means of confirming the clinical diagnosis in choroideremia and is mandatory for the inclusion in gene therapy clinical trials. It also offers a means of identifying carriers and establishing presymptomatic diagnoses in families that carry a pathogenic change. The rate of mutation detection via next generation sequencing has been reported as high as 94% [25]. In cases of unidentified mutations, it is important to request sequencing of the above mentioned deep-intronic and promoter regions, that are not routinely sequenced, to check for pathogenic variations. In addition, functional in-vitro assay that measure levels of REP1 in peripheral blood cells and its prenylation activity [17], can support clinical diagnosis and confirm variants of uncertain pathogenicity. In this regard, choroideremia is different to retinitis pigmentosa, because the unique choroideremia phenotype can justify the additional resources needed to sequence the entire CHM genomic region.

3.1. Genotype–Phenotype Correlation in Choroideremia

Although the clinical phenotype can vary in terms of the age of onset of retinal degeneration and rate of progression, no evidence has been found for genotype–phenotype correlation with regard to onset of symptoms, decline in visual acuity and visual fields [23–25], or in the residual retinal area of fundus autofluorescence [25]. The reasons for this are not fully understood, but the lack of correlation may be due to the near universal absence of REP1 irrespective of the causative mutation that range from single point missense changes to whole gene deletions. The phenotypic variation in choroideremia may in part be explained by the degree to which the absence of REP1 can be compensated by other prenylation proteins such as REP2, which shares 95% of its amino acid sequence with REP1 [26,27].

In addition, genetic modifiers and environmental factors may play roles in the onset and progression of degeneration in choroideremia.

3.2. Molecular Mechanisms of Choroideremia

The molecular mechanisms involved in the pathology of choroideremia have recently been reviewed in great detail [5]. However, some basic concepts are worth re-stating and outlining to aid understanding of the disease. The gene that is disrupted in choroideremia produces REP1 protein. Unlike in many other inherited retinal diseases, this protein is not directly involved in the process of phototransduction or in cellular signalling within the retina. Instead, REP1 is a key player in the addition of prenyl groups (prenylation) to the Rab family of GTPases (Rabs). Such hydrophobic prenyl groups are thought to be necessary to anchor Rabs to the membranes of intracellular organelles and vesicles [28].

In the absence of REP1, there is an observable deficit in the prenylation of several different types of Rabs, and their association with membranes appears to be impaired [29]. Because Rabs themselves act as important regulators of intracellular membrane trafficking, many fundamental cellular processes can potentially be impacted by this deficit. Information from a variety of sources points to a deficit in melanosome trafficking, a delay in phagosome degradation and an accelerated accumulation of intracellular deposits in RPE cells caused by loss of REP1 [4,18,30–33]. The cellular deficits of photoreceptors themselves have been less studied, but it has been suggested that there is mislocalisation of opsin and shortening of photoreceptor outer segments in mice that is independent of RPE degeneration [4].

Fortunately, the absence of REP1 does not appear to be catastrophic for all human cells, which is likely due to the fact that there is a built-in redundancy in this system, provided by the presence of the *CHML* gene [34,35]. The *CHML* gene is thought to be an autosomal retrogene of *CHM*, created by the reverse transcription of the mRNA of the original gene and reinsertion in a new genomic location that occurred sometime during vertebrate evolution. The protein product of *CHML*, known as REP2, appears to be able to largely compensate for the loss of REP1. Although a prenylation deficit of certain Rabs can be detected in several cell types of the body [29,36,37], a single report of a systemic, blood-related, clinical phenotype have not been substantiated [38,39] and loss of REP1 appears to cause cellular dysfunction and death that is limited to specific ocular tissues and manifest as a specific disease of the retina. Differential spatial expression does not provide an obvious answer, as both REP1 and REP2 are expressed ubiquitously.

In truth, the reason why absence of REP1 drives a specific degeneration of the RPE and photoreceptor cells remains a mystery. Perhaps more than other cell types, RPE and photoreceptor cells require acute and sensitive regulation of intracellular membrane trafficking to fulfil their cellular functions. Combined with the fact that there is not any appreciable post-natal replacement of these cells, it may simply be that these cell types are sensitive to the generalised, ongoing prenylation deficit, become 'worn-out' early than usual, and undergo a type of accelerated aging and cell death. Alternatively, it has been proposed that REP1 has a selective affinity to particular Rabs that are of special significance to the cell types affected in the disease. For example, it has been suggested there is a particular requirement for correctly prenylated Rab27a to mediate melanosome trafficking in RPE cells [29,40] and Rab6, 8 and 11 might be important in targeting rhodopsin-bearing vesicles to the photoreceptor outer segment [41,42]. Biochemical assays have suggested that REP1and REP2 have largely overlapping substrate specificities but differences in the association with other catalytic units within the prenylation process might contribute instead [43–45].

3.3. Gene Therapy for Choroideremia

Gene based therapies show great promise for the treatment of inherited retinal disease, including choroideremia [46]. Recent advances have paved a successful progression of gene therapy clinical trials on choroideremia (Table 1). The first phase I/II trial started in Oxford, UK in 2011, using a subretinal delivery of AAV2-REP1 in 14 male patients with choroideremia [9,10]. The two-year trial results were recently reported [11] with median gains in visual acuity (measured by Early Treatment Diabetic Retinopathy Study, ETDRS chart) of 4.5 letters in treated eyes versus 1.5 letter loss in untreated eyes across the cohort at 24 months post treatment. Six treated eyes gained more than 5 ETDRS letters. In two patients with the greatest gains in visual acuity, improvements were noted by 6 months post treatment, and sustained at up to 5 years of follow-up. Two patients in the cohort had complications, one related to surgery (retinal overstretch and incomplete vector dosing) and the other had postoperative inflammation. Both of these events resulted in protocol changes which included developing an automated subretinal injection system and a more prolonged post-operative immunosuppressive regimen.

These encouraging safety and efficacy signals prompted additional trials using the same vector (sponsored by Nightstar Therapeutics, UK) at other international sites including Canada (NCT02077361), USA (NCT02553135) and Germany (NCT02671539) all reporting similar results [12–14], following which a phase III trial started in 2017 at multiple international sites. Independent to the Nightstar led trials, another phase I/II trial (NCT02341807) using a similar AAV vector construct (without the woodchuck hepatitis virus posttranscriptional regulatory element) begun in 2015 in Philadelphia, USA. The results of this trial are expected in the coming years.

The above-mentioned early phase I/II gene therapy clinical trials recruited patients with advanced disease with early efficacy signals suggesting that vision can be restored following treatment. Reassuring safety data, following improvements in the surgical technique, prompted initiation of a phase II trial (NCT02407678) sponsored by University of Oxford that included patients with early central degeneration and normal visual acuity. The REGENERATE trial recently completed recruitment of 30 male patients with choroideremia with prediction that earlier intervention might slow down or halt the degeneration prior to irreversible structural disorganisation.

The solstice study is an observational, long-term follow up study of 100 participants that will evaluate the safety and efficacy of the AAV2-REP1 used in the above-mentioned interventional choroideremia trials.

The outcomes of clinical trials are measured in terms of clearly defined clinical endpoints, which predict the success and ultimately the approval of new treatments. These outcomes must be selected carefully to capture the most sensitive and reliable measures of the disease progression during the course of a clinical trial and will critically depend on the stage of retinal degeneration. In the reported choroideremia trials, the primary endpoint was the change from baseline in best-corrected visual acuity (BCVA) in the treated eye compared to the untreated eye with evidence of gains in vision after gene therapy in treated eyes. This suggests that BCVA can be used as a viable primary outcome in cases of advanced choroideremia, where disease process has already affected the visual acuity. Indeed, the phase III STAR trial is using BCVA as a primary outcome measure. However, in patients with early disease stage with near-normal vision, BCVA may not be the most sensitive outcome measure, especially since the visual loss in choroideremia typically progresses very slowly. Thus, for the REGENERATE trial, secondary endpoints including the measure of central visual field by microperimetry and anatomical measures such as fundus autofluorescence and optical coherence tomography may prove to be additional valuable outcomes. However, measurements of these secondary outcomes may not always be straightforward, and need to be interpreted with caution. For example, the remaining autofluorescence area may not be easily demarcated, even with the use of automated algorithms, which may influence area measurements especially following sub-retinal gene therapy which may differentially affect central (para-foveal) and peripheral areas of the treated island.

4. Should We Treat Female Carriers in the Future?

Heterozygous female choroideremia carriers often show generalized RPE mottling due to random X-inactivation (Figure 3A–F) and are usually asymptomatic or show early deficits in dark adaptation. In some carriers a coarser pattern of degeneration is seen, with patches of atrophy interspersed with normal tissue (Figure 3G–L). Usually, a mild reduction in retinal function is observed with this carrier phenotype. Occasionally, however, female carriers manifest with more severe male-like pattern of retinal degeneration with associated deficit in visual function [47]. This is most likely the result of skewed X-inactivation, or the proportion of cells expressing the mutant X chromosome, which occurs during early retinal development.

Choroideremia gene therapy trials are currently including affected male subjects only. For the majority of female carriers who are mildly affected and asymptomatic or have minor deficits in night vision or visual fields, treatment may not be necessary. Such functional deficits are usually slowly progressing with the majority of cases being able to maintain driving standard vision. However, the more severe female carrier phenotypes, with associated visual field loss and reduction in visual acuity, are likely to benefit from gene therapy and could be included in future clinical trials. Careful characterisation and geneotype-phenotypes correlations will help with the inclusion criteria and give insight into the optimal timing for successful gene therapy.

5. Alternative Therapies

The potential therapy that has been discussed in this review is gene replacement/augmentation therapy. This is the therapy that has advanced the furthest clinically but there are other potential therapies worth considering.

Instead of adding a working copy of the *CHM* gene, it may instead be possible to alter the patient's own copy with gene editing. Techniques to achieve this, such as zinc finger nucleases or Tal-effector nucleases (TALENs), have existed for some time, but the clinical relevance of these techniques has been somewhat limited by the low editing efficiencies generally achieved. The development of CRISPR/Cas (clustered regularly interspaced short palindromic repeats/CRISPR-associated nuclease 9) technology has given gene editing a renaissance for two reasons. Firstly, gene-editing efficiency appears to be generally better, with the potential to be more clinically meaningful. Secondly, in the CRISPR/Cas9 system, most of the investigational medicinal product can remain the same and only a specific RNA guide sequence needs to be developed to target a site within the disease specific gene—this is more attractive in terms of a clinical development pathway. Gene editing therapy is most useful when there is a need to correct or silence a mutated gene, such as when a missense mutation leads to production of dominant negative or toxic gain-of-function protein, which normally manifests as autosomal dominant and semi-dominant disease [48]. Because the vast majority of mutations in choroideremia are effectively null and therefore result in no detectable protein [24] there is no compelling need to develop a gene editing approach, and simply adding a correct copy as an episomal transgene would be sufficient to result in a therapeutic effect. Correcting the genomic copy of the gene might provide higher confidence of a correct and sustained level of expression, given that the gene would be subject to regulation by its normal transcriptional regulation and epigenetic environment. However, there is evidence that expression from a transgene can be sustained for years when using the appropriate delivery vector and expression cassette [49]. For choroideremia, there is no cell type in which ectopic expression may be predicted to cause a problem, as the protein in normally ubiquitously expressed. In terms of the level of expression, we know that the level of restored REP1 expression is inversely proportional to the prenylation deficit, and so far there is no evidence of overexpression causing toxicity [50]. Although it may be theoretically possible to develop a gene editing approach for some mutations that cause choroideremia, using CRISPR/Cas9, the effectiveness of such strategies has not yet been well established in the retina. Therefore, as gene editing might offer only marginal benefits over gene replacement, it is not currently an attractive strategy of treating choroideremia.

Another therapy that has been suggested and developed is the use of drug-stimulated translational read-through (RT) of premature termination codons (PTC). Nonsense mutations arise when a point mutation converts an amino-acid codon into a PTC that can cause premature translational termination of the mRNA, and subsequently inhibit normal full-length protein expression. Occasionally, instead of translational termination, read-through occurs. Here, a partial mispairing of codon–anticodon is successful, an amino acid is incorporated and protein synthesis continues. Small molecule translational read-through inducing drugs (TRIDs) exist that form the basis of the proposed therapy [51]. Nonsense mutations are the cause of choroideremia in over 30% of patients [52], so, although this will not be appropriate for all patients, there is a significant proportion in which it might be used.

Translational read-through inducing drugs have been used in clinical trials for life-limiting congenital diseases, such as Duchenne muscular dystrophy (DMD) and cystic fibrosis. Early trials appeared to successfully suppress premature stop mutations in patients, but there were concerns over toxicity and the need for repeated intramuscular or intravenous dosing. A newer read-through drug, Ataluren (PTC124), showed a good safety profile when administered orally and the clinical benefit shown in DMD has led to its approval in the EU for this disease [53]. Although no adverse effects have been observed so far, even the approximately 48 weeks of administration given in the clinical studies do not approach the decades of treatment that would be necessary for choroideremia. Preclinical work in the lower-vertebrate, zebrafish model has been important in developing the proof-of-concept, as this is currently the only existing model of choroideremia with a nonsense mutation [54,55]. However, absence of the CHML (REP2) gene in zebrafish means that the CHM mutation is lethal—-translational read-through inducing drugs increase the lifespan of the zebrafish model but this is outcome is not directly clinically relevant. The ability of TRIDs to rescue the Rab prenylation defect in fibroblast of a patient with a particular choroideremia nonsense mutation is encouraging, despite the fact that levels of full-length REP1 protein remained below the level of detection [55]. Given the relatively slow disease progression and the potential risks and cost to the patient from long-term administration of TRIDs, it would be judicious to establish that the correction of the prenylation deficit by TRIDs is present in fibroblast from patients with the equivalent nonsense mutations in which treatment will be attempted in any clinical study [56].

It might be argued that systemic or ocular administration of TRIDs has the potential to treat a larger area of retina when compared to gene therapy, as the former might spread by local diffusion while the latter is limited by the extent of the subretinal bleb. However, to our knowledge, the local concentration achieved in the posterior segment of the eye has never been measured when TRIDs are taken orally or administered locally. The effect of TRIDs appears to often follow an inverted u-shaped dose-response curve, so the pharmacokinetics of therapy may be critical important [57]. Until such questions are addressed, it would appear that translational read-through inducing drugs do not represent a superior strategy compared to gene replacement therapy.

Recent work has identified that antisense oligonucleotides (AONs) may also provide another potential therapy for choroideremia [58]. In some cases of choroideremia, deep-intronic mutations can create a cryptic splice acceptor site that results in the insertion of a pseudoexon in the CHM transcript. This disrupts gene function, and specific AONs can be designed to bind to the pre-mRNA and redirect the splicing process, potentially returning it to a normal, working transcript [59,60]. For choroideremia, AONs therapy has shown some promising in vitro results but is further along the clinical development pathway for several inherited disorders, including other forms of inherited retinal dystrophy [59,60]. As AON therapy relies on particular types of mutations, it will not be relevant for all cases of choroideremia and such a strategy is most attractive when conventional gene replacement therapy is not possible because of the large size of the coding sequence of the genes involved, such as in CEP290-associated Leber congenital amaurosis [59,60].

The therapies above aim to slow down or stop the degeneration of the retina and RPE and are obviously the preferred choice. However, it is also worth considering strategies that might restore vision in the late stages of the disease, when the majority of photoreceptors have already been lost. Cell transplantation is an interesting strategy for the treatment of inherited retinal disease, but this might present a significant challenge in late-stage choroideremia, where RPE and choroid have been lost along with the degenerating photoreceptors. A more feasible approach may be to use some form of retinal prosthesis. Although most systems rely on surviving inner retinal layers, with intact ganglion cell nerve conduction, there is no dependence on survival of the RPE, photoreceptors or choroid. The Argus II retinal prosthesis, an epiretinal device approved for commercial use in advanced retinal degeneration in the EU and USA, has been implanted in at least one patient with choroideremia [61]. This device has a very good safety profile and various improvements in visual function have been reported, although these vary widely between individuals [62]. Other devices exist or are in development (44-channel suprachoriodal Bionic Eye Device (NCT03406416) Melbourne, Australia and Intelligent Retinal Implant System, IRIS V1 (NCT01864486) and V2 (NCT02670980) Pixium Vision SA) that could theoretically restore much greater levels of visual function than the Argus II, however, stopping cell loss, even at a late-stage will likely still result in a better functional outcome. Another potential therapy to restore vision in choroideremia is to render the remaining cells of the retina sensitive to light by ectopically expressing light-sensitive ion channels or opsins. This strategy, known as optogenetics, has its own considerations and challenges, which will not be discussed extensively here. Suffice to say, a number of systems are in various stages of pre-clinical development and are beginning to be investigated in clinical trials [63–65]. Again, the level of vision that can be restored by this method is likely to be relatively crude, however, this is likely to be comparable to any retinal prosthesis and may offer specific benefits such as less invasive surgery and potential restoration of a wider visual field.

6. Summary

Molecular mechanisms in choroideremia are well established. Ultimately, the absence or reduced prenylation of REP1 activity disrupts intracellular trafficking pathways leading to accumulation of toxic products and premature degeneration of the retina and vision less. Logically then, replacement of REP1 to the retinal tissue, via gene-based therapy, could restore cellular function and slow down the degeneration. Multiple clinical trials are underway testing this hypothesis. The trials are using subretinal delivery of AAV2-REP1 to target surviving central islands of the retina with promising safety and early efficacy results.

Despite ubiquitous expression of REP1, a robust systemic association with choroideremia has not been identified, although the prenylation defect is visible in assays of the peripheral blood cells. This assay can be used to support the diagnosis of choroideremia. It is not known why the retina is the only part of the body that becomes clinically affected by the lack of REP1 activity. Moreover, the complex interactions between different retinal cell types during the pathogenesis of choroideremia mean that it is difficult to deconvolve the exact order in which RPE, photoreceptors and the choroid degenerate. It appears likely that the RPE is directly affected by the loss of REP1, and is a key driver of pathogenesis, but the importance of primary or secondary degeneration of photoreceptors is less clear. Elucidating these mechanisms may help us to understand what triggers the onset of clinically significant degeneration and how the rate of degeneration in each cell type might be affected following treatment.

Evidence to date has shown no apparent genotype–phenotype correlation within the spectrum of reported CHM mutations, with regard to the onset of symptoms and the rate of functional visual decline. Since variations in male phenotypes cannot be explained by mutations in *CHM* only, genetic modifiers or environmental factors must play a role in the onset and progression of degeneration in choroideremia. Ongoing natural history studies are adding insight into the progression of the disease and the characteristics of the clinical phenotype that will help to establish the optimal therapeutic window for choroideremia. Female carriers should be enrolled into natural history studies with aim to offer gene therapy (under the realm of clinical trials) to those affected by skewed X inactivation.

Author Contributions: Writing: J.C.K. and A.R.B. Revision: J.C.K. and A.R.B. Supervision: R.E.M.

References

1. Cremers, F.P.; van de Pol, D.J.; van Kerkhoff, L.P.; Wieringa, B.; Ropers, H.H. Cloning of a gene that is rearranged in patients with choroideraemia. *Nature* **1990**, *347*, 674–677. [CrossRef] [PubMed]
2. Seabra, M.C.; Brown, M.S.; Goldstein, J.L. Retinal degeneration in choroideremia: Deficiency of rab geranylgeranyl transferase. *Science* **1993**, *259*, 377–381. [CrossRef] [PubMed]
3. Van den Hurk, J.A.; Schwartz, M.; van Bokhoven, H.; Van de Pol, T.J.R.; Bogerd, L.; Pinckers, A.J.L.G.; Bleeker-Wagemakers, E.M.; Pawlowitzki, I.H.; Rüther, K.; Ropers, H.H.; et al. Molecular basis of choroideremia (CHM): Mutations involving the Rab escort protein-1 (*REP-1*) gene. *Hum. Mutat.* **1997**, *9*, 110–117. [CrossRef]
4. Tolmachova, T.; Anders, R.; Abrink, M.; Bugeon, L.; Dallman, M.J.; Futter, C.E.; Ramalho, J.S.; Tonagel, F.; Tanimoto, N.; Seeliger, M.W.; et al. Independent degeneration of photoreceptors and retinal pigment epithelium in conditional knockout mouse models of choroideremia. *J. Clin. Investig.* **2006**, *116*, 386–394. [CrossRef] [PubMed]
5. Patrício, M.I.; Barnard, A.R.; Xue, K.; MacLaren, R.E. Choroideremia: Molecular mechanisms and development of AAV gene therapy. *Expert Opin. Biol. Ther.* **2018**, *18*, 807–820. [CrossRef] [PubMed]
6. Aleman, T.S.; Han, G.; Serrano, L.W.; Fuerst, N.M.; Charlson, E.S.; Pearson, D.J.; Chung, D.C.; Traband, A.; Pan, W.; Ying, G.S.; et al. Natural history of the central structural abnormalities in choroideremia: A Prospective Cross-Sectional Study. *Ophthalmology* **2017**, *124*, 359–373. [CrossRef] [PubMed]
7. Hariri, A.H.; Velaga, S.B.; Girach, A.; Ip, M.S.; Le, P.V.; Lam, B.L.; Fischer, M.D.; Sankila, E.M.; Pennesi, M.E.; Holz, F.G.; et al. Measurement and reproducibility of preserved ellipsoid zone area and preserved retinal pigment epithelium area in eyes with choroideremia. *Am. J. Ophthalmol.* **2017**, *179*, 110–117. [CrossRef] [PubMed]
8. Sun, L.W.; Johnson, R.D.; Williams, V.; Summerfelt, P.; Dubra, A.; Weinberg, D.V.; Stepien, K.E.; Fishman, G.A.; Carroll, J. Multimodal imaging of photoreceptor structure in choroideremia. *PLoS ONE* **2016**, *11*, e0167526. [CrossRef] [PubMed]
9. MacLaren, R.E.; Groppe, M.; Barnard, A.R.; Cottriall, C.L.; Tolmachova, T.; Seymour, L.; Clark, K.R.; During, M.J.; Cremers, F.P.; Black, G.C.; et al. Retinal gene therapy in patients with choroideremia: Initial findings from a phase 1/2 clinical trial. *Lancet* **2014**, *383*, 1129–1137. [CrossRef]
10. Edwards, T.L.; Jolly, J.K.; Groppe, M.; Barnard, A.R.; Cottriall, C.L.; Tolmachova, T.; Black, G.C.; Webster, A.R.; Lotery, A.J.; Holder, G.E.; et al. Visual Acuity after Retinal Gene Therapy for Choroideremia. *N. Engl. J. Med.* **2016**, *374*, 1996–1998. [CrossRef]
11. Xue, K.; Jolly, J.K.; Barnard, A.R.; Rudenko, A.; Salvetti, A.P.; Patrício, M.I.; Edwards, T.L.; Groppe, M.; Orlans, H.O.; Tolmachova, T.; et al. Beneficial effects on vision in patients undergoing retinal gene therapy for choroideremia. *Nat. Med.* **2018**, *24*, 1507–1512. [CrossRef] [PubMed]
12. Dimopoulos, I.S.; Hoang, S.C.; Radziwon, A.; Binczyk, N.M.; Seabra, M.C.; MacLaren, R.E.; Somani, R.; Tennant, M.T.; MacDonald, I.M. Two-year results after aav2-mediated gene therapy for choroideremia: The Alberta experience. *Am. J. Ophthalmol.* **2018**, *193*, 130–142. [CrossRef] [PubMed]
13. Lam, B.L.; Davis, J.L.; Gregori, N.Z.; MacLaren, R.E.; Girach, A.; Verriotto, J.D.; Rodriguez, B.; Rosa, P.R.; Zhang, X.; Feuer, W.J. Choroideremia Gene Therapy Phase 2 Clinical Trial: 24-Month Results. *Am. J. Ophthalmol.* **2019**, *197*, 65–73. [CrossRef] [PubMed]
14. Fischer, M.D.; Ochakovski, G.A.; Beier, B.; Seitz, I.P.; Vaheb, Y.; Kortuem, C.; Reichel, F.F.; Kuehlewein, L.; Kahle, N.A.; Peters, T.; et al. Changes in retinal sensitivity after gene therapy in choroideremia. *Retina* **2018**. [CrossRef] [PubMed]
15. Jolly, J.K.; Xue, K.; Edwards, T.L.; Groppe, M.; MacLaren, R.E. Characterizing the natural history of visual function in choroideremia using microperimetry and multimodal retinal imaging. *Investig. Ophthalmol. Vis. Sci.* **2017**, *58*, 5575–5583. [CrossRef] [PubMed]
16. Hariri, A.H.; Ip, M.S.; Girach, A.; Lam, B.L.; Fischer, M.D.; Sankila, E.M.; Pennesi, M.E.; Holz, F.G.; Maclaren, R.E.; Birch, D.G.; et al. Macular spatial distribution of preserved autofluorescence in patients with choroideremia. For Natural History of the Progression of Choroideremia (NIGHT) Study Group. *Br. J. Ophthalmol.* **2019**, *103*, 933–937. [CrossRef] [PubMed]

17. Patrício, M.I.; Barnard, A.R.; Cox, C.I.; Blue, C.; MacLaren, R.E. The Biological Activity of AAV Vectors for Choroideremia Gene Therapy Can Be Measured by In Vitro Prenylation of RAB6A. *Mol. Ther. Methods Clin. Dev.* **2018**, *9*, 288–295. [CrossRef]

18. Syed, N.; Smith, J.E.; John, S.K.; Seabra, M.C.; Aguirre, G.D.; Milam, A.H. Evaluation of retinal photoreceptors and pigment epithelium in a female carrier of choroideremia. *Ophthalmology* **2001**, *108*, 711–720. [CrossRef]

19. Morgan, J.I.; Han, G.; Klinman, E.; Maguire, W.M.; Chung, D.C.; Maguire, A.M.; Bennett, J. High-resolution adaptive optics retinal imaging of cellular structure in choroideremia. *Investig. Ophthalmol. Vis. Sci.* **2014**, *55*, 6381–6397. [CrossRef]

20. Xue, K.; Oldani, M.; Jolly, J.K.; Edwards, T.L.; Groppe, M.; Downes, S.M.; MacLaren, R.E. Correlation of Optical Coherence Tomography and Autofluorescence in the Outer Retina and Choroid of Patients with Choroideremia. *Investig. Ophthalmol. Vis. Sci.* **2016**, *57*, 3674–3684. [CrossRef]

21. Aylward, J.W.; Xue, K.; Patrício, M.I.; Jolly, J.K.; Wood, J.C.; Brett, J.; Jasani, K.M.; MacLaren, R.E. Retinal Degeneration in Choroideremia follows an Exponential Decay Function. *Ophthalmology* **2018**, *125*, 1122–1124. [CrossRef] [PubMed]

22. Ramsden, S.C.; O'Grady, A.; Fletcher, T.; O'Sullivan, J.; Hart-Holden, N.; Barton, S.J.; Hall, G.; Moore, A.T.; Webster, A.R.; Black, G.C. A clinical molecular genetic service for United Kingdom families with choroideraemia. *Eur. J. Med. Genet.* **2013**, *56*, 432–438. [CrossRef] [PubMed]

23. Freund, P.; Furgoch, M.; MacDonald, I. Genotype—Phenotype analysis of male subjects affected by choroideremia. *Investig. Ophthalmol. Vis. Sci.* **2013**, *54*, 1567.

24. Freund, P.R.; Sergeev, Y.V.; MacDonald, I.M. Analysis of a large choroideremia dataset does not suggest a preference for inclusion of certain genotypes in future trials of gene therapy. *Mol. Genet. Genomic Med.* **2016**, *4*, 344–358. [CrossRef] [PubMed]

25. Simunovic, M.P.; Jolly, J.K.; Xue, K.; Edwards, T.L.; Groppe, M.; Downes, S.M.; MacLaren, R.E. The Spectrum of CHM Gene Mutations in Choroideremia and Their Relationship to Clinical Phenotype. *Investig. Ophthalmol. Vis. Sci.* **2016**, *57*, 6033–6039. [CrossRef] [PubMed]

26. Carss, K.; Arno, G.; Erwood, M.; Stephens, J.; Sanchis-Juan, A.; Hull, S.; Megy, K.; Grozeva, D.; Dewhurst, E.; Malka, S.; et al. Comprehensive rare variant analysis via whole-genome sequencing to determine the molecular pathology of inherited retinal disease. *Am. J. Hum. Genet.* **2017**, *100*, 75–90. [CrossRef]

27. Radziwon, A.; Arno, G.K.; Wheaton, D.; McDonagh, E.M.; Baple, E.L.; Webb-Jones, K.G.; Birch, D.; Webster, A.R.; MacDonald, I.M. Single-base substitutions in the CHM promoter as a cause of choroideremia. *Hum. Mutat.* **2017**, *38*, 704–715. [CrossRef] [PubMed]

28. Zhang, F.L.; Casey, P.J. Protein prenylation: Molecular mechanisms and functional consequences. *Ann. Rev. Biochem.* **1996**, *65*, 241–269. [CrossRef]

29. Seabra, M.C.; Ho, Y.K.; Anant, J.S. Deficient geranylgeranylation of Ram/Rab27 in choroideremia. *J. Biol. Chem.* **1995**, *270*, 24420–24427. [CrossRef]

30. Gordiyenko, N.V.; Fariss, R.N.; Zhi, C.; MacDonald, I.M. Silencing of the CHM gene alters phagocytic and secretory pathways in the retinal pigment epithelium. *Investig. Ophthalmol. Vis. Sci.* **2010**, *51*, 1143–1150. [CrossRef]

31. Tolmachova, T.; Wavre-Shapton, S.T.; Barnard, A.R.; MacLaren, R.E.; Futter, C.E.; Seabra, M.C. Retinal pigment epithelium defects accelerate photoreceptor degeneration in cell type-specific knock-out mouse models of Choroideremia. *Investig. Ophthalmol. Vis. Sci.* **2010**, *51*, 4913–4920. [CrossRef] [PubMed]

32. Wavre-Shapton, S.T.; Tolmachova, T.; da Silva, M.L.; Futter, C.E.; Seabra, M.C. Conditional ablation of the choroideremia gene causes age-related changes in mouse retinal pigment epithelium. *PLoS ONE* **2013**, *8*, e57769. [CrossRef]

33. Flannery, J.G.; Bird, A.C.; Farber, D.B.; Weleber, R.G.; Bok, D. A histopathologic study of a choroideremia carrier. *Investig. Ophthalmol. Vis. Sci.* **1990**, *31*, 229–236.

34. Cremers, F.P.; Molloy, C.M.; van de Pol, D.J.; van den Hurk, J.A.; Bach, I.; Geurts van Kessel, A.H.; Ropers, H.H. An autosomal homologue of the choroideremia gene colocalizes with the Usher syndrome type II locus on the distal part of chromosome 1q. *Hum. Mol. Genet.* **1992**, *1*, 71–75. [CrossRef] [PubMed]

35. Cremers, F.P.M.; Armstrong, S.A.; Seabra, M.C.; Brown, M.S.; Goldstein, J.L. REP-2, a Rab escort protein encoded by the choroideremia-like gene. *J. Biol. Chem.* **1994**, *269*, 2111–2117. [PubMed]

36. Anand, V.; Barral, D.C.; Zeng, Y.; Brunsmann, F.; Maguire, A.M.; Seabra, M.C.; Bennett, J. Gene therapy for choroideremia: In vitro rescue mediated by recombinant adenovirus. *Vis. Res.* **2003**, *43*, 919–926. [CrossRef]

37. Tolmachova, T.; Tolmachov, O.E.; Wavre-Shapton, S.T.; Tracey-White, D.; Futter, C.E.; Seabra, M.C. *CHM/REP1* cDNA delivery by lentiviral vectors provides functional expression of the transgene in the retinal pigment epithelium of choroideremia mice. *J. Gene Med.* **2012**, *14*, 158–168. [CrossRef]

38. Zhang, A.Y.; Mysore, N.; Vali, H.; Koenekoop, J.; Cao, S.N.; Li, S.; Ren, H.; Keser, V.; Lopez-Solache, I.; Siddiqui, S.N.; et al. Choroideremia Is a Systemic Disease with Lymphocyte Crystals and Plasma Lipid and RBC Membrane Abnormalities. *Investig. Ophthalmol. Vis. Sci.* **2015**, *56*, 8158–8165. [CrossRef]

39. Radziwon, A.; Cho, W.J.; Szkotak, A.; Suh, M.; MacDonald, I.M. Crystals and Fatty AcidAbnormalities Are Not Present in Circulating Cells from Choroideremia Patients. *Investig. Ophthalmol. Vis. Sci.* **2018**, *59*, 4464–4470. [CrossRef]

40. Futter, C.E.; Ramalho, J.S.; Jaissle, G.B.; Seeliger, M.W.; Seabra, M.C. The role of Rab27a in the regulation of melanosome distribution within retinal pigment epithelial cells. *Mol. Biol. Cell* **2004**, *15*, 2264–2275. [CrossRef]

41. Kwok, M.C.M.; Holopainen, J.M.; Molday, L.L.; Foster, L.J.; Molday, R.S. Proteomics of photoreceptor outer segments identifies a subset of SNARE and Rab proteins implicated in membrane vesicle trafficking and fusion. *Mol. Cell Proteom.* **2008**, *7*, 1053–1066. [CrossRef] [PubMed]

42. Wang, J.; Deretic, D. Molecular complexes that direct rhodopsin transport to primary cilia. *Prog. Retin. Eye Res.* **2014**, *38*, 1–19. [CrossRef] [PubMed]

43. Larijani, B.; Hume, A.N.; Tarafder, A.K.; Seabra, M.C. Multiple factors contribute to inefficient prenylation of Rab27a in Rab Prenylation diseases. *J. Biol. Chem.* **2003**, *278*, 46798–46804. [CrossRef] [PubMed]

44. Rak, A.; Pylypenko, O.; Niculae, A.; Pyatkov, K.; Goody, R.S.; Alexandrov, K. Structure of the Rab7: REP-1 Complex. *Cell* **2004**, *117*, 749–760. [CrossRef] [PubMed]

45. Köhnke, M.; Delon, C.; Hastie, M.L.; Nguyen, U.T.; Wu, Y.W.; Waldmann, H.; Goody, R.S.; Gorman, J.J.; Alexandrov, K. Rab GTPase prenylation hierarchy and its potential role in choroideremia disease. *PLoS ONE* **2013**, *8*, e81758. [CrossRef] [PubMed]

46. Barnard, A.R.; Groppe, M.; MacLaren, R.E. Gene therapy for choroideremia using an adeno-associated viral (AAV) vector. *Cold Spring Harb. Perspect. Med.* **2014**, *5*, a017293. [CrossRef] [PubMed]

47. Edwards, T.L.; Groppe, M.; Jolly, J.K.; Downes, S.M.; MacLaren, R.E. Correlation of retinal structure and function in choroideremia carriers. *Ophthalmology* **2015**, *122*, 1274–1276. [CrossRef]

48. Diakatou, M.; Manes, G.; Bocquet, B.; Meunier, I.; Kalatzis, V. Genome Editing as a Treatment for the Most Prevalent Causative Genes of Autosomal Dominant Retinitis Pigmentosa. *Int. J. Mol. Sci.* **2019**, *20*, 2542. [CrossRef]

49. Cideciyan, A.V.; Jacobson, S.G.; Beltran, W.A.; Sumaroka, A.; Swider, M.; Iwabe, S.; Roman, A.J.; Olivares, M.B.; Schwartz, S.B.; Komaromy, A.M.; et al. Human retinal gene therapy for Leber congenital amaurosis shows advancing retinal degeneration despite enduring visual improvement. *Proc. Natl. Acad. Sci. USA* **2013**, *110*, E517–E525. [CrossRef]

50. Tolmachova, T.; Tolmachov, O.E.; Barnard, A.R.; de Silva, S.R.; Lipinski, D.M.; Walker, N.J.; Maclaren, R.E.; Seabra, M.C. Functional expression of Rab escort protein 1 following AAV2-mediated gene delivery in the retina of choroideremia mice and human cells ex vivo. *J. Mol. Med.* **2013**, *91*, 825–837. [CrossRef]

51. Nagel-Wolfrum, K.; Möller, F.; Penner, I.; Baasov, T.; Wolfrum, U. Targeting NonsenseMutations in Diseases with Translational Read-Through-Inducing Drugs (TRIDs). *BioDrugs* **2016**, *30*, 49–74. [CrossRef]

52. Moosajee, M.; Ramsden, S.C.; Black, G.C.; Seabra, M.C.; Webster, A.R. Clinical utility gene card for: Choroideremia. *Eur. J. Hum. Genet.* **2014**, *22*, 572. [CrossRef]

53. McDonald, C.M.; Campbell, C.; Torricelli, R.E.; Finkel, R.S.; Flanigan, K.M.; Goemans, N.; Heydemann, P.; Kaminska, A.; Kirschner, J.; Muntoni, F.; et al. Clinical Evaluator Training Group; ACT DMD Study Group. Ataluren in patients with nonsense mutation Duchenne muscular dystrophy (ACT DMD): A multicentre, randomised, double-blind, placebo-controlled, phase 3 trial. *Lancet* **2017**, *390*, 1489–1498. [CrossRef]

54. Moosajee, M.; Gregory-Evans, K.; Ellis, C.D.; Seabra, M.C.; Gregory-Evans, C.Y. Translational bypass of nonsense mutations in zebrafish rep1, pax2.1 and lamb1 highlights a viable therapeutic option for untreatable genetic eye disease. *Hum. Mol. Genet.* **2008**, *17*, 3987–4000. [CrossRef]

55. Moosajee, M.; Tracey-White, D.; Smart, M.; Weetall, M.; Torriano, S.; Kalatzis, V.; da Cruz, L.; Coffey, P.; Webster, A.R.; Welch, E. Functional rescue of REP1 following treatment with PTC124 and novel derivative PTC-414 in human choroideremia fibroblasts and the nonsense-mediated zebrafish model. *Hum. Mol. Genet.* **2016**, *25*, 3416–3431. [CrossRef]

56. Torriano, S.; Erkilic, N.; Baux, D.; Cereso, N.; De Luca, V.; Meunier, I.; Moosajee, M.; Roux, A.F.; Hamel, C.P.; Kalatzis, V. The effect of PTC124 on choroideremia fibroblasts and iPSC-derived RPE raises considerations for therapy. *Sci. Rep.* **2018**, *8*, 8234. [CrossRef]

57. Dabrowski, M.; Bukowy-Bieryllo, Z.; Zietkiewicz, E. Advances in therapeutic use of a drug-stimulated translational readthrough of premature termination codons. *Mol. Med.* **2018**, *24*, 25. [CrossRef]

58. Garanto, A.; van der Velde-Visser, S.D.; Cremers, F.P.M.; Collin, R.W.J. Antisense Oligonucleotide-Based Splice Correction of a Deep-Intronic Mutation in CHM Underlying Choroideremia. *Adv. Exp. Med. Biol.* **2018**, *1074*, 83–89.

59. Collin, R.W.; den Hollander, A.I.; van der Velde-Visser, S.D.; Bennicelli, J.; Bennett, J.; Cremers, F.P. Antisense Oligonucleotide (AON)-based Therapy for Leber Congenital Amaurosis Caused by a Frequent Mutation in CEP290. *Mol. Ther. Nucleic Acids.* **2012**, *1*, e14. [CrossRef]

60. Gerard, X.; Perrault, I.; Hanein, S.; Silva, E.; Bigot, K.; Defoort-Delhemmes, S.; Rio, M.; Munnich, A.; Scherman, D.; Kaplan, J.; et al. AON-mediated Exon Skipping Restores Ciliation in Fibroblasts Harboring the Common Leber Congenital Amaurosis CEP290 Mutation. *Mol. Ther. Nucleic Acids.* **2012**, *1*, e29. [CrossRef]

61. Parmeggiani, F.; De Nadai, K.; Piovan, A.; Binotto, A.; Zamengo, S.; Chizzolini, M. Optical coherence tomography imaging in the management of the Argus II retinal prosthesis system. *Eur. J. Ophthalmol.* **2017**, *27*, e16–e21. [CrossRef]

62. Luo, Y.H.; da Cruz, L. The Argus® II Retinal Prosthesis System. *Prog. Retin. Eye Res.* **2016**, *50*, 89–107. [CrossRef]

63. Simunovic, M.P.; Shen, W.; Lin, J.Y.; Protti, D.A.; Lisowski, L.; Gillies, M.C. Optogenetic approaches to vision restoration. *Exp. Eye Res.* **2019**, *178*, 15–26. [CrossRef]

64. Cehajic-Kapetanovic, J.; Eleftheriou, C.; Allen, A.E.; Milosavljevic, N.; Pienaar, A.; Bedford, R.; Davis, K.E.; Bishop, P.N.; Lucas, R.J. Restoration of Vision with Ectopic Expression of Human Rod Opsin. *Curr. Biol.* **2015**, *25*, 2111–2122. [CrossRef]

65. Eleftheriou, C.G.; Cehajic-Kapetanovic, J.; Martial, F.P.; Milosavljevic, N.; Bedford, R.A.; Lucas, R.J. Meclofenamic acid improves the signal to noise ratio for visual responses produced by ectopic expression of human rod opsin. *Mol. Vis.* **2017**, *23*, 334–345.

8

Mouse Models of Inherited Retinal Degeneration with Photoreceptor Cell Loss

Gayle B. Collin [1,†], Navdeep Gogna [1,†], Bo Chang [1], Nattaya Damkham [1,2,3], Jai Pinkney [1], Lillian F. Hyde [1], Lisa Stone [1], Jürgen K. Naggert [1], Patsy M. Nishina [1,*] and Mark P. Krebs [1,*]

[1]   The Jackson Laboratory, Bar Harbor, Maine, ME 04609, USA; gayle.collin@jax.org (G.B.C.); navdeep.gogna@jax.org (N.G.); bo.chang@jax.org (B.C.); nattaya.damkham@jax.org (N.D.); jai.pinkney@jax.org (J.P.); Lillian.Hyde@jax.org (L.F.H.); lisa.stone@jax.org (L.S.); juergen.naggert@jax.org (J.K.N.)

[2]   Department of Immunology, Faculty of Medicine Siriraj Hospital, Mahidol University, Bangkok 10700, Thailand

[3]   Siriraj Center of Excellence for Stem Cell Research, Faculty of Medicine Siriraj Hospital, Mahidol University, Bangkok 10700, Thailand

*   Correspondence: patsy.nishina@jax.org (P.M.N.); mark.krebs@jax.org (M.P.K.);

†   These authors contributed equally to this work.

Abstract: Inherited retinal degeneration (RD) leads to the impairment or loss of vision in millions of individuals worldwide, most frequently due to the loss of photoreceptor (PR) cells. Animal models, particularly the laboratory mouse, have been used to understand the pathogenic mechanisms that underlie PR cell loss and to explore therapies that may prevent, delay, or reverse RD. Here, we reviewed entries in the Mouse Genome Informatics and PubMed databases to compile a comprehensive list of monogenic mouse models in which PR cell loss is demonstrated. The progression of PR cell loss with postnatal age was documented in mutant alleles of genes grouped by biological function. As anticipated, a wide range in the onset and rate of cell loss was observed among the reported models. The analysis underscored relationships between RD genes and ciliary function, transcription-coupled DNA damage repair, and cellular chloride homeostasis. Comparing the mouse gene list to human RD genes identified in the RetNet database revealed that mouse models are available for 40% of the known human diseases, suggesting opportunities for future research. This work may provide insight into the molecular players and pathways through which PR degenerative disease occurs and may be useful for planning translational studies.

Keywords: visual photoreceptor cell loss; mouse genetic models; retinitis pigmentosa; Leber congenital amaurosis; ciliopathies

1. Introduction

Inherited forms of retinal degeneration (RD) encompass a genetically and clinically heterogeneous group of disorders estimated to cause vision impairment and loss in more than 5.5 million individuals worldwide [1,2], with 282 mapped and identified retinal degenerative disease genes documented in the RetNet human database [3]. Animal models, such as non-human primates [4], dogs [5], mice [6,7], zebrafish [8], and fruit flies [9], have been used to identify candidates for human retinal disease genes, to elucidate pathological mechanisms, and to serve as a resource for exploring therapeutic approaches. As potential therapies for retinal diseases are investigated, the need for animal models increases. Information about the disease onset and rate of progression, the pathogenic pathways involved, and the genetic background in which the disrupted genes are situated are all factors that must be considered when selecting appropriate models for testing therapeutics. These factors will also play a role in interpreting the outcome of treatment studies.

The purpose of this review is to compile a searchable list of mouse models of inherited retinal diseases caused by single gene mutations that specifically lead to the post-developmental rod and/or cone photoreceptor (PR) cell loss. To identify these models, we reviewed mouse-specific data available in the Mouse Genome Informatics (MGI) and National Center for Biotechnology Information (NCBI) databases at The Jackson Laboratory (JAX) and National Institutes of Health (NIH), respectively. We recorded, when available, PR cell loss data from publications describing mutant alleles of the genes identified. We also included representative fundus photographs and optical coherence tomography (OCT) images of selected mouse models from the Eye Mutant Resource (EMR) and the Translational Vision Research Models (TVRM) programs at JAX as examples of the retinal phenotypes found among mouse models that fit our criteria. We attempted to cluster genes based on the function and then compared the progression of PR cell loss among these clusters to provide potential insights into disease mechanisms. We also compared our list of mouse genes associated with PR cell loss with the RetNet gene list, to highlight mouse models for specific retinal diseases, to reveal opportunities to create novel models, and to identify candidate genes within human loci for which a causative gene is currently unknown. Finally, we coordinated with the MGI team to incorporate our annotations into the MGI database, which will allow future analyses using tools available through that platform. It is hoped that our work will be useful as a resource for investigators to assist in the selection of appropriate mouse models within and across functional clusters in new studies to understand and develop treatments for human retinal degenerative disease.

In the three decades since the genes linked to PR loss phenotype were first identified in the mouse and human [10–12], rapid progress in understanding the genetic basis of inherited RD has been summarized in many excellent reviews. Many of the topics presented in the current article have been discussed previously in reviews of mouse RD models [6,7,13,14] and in summaries of our work at JAX [15–21]. Although we have made every effort to acknowledge the many contributions to this field, we note that there is a large body of relevant literature and apologize in advance to authors whose reviews or articles we may have inadvertently overlooked.

2. Background

2.1. Photoreceptor (PR) Cell Structure

PR cells are sensory neurons within the retina that detect light and signal this event to other cells. Since PR cells are essential for vision, their loss can dramatically and negatively affect the quality of life. PR cells include rod and cone cells (Figure 1a,b) that occupy the outermost layers of the neurosensory retina. Although intrinsically photosensitive retinal ganglion cells have also been described as photoreceptors [22], we did not include them in this review, as their contribution to RD is unknown. Rod and cone photoreceptors possess unique structures that serve to compartmentalize processes that are critical for cell function and maintenance.

- The outer segment (OS), which is cylindrical in rod PR cells and tapered in cones, contains phototransduction proteins that sense light and amplify the ensuing signal, culminating in PR cell hyperpolarization (Figure 1c). Much of the phototransduction apparatus is localized to double-bilayer discs formed by evagination of the plasma membrane at the base of the OS. These discs are largely internalized in rods except at the base of the OS, but remain contiguous with the plasma membrane in cones to yield a highly convoluted OS surface [23].
- The OS is stabilized by a ciliary axoneme, which runs through much of its length (Figure 1d; Ax). At the proximal end of the axoneme, the connecting cilium, analogous to the transition zone in other cilia (Figure 1d; CC-TZ), serves as a conduit through which all membrane and protein components destined for the OS are thought to pass. At the base of the connecting cilium lies the basal body (Figure 1d; BB), a cylindrical organelle derived from the mother centriole. Altogether

these structures represent a modified primary cilium that encompasses an extensive network of protein complexes that transport proteins and lipids and shares characteristics with primary cilia in many other cell types. The ciliary networks also function to prevent the flow of OS components to other parts of the cell and may associate with the intracellular trafficking apparatus to ensure the directed movement of needed components to the OS.

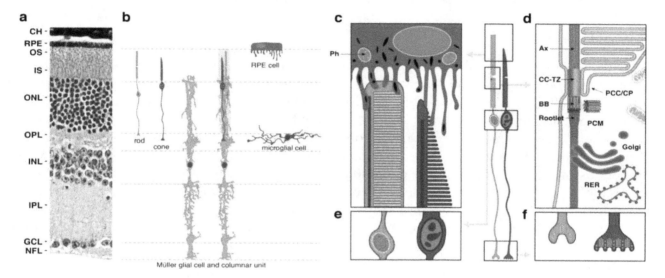

Figure 1. Retinal tissue organization emphasizing cell types and subcellular structures that may be sites of pathological processes in mouse models of photoreceptor (PR) cell loss. (**a**) A radial section of the posterior eye stained with hematoxylin and eosin shows the layered structure of the retina. CH, choroid; RPE, retinal pigment epithelium; IS, inner segment; OS, outer segment; ONL, outer nuclear layer; OPL, outer plexiform layer; INL, inner nuclear layer; IPL, inner plexiform layer; GCL, ganglion cell layer; NFL, nerve fiber layer. (**b**) Two PR cell types (rods and cones) and additional cell types that may be the target of processes implicated in PR cell loss. Dashed lines indicate alignment with retinal layers in (**a**). A columnar unit consisting of one cone and one Müller cell and roughly 20 rod cells is shown. (**c–f**) Details of PR and RPE cells. (**c**) PR cell OSs contain flattened discs (rod, left) or incomplete discs (cone, right) where the light sensing apparatus is located. OS tips engulfed by RPE cell apical processes are digested in phagolysosomes (Ph). (**d**) The base of the OS, the connecting cilium, and the apical portion of a rod cell IS (adapted with permission from [24]). The axoneme (Ax) and rootlet provide physical stability to the cilium. BB, basal bodies; CC-TZ, connecting cilium-transition zone; PCM, pericentriolar matrix; PCC/CP, periciliary complex/ciliary pocket; RER, rough endoplasmic reticulum. (**e**) The PR cell soma is largely occupied by the nucleus. (**f**) Rod and cone synaptic termini include presynaptic ribbons and associated neurotransmitter vesicles.

- The inner segment (IS) contains the biosynthetic machinery and energy sources needed to produce and assemble newly synthesized phototransduction proteins and their associated membranes (Figure 1d). The capacity of this cellular factory is impressive, as up to 10% of the OS is shed daily and removed via phagocytosis by the retinal pigment epithelium (see below) and must be renewed. Most protein and lipid components are synthesized de novo, but the IS also has an extensive recycling machinery that can reassemble components provided from outside the cell.

- The cell body or soma includes the nucleus, which is highly condensed in rod PR cells, but is larger in cones and includes patches of heterochromatin (Figure 1e). To increase the density of rod and cone OSs in the retina, the somas are stacked in columns within the outer nuclear layer (ONL). This arrangement necessitates thin cell extensions reaching from the soma to the IS or to the synapse. PR cell loss is measured by counting ONL nuclei, which are prominently stained in retinal sections (Figure 1a), or in the case of rods, which are more abundant than cones, by measuring ONL thickness from micrographs or by OCT.

- The PR cell terminus contains ribbon synapses close to the presynaptic membrane loaded with vesicles containing the excitatory neurotransmitter glutamate (Figure 1f). In the dark, a steady-state level of glutamate is released at the synapse, which is reduced when the cells are hyperpolarized in the light. Changes in glutamate levels at the synapse signal postsynaptic secondary neurons in the inner nuclear layer, which communicate with ganglion cells on the vitreal surface of the retina that connect through long axons to the visual cortex of the brain.

2.2. Neighboring Cells

Müller glia are radial cells that span much of the neurosensory retina, reaching from the internal limiting membrane at the vitreal surface of the retina to the external limiting membrane on the scleral edge of the ONL [25]. Within the ONL, fine Müller cell extensions appear to ensheath the PR cell soma. As they also interact with vascular layers within the retina, Müller cells may provide essential nutrients to PR cells, which do not directly contact the circulation. They also regulate extracellular volume, ion and water homeostasis, serve to modify neuronal activity through release of neuroactive compounds, and modulate immune and inflammatory responses [26]. At the external limiting membrane, Müller cell endfeet engage rod and cone cell ISs in intercellular adhesion interactions, including tight junctions, which create a diffusion barrier. Notably, the arrangement of an Müller cell, rods, and a cone cell has been proposed to form a columnar unit (Figure 1b), which may result in physiological and functional coordination of these cell types.

RPE cells (Figure 1b,c) constitute an epithelial monolayer that lies between the retina and a capillary bed, the choriocapillaris. The flow of water, ions, small molecules, and metabolites from the blood to the outer retina is thus regulated by RPE cells. Their apical surface features microvilli and microplicae (Figure 1b,c) that contact roughly the outermost third of OSs and play important roles in recycling molecules needed for PR renewal. These apical processes also mediate initial steps in the daily phagocytosis of OS tips. As an epithelium with high-resistance intercellular junctions [27], the RPE performs an important barrier function, disruption of which may cause PR degeneration.

Microglial cells form ramified networks within the same retinal layers as the retinal vasculature, which includes the superficial, intermediate and deep vascular beds. Microglia at the level of the outer plexiform layer in healthy retinas extend dendritic arms into the ONL (Figure 1b), where they contact PR soma as part of a dynamic survey process. During development and in rare events that occur in healthy retinas, these cells engulf and phagocytose PR soma, presumably in response to a defect in PR function.

PRs form synaptic connections in the outer plexiform layer with secondary neurons, including bipolar and horizontal cells. Although these connections are critical for signal transmission, they are not as extensive as the contacts made between PRs and Müller glia, RPE cell apical processes, or the dynamic extensions on microglial cells, and were therefore omitted from the summary diagram in Figure 1. Nevertheless, perturbation of the interactions among these cells may lead to PR degeneration, conceivably due to an alteration of signal transmission.

2.3. Inherited Diseases that Cause PR Cell Loss

Major monogenic inherited RDs in which PR cells are lost include: retinitis pigmentosa [28], Leber congenital amaurosis [29], and syndromic disorders that manifest disease in multiple organs, including the eye, particularly ciliopathies, such as Joubert [30], Bardet–Biedl [31], or Usher [32] syndrome. The remarkable success of gene augmentation therapy for a form of Leber congenital amaurosis has invigorated research efforts to treat these diseases [33].

3. Methods

3.1. Public Database and Literature Searches

The search strategy employed in this review is summarized in Figure 2. Initially, the MGI database [34] was queried to identify mutant protein-coding genes associated with a mammalian disease phenotype indicating a loss of PR cells. MGI is a curated database that includes expert annotation based on full-text searching of 148 selected journals, which is limited compared to literature databases, such as PubMed. Typically, only the first paper describing a new allele is fully curated for phenotype data in the database due to resource constraints. Although our analysis yielded 159 mutant genes that were associated with PR cell loss, a number of mutant genes known to cause this phenotype were absent or not annotated, possibly due to these aforementioned limitations.

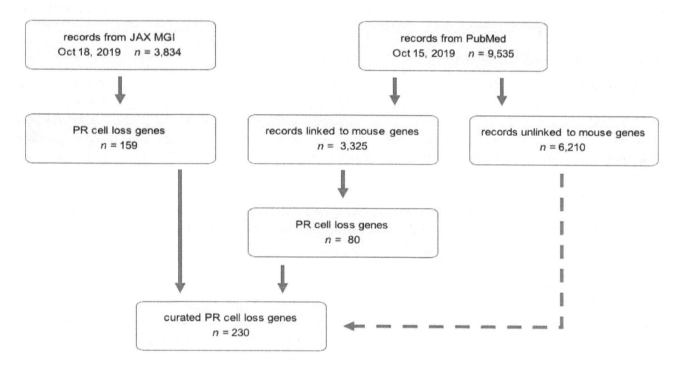

Figure 2. Flow chart depicting the progression of the search strategy utilized in this review. The number of records or genes identified from them is indicated at each stage of the process. The dashed line indicates that some genes were identified from records that remain to be systematically screened.

To expand the search, we used NCBI databases, including PubMed [35] and Gene. We refined a PubMed query by searching with keyword phrases to generate article lists, using the Gene option of Find Related Data to yield mouse genes linked to the articles, and then assessing whether these genes were on our MGI list. The goal was to develop a broad query that included as many genes from the MGI list as possible but also included additional hits. The most successful was: (ONL OR "outer nuclear layer" OR retina* OR PR OR rod OR rods OR cone*) AND (degener* OR loss OR thin* OR thick*) AND (mouse OR mice OR murine), which captured >97% of the MGI list. Restricting this query to entries posted to PubMed on or before October 15, 2019, yielded 9535 articles. To review these articles efficiently we tried two approaches, the first generating a spreadsheet containing hyperlinks in which each linked gene symbol was combined with the Boolean query, and the second using mouse gene identification numbers corresponding to the linked genes and applying an Entrez script that accessed the Gene and PubMed databases to find all articles satisfying the Boolean query for each linked gene.

3.2. Search Strategy

Each MGI database-derived entry was curated manually or automatically to identify candidate models that reported PR degeneration as a phenotype, as described above. In the case of PubMed entries, although the automated approaches were useful for quickly identifying genes that satisfied our criteria, neither was comprehensive, and additional candidate models were identified by review of the title and abstract from some of the remaining articles in the full collection of 9535 articles. Subsequently, an independent coauthor identified an original publication for each candidate gene and determined if PR cell loss was reported. If sufficient evidence for PR cell loss was obtained, the gene and mouse model was assigned to one of 11 categories. Genes within each category were curated further by coauthors who identified alternate alleles and extracted information regarding the disease phenotype induced by the disruption of a gene. Each entry in Table S1 is the result of the examination of an original article (indicated by PubMed ID numbers, PMIDs) and data from MGI to capture information such as mutation type, associated human diseases, and disease onset and progression.

3.3. Comparative Analysis and Updating the MGI Database

Once our final list was completed, we used tools in Excel to compare it to a list constructed from online tables downloaded on 8 December 2019, from RetNet, a public compilation of human genes linked to inherited RD. We also provided our data to the MGI team at JAX, who assigned allele nomenclature, added strain information for newly described mutants, and updated phenotype data for alleles that were present in the MGI database but not yet annotated with respect to PR cell loss. This review has been referenced at MGI so that the alleles documented in the article can be examined using MGI tools or downloaded in tabular format for analysis with other software. The collaborative approach between mouse phenotyping experts and the MGI team may be attractive for ensuring that this useful resource remains current in the face of limited funding, personnel, and time.

3.4. Inclusion/Exclusion Criteria

Monogenic models generated from a variety of sources were included in Table S1. However, in the case of conditional models, only those for which a germline null allele was reported in the MGI database that resulted in embryonic, prenatal, or postnatal lethality were included. We excluded the following models from Table S1: those for which a causative gene had yet to be identified and for which complementation tests were unavailable; those requiring multiple genes for the presentation of the disease phenotype; those based on overexpressing transgenes; and those in which PR degeneration depended on experimental interventions, such as an altered diet, drug treatment, or exposure to bright illumination. Environmental influences on retinal diseases are very important and may affect the progression of PR cell loss, but models that depend on environmental conditions are challenging to compare because of the significant variation among the types of environmental perturbations and the methods used to apply them. We also excluded models that exhibited a reduction in the PR cell number during development but not a progressive loss with age, and those where IS and/or OS dysmorphology or reduction in length was observed without a loss of PR cells, as indicated by a reduction in nuclei number or ONL thickness within the time frame reported in the papers. Although these models were excluded from Table S1, examples are included in the Results.

3.5. Heterogeneity of Data

The type and frequency of data gathered varied greatly among the studies reviewed. In some papers, only one figure with one retinal section was offered as evidence for PR degeneration, while other papers showed extensive quantitation of their data. To document potential sources of variability in the data, we indicate the method by which the degree of degeneration was determined, either by measuring ONL thickness or by count of nuclei in the ONL, typically the number of rows of nuclei spanning the ONL but sometimes a total count of ONL nuclei in a fixed area of a retinal micrograph.

In some instances, when data was quantified in spider plots or bar graphs, mean values obtained from the central retina were used in estimating the PR loss. We normalized the data among studies by recording the percent degeneration as determined by dividing the mutant values by the corresponding values from age-matched controls as reported in each publication.

3.6. Comparison of Progressive PR Cell Loss

To compare progressive PR cell loss among models, we fit normalized data from each article to an exponential decay that includes a delay, or offset [36]. Ranges of either age or photoreceptor numbers, if reported, were averaged. Fitting was performed in Excel Visual Basic using a piecewise equation that modeled the delay with a straight line at 100% and the remaining points with a monoexponential decay to 0%. Two adjustable parameters, the delay and the decay rate constant, were optimized. We calculated the age at which PR cell numbers reached 50% of control values (D_{50}) as a measure of progression. Roughly one third of the datasets contained only a single point within the exponential regime, which was insufficient to calculate D_{50}. In these cases, D_{50} was calculated at the extremes of zero delay and infinite rate, and the mean of these values was used as a D_{50} estimate.

3.7. Generation of Primary Data Using Fundus Imaging and OCT Scans

Fundus photographs of EMR mutants were taken in unanesthetized mice treated with 1% cyclopentolate to dilate or enlarge the pupil with an in vivo bright field retinal imaging microscope equipped with image-guided OCT capabilities (Micron III; Phoenix Laboratories, Inc., Pleasanton, CA, USA) as previously described [20]. This system allows for the visualization of the location of the OCT scan using the real-time Micron III bright-field image. A superimposed line placed directly on the image over the retinal feature being examined delivers precise cross-sectional information, allowing for the assessment of changes in layer thickness and morphological alterations.

Fundus photodocumentation for TVRM mutants and C57BL/6J control mice was performed using a Micron III or IV retinal camera (Phoenix Laboratories, Inc., Pleasanton, CA, USA) as described [37], except that 1% cyclopentolate or 1% atropine was used as a dilating agent, and in some cases, mice were anesthetized with isoflurane. OCT imaging to assess retinal layer thickness in $Nmnat1^{tvrm113}$, $Ctnna1^{Tvrm5}$, and C57BL/6J control mice was performed using a Bioptigen ultrahigh-resolution (UHR) Envisu R2210 spectral domain OCT (SDOCT) imaging system for volume scanning as described [37,38] with ketamine/xylazine (1.6 mL ketamine (100 mg/mL), 1.6 mL xylazine (20 mg/mL), and 6.8 mL sodium chloride (0.9% w/v)) as an anesthetic. A representative B-scan through the optic nerve head was derived from the OCT volume dataset. $Rpgrip1^{nmf247}$ and $Alms1^{Gt(XH152)Byg}$ were assessed on the same OCT system by obtaining a linear B-scan with the following parameters: length, 1.9 mm; width, 1.9 mm; angle, 0 degrees; horizontal offset, 0 mm; vertical offset, 0 mm; A-scans/B-scan, 1000 lines; B-scans, 1 line; frames/B-scan, 20 frames; and inactive A-scans/B-scan, 80 lines. Linear scans were registered and averaged in the InVivoVue program to merge the 20 frames into a single image.

4. Results

4.1. Summary of Studies that Report PR Cell Loss

The combined searches of MGI and PubMed databases yielded a total of 230 genes associated with PR cell loss. Ultimately, 3834 reports at MGI and 3325 at PubMed, which most typically characterized one mutant gene but on rare occasions described more than one, were used in the present review. The distribution of retrieved publications sorted by functional categories is summarized in Table S1. The genes identified in these models are summarized in Figure 3. Descriptions of gene and protein symbols used in the text, figures, and Table S1 are provided in Table S2.

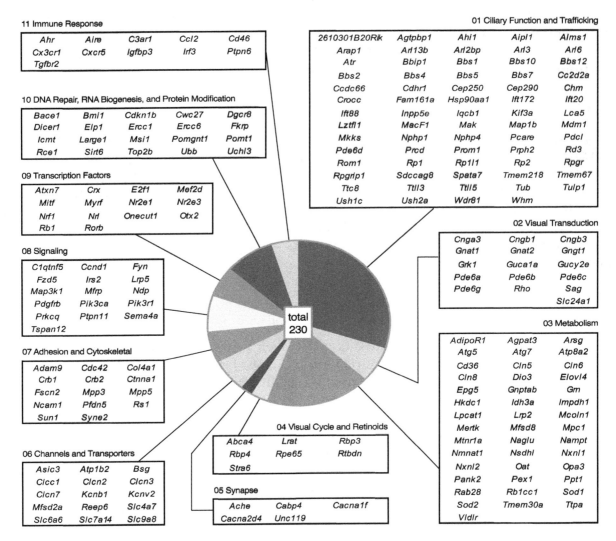

Figure 3. Genes associated with PR cell loss in monogenic mouse models of retinal degeneration (RD). Genes identified by combined review of the Mouse Genome Informatics (MGI) database and articles from a PubMed query were assigned to the indicated functional categories as described in the text. Genes for which mutant alleles are available only in the conditional form are displayed in red. Conditional alleles were included only in instances where germline null alleles resulted in embryonic, prenatal or postnatal lethality. For additional details on inclusion/exclusion criteria, see Section 3.4.

4.1.1. PR Cell Loss Models

The mouse models described in Table S1 were either spontaneous (12%) or chemically induced mutants (11%), or those produced through genetic engineering approaches (77%). This latter group, which was by far the largest, utilized standard homologous recombination, gene-traps, nuclease mediated approaches such as CRISPR/Cas9, and conditionals to mediate genomic changes. Additionally, four models of inadvertent transgene insertion into a unique gene, whose disruption led to PR degeneration, were included within this group. Interesting examples of differences in the disease onset or rate of progression were demonstrated in different models of the same gene (e.g., *Aipl1*) that may be related to allelic differences, null versus missense mutations, or genetic background effects [21,39,40]. Most of the genetically engineered models in Table S1 tended to be in mixed, segregating genetic backgrounds that might impact phenotypic expression (discussed below).

Within the genetically engineered category, a relatively large group of models, 16%, were conditional models, representing 39 genes (Figure 3; red). Generation of conditional mutants is based on the Cre-Lox recombination approach, which requires a floxed gene and a cre-driver to excise the targeted genomic region in a spatial (e.g., cell/tissue specific) or temporal manner (e.g., induction by chemicals such as doxycycline). Since 30% of all null mutations lead to embryonic lethality, as they represent genes that are essential during development, conditionals are often used to examine the adult function of genes [41]. This was the case in 92% of the conditional models described here, as standard organism-wide removal of the genes was reported to be embryonic, perinatal, or postnatal lethal. Thus, conditionals allow us to learn the function of a gene post-developmentally. Conditionals are also sometimes used to determine the cellular contributions to a disease phenotype. If a gene is expressed in multiple retinal cell types, by removing them systematically and examining the consequent phenotype, one can learn how the loss of function of the gene within particular cell types affects the disease phenotype. For example, removal of *Arl3* from rod PRs using a Rho-icre driver shows a later and slower rate of degeneration than that found with Six3-cre, a Cre driver that expresses in early retinal development. This suggests that *Arl3* in rods is necessary for PR survival but that *Arl3* function in other retinal cell types also affects PR survival [42]. The most widely used Cre models include: for targeting retinal progenitor cells, Tg(rx3-icre)1Mjam, Tg(Six3-cre)69Frty, Tg(Chx10-EGFP/cre,-ALPP)2Clc, Tg(Crx-cre)1Tfur, and Tg(Pax6-cre,GFP)2Pgr; for targeting rods, Tg(Rho-icre)1Ck, Tg(RHO-cre)8Eap, and *Pde6g^{tm1(cre/ERT2)Eye}*; for targeting M-cone PRs, Tg(OPN1LW-cre)4Yzl (also known as HRGP-cre); for targeting PRs, Tg(Rbp3-cre)528Jxm (also known as IRBP-cre); for targeting RPE, Tg(BEST1-cre)1Jdun, Tg(BEST1-rtTA,tetO-cre)1Yzl and *Foxg1^{tm1(cre)Skm}*; and for targeting adult tissues using tamoxifen, Tg(CAG-cre/Esr1*)5Amc.

4.1.2. Mouse Models from Phenotyping Programs

The models listed in Table S1 come from many sources. In addition to individual investigator-initiated efforts, currently the largest contributor to ocular models is the International Mouse Phenotyping consortium, in which 19 phenotyping centers from 11 countries participate to systematically characterize knockout mice generated in a standardized manner [41,43]. All centers do some eye phenotyping, thus providing a window into potential models. Although only a few models from this program are included in Table S1, as most are not yet fully characterized, it is anticipated that this consortium will provide a wealth of models for individual laboratories to study. For example, in the MGI database, 39 IMPC models were identified with "reduced retinal thickness" that with further characterization may reveal PR degeneration.

At The Jackson Laboratory, the Eye Mutant Resource (EMR) and the Translational Vision Research Models (TVRM) programs are dedicated to screen for or generate mouse models with ocular diseases. The EMR has been screening retired breeders by slit lamp biomicroscopy, indirect ophthalmoscopy, and electroretinography since 1988. Retired breeders from the production and genetic resources colonies are screened. Heritable mutants are phenotypically and genetically characterized and the spontaneous mutants are distributed worldwide. The TVRM program arose from the JAX Neuromutagenesis Facility. Mice for this program are generated by chemical mutagenesis or genetic engineering. Carefully characterized mutants are also distributed. Examples of mutants from the EMR and TVRM programs are shown in Figures 4 and 5, respectively.

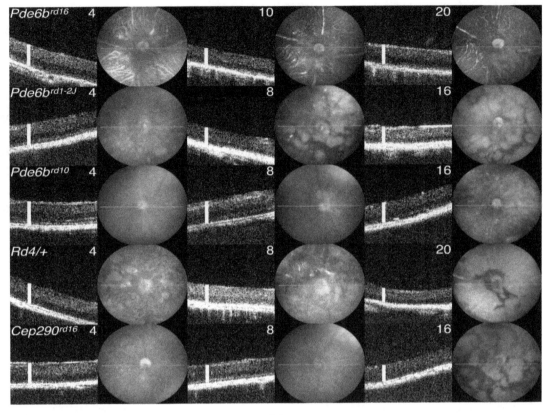

(a)

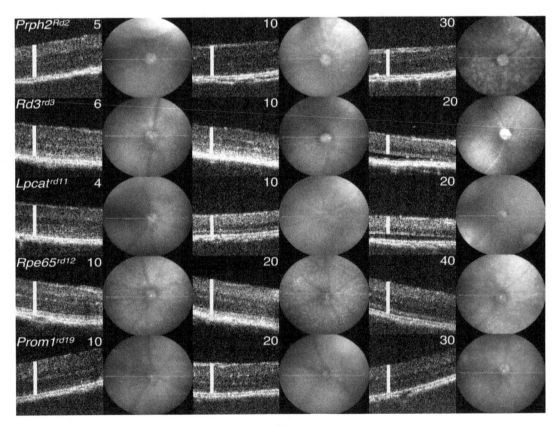

(b)

Figure 4. *Cont.*

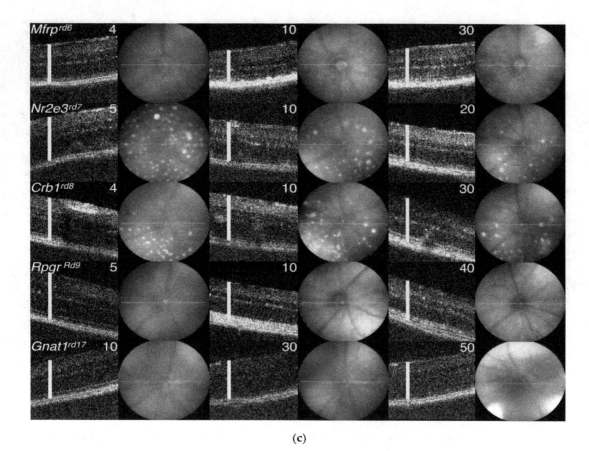

(c)

Figure 4. (**a**) Characterization of mouse models from the Eye Mutant Resource (EMR) program at JAX. Example optical coherence tomography (OCT) and fundus images were taken from rapid RD models: *Pde6b^{rd1}* (B6.C3-*Pde6b^{rd1}* Hps4^{le}/J, Stock No: 000002), *Pde6b^{rd1-2J}* (C57BL/6J-*Pde6b^{rd1-2J}*/J, Stock No: 004766), *Pde6b^{rd10}* (B6.CXB1-*Pde6b^{rd10}*/J, Stock No: 004297), *Rd4/+* (STOCK In(4)56Rk/J, Stock No: 001379) and *Cep290^{rd16}* (B6.Cg-*Cep290^{rd16}*/Boc, Stock No: 012283) (**b**) Example images from slower RD models: *Prph2^{Rd2}* (C3A.Cg-*Pde6b$^+$* *Prph2^{Rd2}*/J, Stock No: 001979), *Rd3^{rd3}* (B6.Cg-*Rd3^{rd3}*/Boc, Stock No: 008627), *Lpcat1^{rd11}* (B6.Cg-*Lpcat1^{rd11}*/Boc, Stock No: 006947), *Rpe65^{rd12}* (B6(A)-*Rpe65^{rd12}*/J, Stock No: 005379) and *Prom1^{rd19}* (B6.BXD83-*Prom1^{rd19}*/Boc, Stock No: 026803). (**c**) Examples from slow and very slow RD models: *Mfrp^{rd6}* (B6.C3Ga-*Mfrp^{rd6}*/J, Stock No: 003684), *Nr2e3^{rd7}* (B6.Cg-*Nr2e3^{rd7}*/J, Stock No: 004643), *Crb1^{rd8}* (STOCK *Crb1^{rd8}*/J, Stock No: 003392), *Rpgr^{Rd9}* (C57BL/6J-*Rpgr^{Rd9}*/Boc, Stock No: 003391), and *Gnat1^{rd17}* (B6.Cg-*Gnat1^{irdr}*/Boc, Stock No: 008811). *Yellow bars* indicate full retinal thickness. Values correspond to the mouse age at the time of imaging (weeks).

5. Analysis

5.1. Progression of PR Cell Loss

While a host of effects can occur as a result of disruptions in genes expressed in PRs and ancillary cell types that functionally impair vision, such as night blindness, or color vision defects, the focus of the models described here are those that bear single gene mutations that lead to actual PR cell loss. From a review of the models in Table S1, significant PR cell loss is reported as early as postnatal day 7 (P7) and can extend throughout the lifetime of animals examined. The progression of PR cells loss is also highly variable and includes models that progress rapidly with complete ablation within several weeks to models with extremely slow progression where only <10% PR cell loss is noted over the span of time in which animals were examined. Generally, while rapid to moderate progression led to almost complete PR ablation, slow and very slow progression, or degeneration in models that primarily affect cone PRs left a substantial number of PR cells intact.

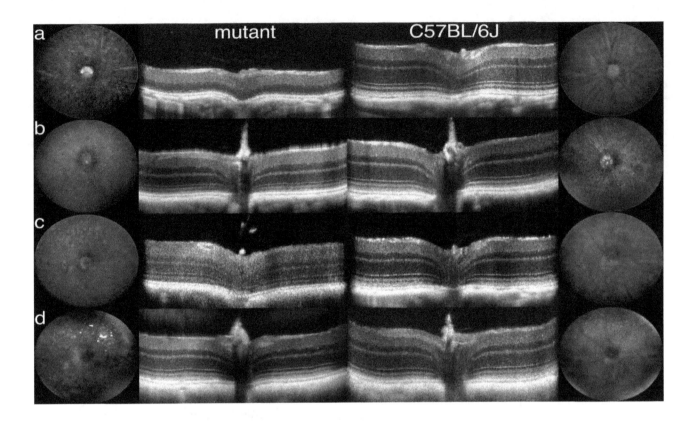

Figure 5. Characterization of mouse models from the Translational Vision Research Models (TVRM) program at JAX. A fundus image (circular panels) and corresponding OCT B-scan are shown for homozygous (**a**) $Rpgrip1^{nmf247}$, at one month of age; (**b**) $Nmnat1^{tvrm113}$, at two months; (**c**) $Alms1^{Gt(XH152)Byg}$, at one year; and (**d**) $Ctnna1^{Tvrm5}$, at two years. Age-matched OCT and fundus images for C57BL6/J control mice are shown to the right of the mutant images. PR cell loss is indicated by a decreased ONL thickness. Fundus images were acquired using a Micron III or IV retinal camera. The vertical dimension of OCT images was doubled to emphasize changes in retinal layer thicknesses.

To compare cell loss among functionally similar genetic models, models in each category of Table S1 were sorted based on the estimated age at which the PR cell population had degenerated by 50% compared to control values, defined as D_{50} (Figure 6). This quantity represents neither the rate of PR cell loss nor the delay before loss commences, although both parameters are used to calculate it. Rather, D_{50} provides a common measure of progression that allows both complete and sparse datasets to be evaluated. With sufficient data, delay, and exponential decay constants were calculated and are reflected by the shaded bars in Figure 6. Many datasets with fewer measurements, some containing a single point, allowed only an estimate of D_{50} (Figure 6; filled circles, range lines indicate estimated limits). Figure 6 may be used to identify models in which overall PR cell loss progresses at an earlier age (lower D_{50}), proceeds at a higher rate once initiated (shorter bar), or is accompanied by a substantial delay (bar starts farther to the right), which may aid in experimental design. Values for D_{50}, the exponential decay constant k, and the delay, when available, are also included in Table S1. We relate qualitative descriptions of progression to D_{50} as follows: rapid, <2 months; moderate, 2 to <6 months; slow, 6 to <12 months; and very slow, ≥12 months.

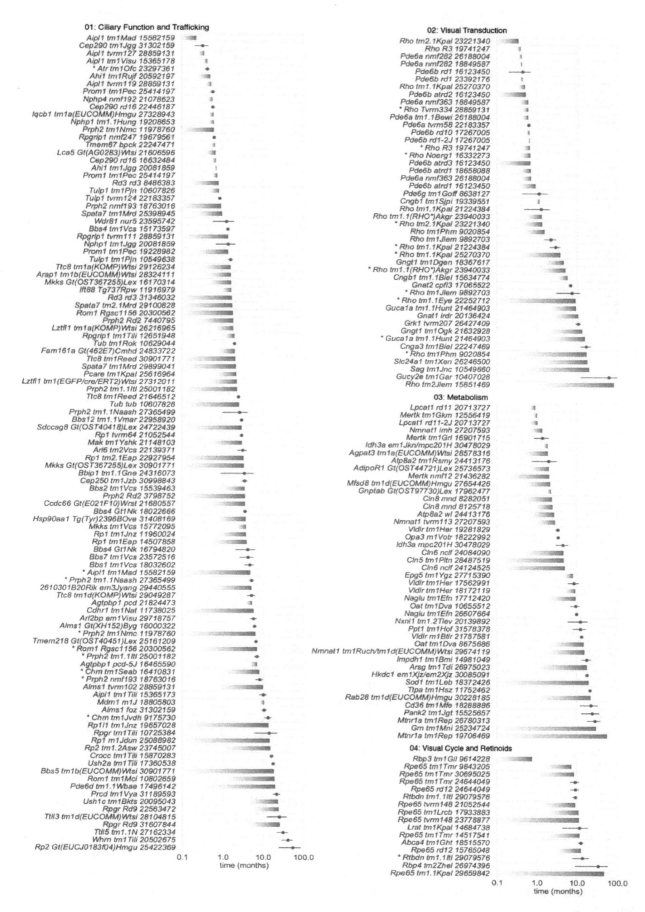

Figure 6. *Cont.*

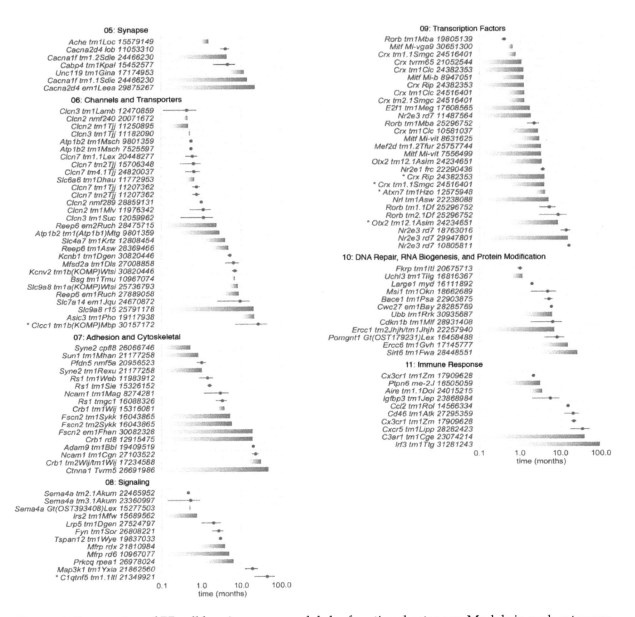

Figure 6. Progression of PR cell loss in mouse models by functional category. Models in each category were sorted by the age at which the estimated number of PR cells reached 50% of wild-type (D_{50}) as determined by fitting reported data to an exponential decay function combined with a delay. Models are identified by gene symbol, MGI allele symbol, and PMID. Models are homozygous except as indicated by * (heterozygous) or by the presence of two allele symbols (compound heterozygous). Left- and right-hand margins of shaded bars represent the delay and D_{50} values, respectively. Bars with a delay value of ≤0.1 month derive from datasets in which no values at 100% of wild type were reported. The midpoint and range of estimated D_{50} values for datasets with only one point in the 5–95% range is indicated by closed circles and range lines, respectively. In cases where the dataset consisted of a single point at 50%, no estimate was needed.

Figure 6 does not include models in which the age of the animal at the time of measurements was not provided, or was reported as "adult", although these models were included in Table S1. We also omitted models where only cone PR cell degeneration was reported, as limited data and a lack of cone nuclei counts made mathematical modeling of cell loss unreliable. Finally, we omitted all conditional alleles from Figure 6, as the efficiency and specificity of inactivation of genes, as well as the temporal expression of different transgenic Cre drivers utilized varies, making comparison of these alleles difficult.

5.2. Biological Processes Affected by Mutations

Categorization of PR cell loss genes (Figure 3) relied on current functional knowledge, similarity to other genes, and localization, if known. Genes are often expressed in multiple cell types and serve different functions within the retina. We placed genes in categories that were most pertinent to their roles in the PR or effect on PR survival. The data in Table S1 can be explored after reassigning models to different categories if desired. In the descriptions below, we provide an overview for the first three categories and then a detailed description of the effect of gene disruptions on biological functions included in these categories. Subsequent categories are described without overview.

5.2.1. Category 01: Ciliary Function and Trafficking

Overview. Disruptions in a vast number of genes associated with PR sensory cilia result in RD [24,44]. The onset and rate of PR cell loss may vary depending on the role of a given gene in maintaining ciliary structural integrity and function during early PR development and maintenance in adulthood. Retinal defects within any one of the key ciliary structures and/or processes such as ciliogenesis, OS morphogenesis, or PR homeostasis may result in the loss of rod and cone PR cells. Understanding the pathophysiological mechanisms involved in PR cell loss requires a detailed examination of the components and functionalities of the PR sensory cilium.

The mouse PR sensory cilium is a specialized structure comprised of a tubulin-rich axoneme with a symmetrical "9+0" arrangement of microtubular doublets [45]. The connecting cilium (CC) is akin to the transition zone (TZ) of primary cilia [46,47] and serves as a passageway for the movement of proteins from the organelle-rich IS to the photosensory OS. The OS is composed of an elongated distal axoneme with adjacent stacked membranous discs decorated with proteins necessary for phototransduction. It has been hypothesized that extension of the PR plasma membrane towards the apical RPE provides a convenient sink in the OS for the storage of a large number of membrane proteins [48]. In the CC-TZ, axonemal microtubule doublets interconnect the distal axoneme and basal body, and also connect to the periciliary membrane via Y-linkers. The CC-TZ harbors membrane-associated and soluble proteins that coordinate as gatekeepers to regulate the entry, retention, and exit of proteins in and out of the OS [47,49,50]. At the axonemal base, the ciliary membrane is anchored by the nine microtubular triplets of the basal body and its associated appendages.

In developing murine PRs, the connecting cilium and OSs assemble through a series of coordinated events. Shortly after cell cycle exit of retinal progenitor cells, the mother centriole docks to a primary ciliary vesicle initiating its expansion and fusion with the plasma membrane. Concurrently, the microtubular axoneme elongates towards the apical end of the neuroblastic layer [51]. In rod PRs, ciliogenesis typically begins shortly after birth with the appearance of a mature centriolar-bound ciliary vesicle at around P4 [52]. Subsequently, OS biogenesis occurs asynchronously between P8 and P14 [52–54] while axoneme and PM extension continue until OS maturation around P19–25 [52,53]. During this process, intraflagellar transport (IFT) provides an efficient mechanism for the movement and delivery of crucial proteins to the developing OS [55,56], as discussed in greater detail below.

Over the past several decades, two disparate mechanisms of rod disc morphogenesis have been debated, a vesicular fusion model [57,58], which postulates that membrane discs originate from rhodopsin bearing vesicles that undergo intracellular membrane fusion, and the classic evagination model [59], which proposes that new discs result from the evagination of the plasma membrane at the base of the OS. Recent ultrastructural studies in mouse rod PRs have provided compelling evidence that support the classic evagination model. By high resolution microscopy, several groups demonstrated the plasma membrane origin of the evaginated rod disc membranes [60], which subsequently flatten, elongate, and become enclosed [52,60,61].

OS membranous discs undergo a rapid and continuous turnover with approximately 75 rod discs being shed daily, corresponding to 10% of the OS [53,62]. At the ciliary tip, aged discs are removed by the adjacent RPE through phagocytosis. Consequently, OS renewal requires a continuous flow of new proteins from IS to the OS through the connecting cilium, a process that requires careful regulation.

For the CC-TZ gate to function properly, efficient mechanisms are needed to prevent the entry of undesired proteins and to remove the non-OS proteins improperly targeted to the OS. At the base of the CC-TZ lie transition fibers, which act as a barrier in conjunction with other CC-TZ components, such as the membrane-associated Meckel syndrome (MKS) complex. The BBSome, an octameric coat complex, is thought to coordinate the delivery and removal of proteins from the OS during ciliary formation and maturation [63,64].

Finally, protein trafficking through the CC-TZ is important for PR development and maintenance [51,65,66]. The movement of protein cargo from the IS to the OS requires a highly regulated passage of vesicles along microtubules that dock and fuse with the periciliary membrane to deliver their cargo at the CC base. Movement of targeted proteins through the cilia to the OS may be facilitated by IFT transport machinery [65] or by a lipidated protein trafficking system [67,68]. During IFT, protein cargo associate with IFT particles that attach to kinesin and dynein motors and move along the axonemal microtubules in both anterograde and retrograde directions, respectively. The BBSome is known to associate with IFT particles and may provide a mechanism for the removal of non-targeted protein accumulation in the OS [69].

Ciliogenesis. As the ciliary axoneme serves as an important conduit for the IFT movement of signaling molecules, it comes as no surprise that the disruption of ciliogenesis genes may result in significant developmental abnormalities causing early lethality and/or rapid PR degeneration. Genes essential for the elongation of the proximal axoneme (A and B tubules) include *Kif3a* [70], which encodes a subunit of kinesin 2, *Iqcb1* [71], *Arl3* [42], and *Arl13b* [72]. While patients with missense mutations in *ARL13B* present with Joubert-associated features [73], a null mutation, *Arl13b^hnn*, results in embryonic lethality in mice [74]. Axonemal disturbances and a failure to form OS discs are observed in developing retinas with conditional *Arl13b* disruption [72].

Axonemal and ciliary membrane extension. Disruptions in genes that affect ciliary extension include *Rp1/Rp1l1/Spata7* (distal axoneme), *Mak*, and *Pcare* (*C2orf71*; ciliary membrane). Mice with knockout alleles of *Rp1* (*Rp1^tm1Eap* and *Rp1^tm1Jnz*) and *Spata7* (*Spata7^tm1Mrd*) show a progressive, moderate loss in PR cells through the first year of life. *Rp1^m1Jdun* mice homozygous for a Leu66Pro missense mutation experience a much slower degeneration with 30% of PRs left at 26 months of age. Conditional ablation studies of *Spata7* in PRs and in the RPE have shown that the disruption of SPATA7 in rod and cone PRs, but not in the RPE, is the molecular basis of the retinal degenerative phenotype [75].

Ciliary Gate and the CC-TZ. Sensory/primary cilia and their gatekeepers (CC-TZ) are found abundantly in most cell types [76]. Thus, the disease spectrum of ciliary proteins is extensive given their roles in ciliary trafficking, signaling, and development. Disruptions in CC-TZ genes may result in isolated cases of inherited retinal dystrophies such as Leber congenital amaurosis or in multisystemic, ciliopathies such as Joubert, Meckel, or Senior-Løken Syndrome. Such syndromic ciliopathies may include a multitude of disease phenotypes such as brain malformations, renal cysts, nephronophthisis, and retinal dystrophy.

Within the CC-TZ reside MKS and NPHP modules that closely interact and form multiple distinct protein complexes [47,50,77–79]. The MKS complex includes membrane-associated proteins, such as MKS1 and TMEM67, while NPHP complex proteins, such as NPHP1 and NPHP4, associate in closer proximity to the ciliary axoneme. Mice harboring mutations in genes coding for these complex-associated proteins form normal cilia, however, display early abnormalities in OS morphogenesis. After ciliary biogenesis, retinas in these mutant mice quickly degenerate, eliminating most PRs by 3–4 weeks of age. Genes whose disruptions affect the ciliary gate functions of the CC-TZ and cause rapid degeneration include *Nphp1*, *Nphp4*, *Ahi1*, *Iqcb1*, *Tmem67*, and *Cep290*. In humans, mutations in *CEP290* can lead to primarily single-organ diseases such, as retinitis pigmentosa and nephronophthisis, or pleiotropic diseases, such as the Joubert, Meckel, and Bardet–Biedl syndromes. The most studied allele is *rd16*, which harbors a 297 basepair in-frame deletion in *Cep290*. Compared to *Cep290^tm1.1Jgg* knockout mice, which show a rapid 78% loss at P14, *Cep290^rd16* homozygotes have a longer disease progression with a 60% ONL loss at three weeks of age.

Basal bodies and associated pericentriolar material (PCM). The basal body is a structure derived from the mother centriole and resides at the base of the cilium along with the daughter centriole, neighboring centriolar satellites and other related PCM. Proteins positioned at the ciliary base can also be seen in centrosomes of dividing cells (ALMS1, CEP250, and C8ORF37). Specifically, ALMS1 and CEP250 (CNAP1) localize in close proximity to each other at the proximal ends of centrioles [80]. *ALMS1* encodes a 460kDa protein that when disrupted results in the Alström syndrome (ALMS) [81,82]. Mice with a gene trap, frameshift, and nonsense mutations recapitulate human ALMS disease features such as obesity, diabetes, and neurosensory deficits [21,83,84]. The proper formation of the connecting cilium and the slow progression of PR cell loss in *Alms1*$^{Gt(XH152)Byg}$ [83], *Alms1*^{foz} [84], and *Alms1*^{tvrm102} [21] models suggests that ALMS1 is not essential for ciliary biogenesis but necessary for overall PR homeostasis.

The ciliary base contains supportive structures necessary for the proper docking of cargo to the ciliary membrane. Targeted *Macf1* null mutants fail to develop the ciliary vesicle needed for basal body docking while conditional ablation of *Macf1* in the developing retina disrupts retinal lamination and maturation [85]. Mutations in *Cdcc66*, which encodes a component of centriolar satellites and *Sdccag8*, which encodes a recruiter of PCM, result in an early onset but slow-moderately progressive disease [86,87]. The slower RD makes these alleles attractive models for therapeutic investigations.

Genetic mutations in *CC2D2A*, which encodes a component of the subdistal appendages of mother centrioles and basal bodies [88], have been observed in patients with Meckel Syndrome [89], Joubert Syndrome [90], and non-syndromic rod-cone dystrophy [91]. Mice with null mutations in *Cc2d2a* experience embryonic lethality due to the absence of subdistal appendages and nodal cilia [88]. The retinas of adult mice with tamoxifen-induced deletion of *Cc2d2a* in PRs have a significantly diminished ONL (2–3 layers) 12 weeks post-injection [92], suggesting that CC2D2A is necessary for ciliary homeostasis.

Periciliary membrane complex. At the periciliary membrane complex of PRs lies an Usher protein interactome complex that provides a scaffold for the anchoring of fibers to the periciliary membrane [93]. Mutations in genes encoding members of this complex, *Ush1c*, *Whrn*, and *Ush2a*, result in Usher syndrome, a disease that results in progressive hearing and vision loss. Multiple forms of Usher syndrome exist resulting in different degrees of the onset and severity of disease symptoms. In the mouse, targeted mutations in Usher genes results in a late-onset and very slow progression of PR degeneration. Homozygous *Ush2a*^{tm1Tili} mice have normal retinas at 10 months of age and lose 70% of their PRs by 20 months of age [94]. PR degeneration in *Whrn*^{tm1Tili} retinas is protracted with only 30% loss observed at 28 months of age [95].

Disc morphogenesis. Although the molecular mechanisms involved in OS disc morphogenesis are not completely understood, there has been considerable progress within the past decade with the emergence of refined ultrastructural methods. The OS protein, peripherin-2 (PRPH2), localizes to the rims of rod and cone discs and functions to establish and maintain the membrane rim curvature during disc formation and maintenance [96,97]. Recent investigations using the *Prph2*^{Rd2} (*rds*) mouse model [10] have suggested another role for PRPH2 during disc morphogenesis [52]. Using transmission electron microscopy, Salinas et al. [52] demonstrated that like other forms of cilia [98,99], PR sensory cilia have an innate ability to spew off ectosomes at the OS base. During normal development of the OS, ectosome release is inhibited and the retained membrane at the CC-TZ is transformed into discs upon membrane evagination. In the homozygous *Prph2*^{Rd2} mice, discs fail to form resulting in the accumulation of ectosomes at the OS base. This finding led the authors to propose that PRPH2 may play a role in inhibiting ectosome release during normal rim formation [52].

Knock-in mice carrying heterozygous alleles of *Prph2* (Tyr141Cys [100] and Lys153Δ [101], mimic the dominant RP disease observed in human patients. It is interesting that PR degeneration rates vary among *Prph2* mutant alleles. While homozygous *Prph2*^{Rd2} mice gradually lose their PRs within the first year [102,103], mice harboring a homozygous null mutation, *Prph2*^{tm1Nmc} undergo a faster degeneration with most PRs lost by 4 months of age [104]. Heterozygous *Prph2*^{tm1Nmc} mice also experience PR loss, however the rate of decline is much slower [104]. Comparative studies of $Prph2^{Rd2}$ with rhodopsin double-knockout mice have suggested that abnormal accumulation of mislocalized rhodopsin may contribute to PR degeneration in $Prph2^{Rd2}$ [105]. Hence, the zygosity differences in degeneration rates may be a result of varying rhodopsin: PRPH2 ratios. In addition, the onset and severity of the disease may be influenced by the location of the mutation, as different PRPH2 domains have been implicated in dual roles during disc morphogenesis, the tetraspanin core in rim membrane curvature, and the C-terminal domain in ectosome release suppression [52].

ROM1 is thought to be involved in the regulation of OS disc formation. PRPH2 and ROM1 are closely associated at the disc rims in the OS. In humans, a double heterozygous disruption in both *ROM1* (a PRPH2-interacting protein) and *PRPH2* results in digenic RP [106]. While it is not clear whether defects in ROM1 alone causes RP in humans, mice with a monogenic *Rom1* disruption show signs of dominant RP. At one month of age, *Rom1* knockout OS discs are visible but appear enlarged and slightly disorganized [107]. PRs slowly degenerated, reducing the ONL by 34% at 1 year of age. In contrast, $Rom1^{Rgsc1156}$ mice with a heterozygous missense mutation, p.W182R, show a 55% loss of PRs at 35 weeks of age [108]. Furthermore, RD was more pronounced in homozygous mice. The degeneration in $Rom1^{Rgsc1156}$ mice may be a consequence of an early reduction in endogenous PRPH2 and ROM1 levels, which may interfere with PRPH2-mediated stabilization of disc outer rims.

PRCD, progressive rod-cone degeneration, is a rhodopsin-binding protein [109] that localizes to the OS disc rims [110]. Patients and canines with $PRCD^{C2Y}$ mutations have a slowly progressive form of rod-cone degeneration [111]. The Cys2Tyr mutation results in mislocalization of PRCD from the OS to the ONL where it is actively degraded [109]. In the PRs of mice with homozygous $Prcd^{tm1Vya}$ mutations, loss of PRCD results in the formation of bulging discs that do not properly flatten and in the accumulation of extracellular vesicles that originate at the OS base [112]. Interestingly, mutant PRs are able to form membrane discs and the distribution of OS proteins and light response do not appear to be perturbed. While activated microglia infiltrate the interphotoreceptor space to remove extracellular vesicles and debris, removal is insufficient and PRs undergo a very slow degeneration. Homozygous $Prcd^{tm1Vya}$ mice show only 36% ONL loss at 17 months [112] while in $Prcd^{tm1(KOMP)Mbp}$ homozygotes a similar loss is observed at 30 weeks of age [110]. Both models are knockout alleles that target the 5' end of *Prcd* but are on different genetic backgrounds. Further investigations are necessary to determine whether gene modifiers affect progressive PR cell loss in these two models.

IFT trafficking. IFT is essential for ciliogenesis in mammals [113] and disruption of this process often leads to abnormalities in embryonic development. In the mouse, null mutations in genes encoding subunits of the IFT-A (*Ift122* [114], *Ift88* [115], and *Ttc21b* [116]) and IFT-B (*Ift172* [117], *Ift80* [118], and *Traf3ip1* [119]) complexes result in embryonic lethalities, many of which are attributable to ciliary-related disturbances in hedgehog signaling [120,121]. These findings further highlight the integral role of cilia and IFT machinery during embryogenesis.

Hypomorphic and conditional alleles have been useful for elucidating the roles of IFT components in retinal disease. The hypomorphic allele, $Ift88^{Tg737Rpw}$, contains a transgenic insertion resulting in a 2.7 kb intronic deletion. Homozygous $Ift88^{Tg737Rpw}$ mice exhibit disorganized OSs as early as P10 and a progressive degeneration of PRs that reduces the ONL to one layer at P77 [66]. Rod-specific ablation of *Ift172* [122] leads to mislocalization of rhodopsin, RP1, and TTC21B (IFT139) and rapid degeneration of PRs. Conditional depletion of *Ift20* in M cones and mature rods both results in opsin mislocalization suggesting that proper opsin trafficking hinges on functional IFT components [123]. To gain a clearer understanding of the roles that IFT molecules play in both rod and cone PRs, additional studies using conditional models are warranted to elucidate the contributions of impaired IFT components to PR cell loss.

Lipidated protein trafficking. Lipid modification of proteins, such as prenylation or acylation, helps direct intracellular protein targeting and regulates protein activity [124]. These hydrophobic modifications help tether their protein partners to the surface of specific membranes throughout the cell, such as the ER, Golgi, transport vesicles, or plasma membranes. Improper trafficking of lipidated proteins can result in RD. RP2 is a GTPase activating protein that interacts with ARL3 to regulate assembly and movement of membrane-associated protein complexes [125]. Homozygous mice with mutations in the gene encoding RP2 exhibit a slowly progressive rod-cone degeneration [126,127]. ARL3, a small GTPase, traffics lipidated membrane-associated proteins to the rod OS [128]. Although *Arl3* knockout mice exhibit early postnatal lethality and Joubert-like features [42], mice with hypomorphic mutations survive to post-wean and display OS abnormalities as early as P9 [129]. Conditional ablation of *Arl3* in the developing retina results in the absence of cilia, and therefore PR cells are rapidly lost [42]. In contrast, depletion of *Arl3* in mature rods leads to mislocalization of lipidated OS proteins, shortened OS, and a moderate progressive PR loss. These results are consistent with roles for ARL3 in ciliogenesis during development and cargo displacement during lipidated protein trafficking.

The ciliary TZ-associated protein, RPGR, binds and directs the ciliary targeting of INPP5E [130], a phosphoinositide phosphatase that is important for ciliogenesis [131]. Ciliary localization of RPGR itself requires modification with a prenyl group, which interacts with PDE6D [130], a prenyl-binding protein first discovered as a copurifying component of cGMP phosphodiesterase 6 (PDE6) [132]. Like $Rpgr^{rd9}$ [133] and $Rpgr^{tm1Tili}$ knockout mice [134], mice with $Pde6d^{tm1.1Wbae}$ null mutations [135] undergo a very slow degeneration with at least 50% of PR cells remaining at 20 months of age. Rao et al. have demonstrated reduction of INPP5E in RPGR-deficient axonemal OSs [130]. Altogether, these observations validate RPGRs role in ciliary trafficking and homeostasis and suggest that other players may be involved in ciliary targeting of INPP5E.

Mutations in *Aipl1* result in early and rapid loss of PR cells (Table S1). $D_{50} < 0.55$ months for the four germline alleles shown in Figure 6, $Aipl1^{tm1Mad}$, $Aipl1^{tvrm127}$, $Aipl1^{tm1Visu}$, and $Aipl1^{tvrm119}$ [21,39,136]. AIPL1 is a protein chaperone that mediates the folding of phosphodiesterase 6 (PDE6), a key component of the visual transduction pathway that regulates cGMP levels (see Section 5.2.2. below) [137]. AIPL1 binding is promoted by prenylation of PDE6 subunits [137]. In *Aipl1* mutants, PDE6 subunits are greatly diminished [136], providing further evidence for the importance of lipid modification in PR viability and vision.

BBSome assembly and regulation. Disruptions in the octameric BBSome complex or associated chaperonins may cause syndromic ciliopathies such as the Bardet–Biedl syndrome and McKusick–Kaufman syndrome. In mice, most gene disruptions that affect the BBSome [138] (BBS1, BBS2, BBS4, BBS7, BBIP1, TTC8, and ARL6), and its regulators (LZTFL1, MKKS, BBS10, and BBS12) result in a moderate degeneration of PRs. For instance, PRs in homozygous mice harboring gene trap or null mutations of *Bbs4*, $Bbs4^{Gt1Nk}$ [139], and $Bbs4^{tm1Vcs}$ [140] appear to progressively decline after maturation with >90% loss at 7 months of age. The delay and lack of ciliogenesis defects suggests that there may be some functional redundancy amongst components of the BBSome.

5.2.2. Category 02: Visual Transduction

Overview. Mutant alleles of genes encoding proteins responsible for light detection comprise a second category of models (Category 02: Visual Transduction; Figure 1c, Table S1). The multistep phototransduction process that detects light and amplifies this signal is similar in rod and cone cells, but the specific proteins that catalyze many of the steps are often unique to each cell type [141]. Phototransduction is initiated by the response of opsin-based light-sensitive G protein coupled receptors that are covalently linked to vitamin A retinal as a cofactor. The receptor rhodopsin (RHO) is expressed exclusively in rod cells and is optimized to detect dim green light. Cone pigments that detect short or medium wavelength visible light (OPN1SW and OPN1MW, respectively) are exclusively expressed in cone cells, in some retinal regions coordinately within the same cell. These receptors constitute >90% of OS protein and are localized to the disc membranes.

Light activation of RHO or cone pigments causes the bound retinal to isomerize from an 11-*cis* to an all-*trans* configuration, ultimately leading to its release from the receptor by hydrolysis. Isomerization results in a conformational change in the protein that alters its interaction with a bound heterotrimeric G protein, transducin, activating the exchange of GTP for GDP bound to the α subunit of this protein.

In turn, activated α transducin-GTP binds the inhibitory γ subunits of phosphodiesterase 6, releasing it from the α and β subunits of this complex, which are thereby activated to catalyze the conversion of cGMP to GMP. The ensuing reduction in cGMP levels in the OS closes the cGMP-gated cation channel, slowing the influx of Na^+ and Ca^{2+} ions, which hyperpolarizes the plasma membrane of the OS and, ultimately, the entire cell. Hyperpolarization causes Ca^{2+} channels to close at the cell synapse, which leads to a decrease in the calcium-dependent release of glutamate-containing vesicles into the synapse and activates postsynaptic bipolar neurons.

The process is regulated to ensure the highest sensitivity to illumination. Following its activation, rhodopsin is quenched by the action of arrestin, which binds to bleached opsin molecules that are phosphorylated by rhodopsin kinase. Resetting of the cell following the light flash requires the formation of cGMP from GTP, catalyzed by a membrane-bound guanylate cyclase, the subsequent closing of the cGMP-gated cation channel, and the restoration of electrolyte distribution across the plasma membrane as achieved by ion pumps and transporters. Hydrolyzed retinal is passed from the OS to the RPE as part of the visual cycle (see below), where it is re-isomerized and returned to the PR cell to regenerate bleached opsin. An additional visual cycle involving Müller cells contributes to the regeneration of cone pigments.

Visual pigments. Profound effects on PR viability are observed due to mutations that affect rod cells, which represent 97% of the PR population. Mouse models bearing *Rho* alleles exhibit semidominant and recessive rod cell loss phenotypes that vary greatly in the onset and rate, consistent with the variety of possible disease mechanisms that have been proposed for RHO mutations over decades of study. For example, some missense alleles in Table S1, such as those that encode the Pro23His, Cys110Tyr, Tyr178Cys, and Cys185Arg variants [21,142–146] may support a hypothesis that excessive RHO misfolding in the endoplasmic reticulum induces cellular stress pathways that lead to PR cell loss [147]. Although the pathways linking misfolded RHO to cell death are not fully resolved, recent studies of the Pro23His variant in cultured cells and in rats [148] or mice [145,146] suggest that stress pathways induced by the unfolded protein response are protective, and raise the possibility that increased intracellular calcium due to ER stress may cause cell death [146]. Misfolding may also explain the partial mislocalization of RHO Glu150Lys to the IS [149]. However, in this mutant, much of the protein appears to be correctly exported to the OS, where it leads to irregularly shaped and disorganized discs, possibly due to a defect in higher-order RHO organization [149]. Pro23His RHO also disrupts the orientation of discs during their morphogenesis, possibly through similar effects on higher-order structure [150].

By contrast, the effect of the Gln344Ter variant (Table S1), which is correctly folded but includes sequence extensions at the C-terminus that interfere with export to the OS [151], as well as the graded effect of heterozygous or homozygous knockout alleles *Rho^{tm1Jlem}* and *Rho^{tm1Phm}* [152,153] or the premature truncation mutant Arg107Ter (Table S1), provides evidence that a steady flow of RHO to the OS is essential for PR cell viability. These observations fit an emerging view that a proteostasis network, incorporating not only cellular stress pathways but also protein trafficking and degradation, regulates the cellular protein balance to ensure viability [147,154]. According to this view, a failure to sort vesicles bearing RHO from the Golgi to the periciliary membrane, or a partial or complete loss of the protein, leads to protein imbalance in the IS. This imbalance may induce cellular stress responses and also affect the trafficking of other molecules destined for the OS, such as other phototransduction proteins, lipids, and vitamin A, resulting in cellular toxicity. Finally, the RHO Asp190Asn variant (Table S1) appears to traffic properly to the OSs but may have structural defects that lead to constitutive signaling [155], which has been linked to PR degeneration [156]. The same mechanism may account for the effect of *Rho* mutants that result in rapid degeneration upon bright illumination [157] but were not included in Table S1 due to the dependence of the mutant phenotype on an environmental perturbation (see Discussion). Future studies of these and other models may resolve or converge the many proposed hypotheses to explain RHO-associated RD.

Based on the often profound effect of *Rho* variants on rod cell viability, it might be expected that cone pigment variants would similarly cause cone PR cell loss. However, cones remain viable for more than 1.5 years in homozygous *Opn1sw^{tm1Pugh}* mice, which show a 1000-fold decrease in transcript and produce no detectable OPN1SW by immunoblotting, histochemistry, or single-cell recording of light responses [158]. Likewise, cones are viable for at least 10 months in homozygous *Opn1mw$^{tm1a(EUCOMM)Wtsi}$* knockout mice, despite an absence of OPN1MW in immunoblotting and immunohistochemical studies [159]. These studies suggest fundamental differences in the cellular sensitivity of rod and cone cells to visual pigment deficiency. They also highlight the concern that reactivity to antibodies against cone opsins or other cone cell markers may be abolished even though the cells remain viable, and therefore may not be as reliable as counting cone nuclei [160] to assess cell loss.

Transducins.   Rod transducin subunits α, β, and γ (encoded by *Gnat1*, *Gnb1*, and *Gngt1*, respectively) form the heterotrimeric G protein complex that is essential for propagating the signal from light-activated rhodopsin. *Gnat1* knockout mice have attenuated rod responses and model congenital stationary night blindness (CSNB) [161]. Although slow PR loss was reported for this model, our measurement of ONL thickness at four weeks of age based on reported images yielded a value of 90% of wild type, matching the author's value at 13 weeks [161] and suggesting an early developmental difference rather than progressive cell loss. In support of this finding, others using the same strain reported ONL thickness was 85% of wild type at eight weeks of age with no evidence of significant cell loss up to 52 weeks of age [162]. By contrast, IRD2 mice, which are homozygous for a *Gnat1^{irdr}* allele predicted to yield a prematurely truncated polypeptide, exhibit significant rod PR cell loss (Table S1) accompanied by late cone cell loss and reduced rod-specific ERG responses [163]. Homozygous *Gnat1^{irdr}* mice may recapitulate recessive rod-cone dystrophy, which has recently been linked to human *GNAT1* variants predicted to encode prematurely truncated proteins [164–166]. The *Gnat1^{irdr}* allele was discovered independently in *rd17* mice at JAX, suggesting a founder effect [167,168].

Gnb1 knockout mice have not been studied due to embryonic and perinatal lethality. However knockout alleles of the gene encoding rod γ transducin, *Gngt1^{tm1Dgen}* and *Gngt1^{tm1Ogk}*, result in PR loss that is more rapid than in *Gnat1* mutants [169,170]. In these strains, GNGT1 deficiency is accompanied by a 6- to 50-fold post-translational reduction of GNAT1 and GNB1, indicating a key role of the transducin γ subunit in complex assembly. *Gngt1^{tm1Dgen}*-associated degeneration is rescued by heterozygous *Gnb1$^{Gt(prvSStrap)4B8Yiw}$* mice [171], which express retinal GNB1 at 50% of wild type levels. This result suggests that the toxicity of GNGT1-deficiency is due to an excess of improperly assembled GNB1, which is targeted for degradation but exceeds the capacity of the proteasome [171]. This observation supports the proteostasis network model of PR degeneration [154].

Among genes encoding cone transducin subunits α, β, and γ (*Gnat2*, *Gnb3*, and *Gngt2*), only *Gnat2* alleles have been reported to cause PR loss. A progressive reduction of cone cell ERG responses and a 27% decrease in PNA-positive cells at 12 months of age in homozygous *Gnat2^{tm1Erica}* mice (Table S1) is consistent with cone PR loss [172]. However, cone nuclei were not counted directly, so it is possible that cone cell loss is less pronounced than reported. The predicted GNAT2 Asp173Gly substitution in this model may alter guanine nucleotide binding [172], although how this change might cause cell loss is unresolved. Interestingly, mislocalized cone opsin OPN1MW in this model suggests endoplasmic reticulum stress, which is often associated with PR degeneration. *Gnat2^{cpfl3}* mice (Table S1) show no cone cell loss for at least 14 weeks but exhibit a slow loss of rod cells [173]. In contrast to these models, a recently developed *Gnat2* knockout strain abolishes GNAT2 function without PR loss or dysmorphology in the oldest mice examined at 9 months of age [174]. Although human *GNAT1*-variants are a rare cause of achromatopsia [175], a stationary congenital colorblindness, the clinical presentation is variable and some cases are associated with a reduction in visual acuity with age [176] that may suggest progressive cone cell loss. The available mouse alleles may help to identify disease mechanisms that contribute to this phenotypic variability.

Phosphodiesterase 6. Rod phosphodiesterase 6 consists of a catalytic $\alpha\beta$ complex encoded by *Pde6a* and *Pde6b* and two inhibitory γ subunits encoded by *Pde6g*. The control of cGMP levels by this enzyme is expected to affect both PR function and viability, as cGMP has a central role in the phototransduction cascade and PR cell metabolism [177], and elevated cGMP levels have been linked to PR cell loss [178]. Indeed, *Pde6a* and *Pde6b* mutants show depressed ERG responses at an early age and rapid PR loss with D_{50} values of 11–30 days (Figure 6, Table S1). A study of *Pde6a* mutations on the same strain background made use of an allelic series that varied in disease severity [179]. The order of disease progression due to the alleles reported in this study, *nmf282* (Val685Met; fastest) > *tm1.1Bewi* (Arg562Trp) > *nmf363* (Asp670Gly; slowest), is the same as assessed by D_{50} (Figure 6). This allelic series led to a correlation of more rapid PR degeneration with an increased number of cGMP-positive PR cells [179]. The same trend in the progression of disease in *Pde6a^{nmf282}* and *Pde6a^{nmf363}* mice was found earlier [180], but an opposite cGMP result was obtained, possibly due to the assessment of total retinal cGMP rather than a count of cGMP-positive PR cells [179] (a 0.1-month difference in the D_{50} of *Pde6a^{nmf363}* mice measured in the two studies may reflect strain differences that might also contribute to the difference in findings). The later study also combined two alleles that matched human *PDE6A* variants to create a compound heterozygote [179], mirroring the more typical situation in human genetic disease. Further, the allelic series highlighted a non-apoptotic cell death mechanism involving calpain rather than the expected caspase-mediated apoptotic process [179]. Both elevated cGMP and calpain activation have been observed in other mouse RD models [181]. Thus, allelic series as used in these studies are informative for assessing disease mechanisms and identifying potential differences in treatment efficacy that may reflect disease severity.

Of the *Pde6b* alleles described, *Pde6b^{rd1}* and *Pde6b^{rd10}* have been used most extensively as PR degeneration models. *Pde6b^{rd10}* disease develops later, providing a longer window of opportunity to test therapeutic efficacy (Figure 6). The *Pde6b^{atrd1}* model has an even slower progression (D_{50} = 0.71) than *Pde6b^{rd10}* mice (D_{50} = 0.65), which may make it more attractive for assessing the variation in treatment with disease severity (Figure 6, Table S1). Finally, loss of the inhibitory subunit in homozygous *Pde6g^{tm1Goff}* mice did not lead to an expected increase in catalytic activity; instead PDE6G was found to be essential for activation and possibly stable assembly of the holoenzyme [182].

Cone phosphodiesterase 6 includes two catalytic α subunits encoded by *Pde6c* and two inhibitory γ subunits encoded by *Pde6h*. The *Pde6c^{cpfl1}* mutation leads to severely reduced cone ERG response at three weeks and progressive cone PR loss with age [15] as determined by counting cone nuclei (Bo Chang, unpublished data, presented in Table S1). This model mimics achromatopsia in humans, which is sometimes accompanied by cone PR cell loss [183]. Surprisingly, *Pde6h* knockout mice show no detectable functional cone loss or degeneration, likely due to the expression of the *Pde6g* subunit in mouse cones, which may compensate for PDE6H loss [184]. Variants in human *PDE6H* cause achromatopsia [185,186] but cone cell loss has not been reported.

Cyclic nucleotide gated channels and cation exchanger. The decrease in cGMP levels resulting from PDE6 activation leads to the closing of cyclic nucleotide cation channels in the OS plasma membrane of both rods and cones. Channel closing diminishes the inward flux of Na$^+$ and Ca^{2+} ions that maintain the PR cell in a hyperpolarized state. The rod protein encoded by *Cnga1* and *Cngb1* is an $\alpha_3\beta_1$ heterotetramer, in which the β subunit is a long isoform, CNGB1a [187,188]. *Cnga1* mutations have not yet been described. Rod OSs of homozygous *Cngb1^{tm1.1Biel}* mice yield no detectable CNGB1a or CNGA1, and rapid PR loss is observed [189]. Together with evidence that CNGA1, but not CNGB1a, is capable of self-oligomerizing in heterologous expression systems, this result suggests that CNGB1 plays a critical role in stabilizing CNGA1 for channel assembly during synthesis in the secretory pathway and/or subsequent transport to the OS. Although the mechanisms leading to PR cell loss are unknown, low intracellular Ca^{2+} may overactivate guanylyl cyclase and cause toxicity due to elevated cGMP [189].

The cone channel encoded by *Cnga3* and *Cngb3* functions as an $\alpha_2\beta_2$ tetramer. Due to the absence of downstream synaptic signaling associated with channel defects, mutations in both genes result in a loss of cone ERG responses modeling achromatopsia. In addition, the alleles included in Table S1, $Cnga3^{cpfl5}$, $Cnga3^{tm1Biel}$, $Cngb3^{cpfl10}$, and $Cngb3^{tm1Dgen}$ result in cone PR degeneration as assessed by marker analysis, although confirmation of cell loss by a direct nuclear count was lacking in some studies. The mechanism of cell death is unknown in these models, but by analogy may involve elevated cGMP as hypothesized in rods.

A critical component of phototransduction is SLC24A1 (also called NCKX1), which exports sodium and calcium ions in exchange for potassium. This activity is responsible for the decrease in intracellular Ca^{2+} upon closing of the cGMP-gated channels. Homozygous $Slc24a1^{tm1Xen}$ mice exhibit slow degeneration, possible due to malformation of OS discs [190].

Guanylyl cyclase and activating proteins. Photoreceptor guanylyl cyclases function as homodimers encoded by two genes in mice, $Gucy2e$, and $Gucy2f$. In the homozygous $Gucy2e^{tm1Gar}$ model, D_{50} was >12 months (Figure 6), indicating very slow rod PR cell loss, while cone cell numbers decreased rapidly to 33% of controls in 5 weeks [191]. Cone loss with rod preservation has been observed in Leber congenital amaurosis cases linked to variants of the human $Gucy2e$ ortholog, GUCY2D [192]. However, $Gucy2e^{tm1Gar}$ mice are not considered to model this disease because rod ERG function, though diminished, is still detectable [191]. Although $Gucy2f$ knockout did not cause PR cell loss, double knockout of both guanylyl cyclase genes resulted in moderate degeneration [193]. Rod and cone ERG responses were abolished in this model, suggesting that the residual function in $Gucy2e^{tm1Gar}$ mice was due to compensatory activity expressed from $Gucy2f$. The mechanism of PR cell loss in these models is unlikely to involve elevated cGMP as the enzymes needed for its production are ablated. The post-translational downregulation of other phototransduction proteins in double-knockout mice [193] may indicate a disruption of the proteostasis network that could explain PR cell loss.

Guanylyl cyclase activator proteins provide a feedback loop to restore cGMP levels. When intracellular Ca^{2+} is high, these proteins inhibit guanylyl cyclase; when Ca^{2+} levels are low, they switch to an activating Mg^{2+}-bound conformation that promotes cGMP synthesis. This Ca^{2+}-sensitive regulation permits PR cells to reestablish cGMP levels following light exposure due to lowered intracellular Ca^{2+}, thereby resetting the cell for another stimulus. Double knockout of $Guca1a$ and $Guca1b$, which encode the activator proteins in both rods and cones, had no detectable effect on retinal morphology up to eight months of age [194]. However, homozygous $Guca1a^{tm1.1Hunt}$ mice, which have a Glu155Gly missense substitution identical to one found associated with a severe dominant cone dystrophy [195], result in rapid loss of cones and subsequently rods (Figure 6, Table S1). This mutation, like others associated with the human disease, may constitutively activate guanylyl cyclase due to a defect in calcium sensing [196], leading to cytotoxic accumulation of cGMP.

Recovery from light stimuli. Mechanisms to terminate the phototransduction cascade and recover the PR cell for additional stimuli include the phosphorylation of activated RHO by a $Grk1$-encoded kinase and the binding of Sag-encoded arrestin to the phosphorylated RHO. The binding of SAG limits transducin access to RHO and thereby prevents further activation of transducin and downstream processes. Significantly, defects in either gene induce photoreceptor cell loss, likely due to the accumulation of excess cGMP arising from unregulated active RHO. Early studies aimed at elaborating the role of the SAG or GRK1 proteins used mice raised in the dark [197,198], as typical vivarium cyclic light–dark rearing conditions were described as leading to rapid degeneration. Subsequent studies of homozygous Sag^{tm1Jnc} [199] or homozygous $Grk1^{tvrm207}$ mice [200] reveal slow PR cell loss with D_{50} > 10 months under normal rearing conditions.

5.2.3. Category 03: Metabolism

Overview. Inborn errors of metabolism constitute a heterogeneous group of disorders that affect metabolic pathways due to underlying genetic defects [201] and result in abnormalities in the synthesis or catabolism of biomolecules [201,202]. Many such inborn errors of metabolism are known to be associated with PR cell loss, manifested either as a primary ocular defect or as part of a systemic disease [201]. PR cells, with their high metabolic activity, are particularly vulnerable to defects in metabolism of biomolecules such as lipids, carbohydrates, nucleotides, and proteins, which provide energy and serve many other functions described below. Additionally, since organelles such as mitochondria and lysosomes are the major sites for cellular energy production and homeostasis, defects in organellar metabolism and function are also known to cause PR degeneration. The PR cell loss associated with different metabolic diseases varies in the age of onset, severity, and rate of progression (Figure 6, Table S1) and the underlying genetic defects can be categorized based on the type of biomolecular metabolism or the subcellular location of the pathways affected.

Biomolecular metabolism: lipids. PRs are extremely rich in lipids, which make up to 15% of their cellular wet weight as compared to 1% in most other cell types [203,204]. Phospholipids and cholesterol represent 90–95% and 4–6% (w/w) of total lipids, respectively [205]. The major phospholipids in rod outer segments include phosphatidylethanolamine, phosphatidylcholine, large amounts of phosphatidylserine, along with small amounts of sphingomyelin, phosphatidylinositol, and phosphatidic acid [205]. It has been suggested that the phospholipids in OS membranes are metabolically active and involved in generation of physiological mediators, and changes in metabolism of glycerolipids have been associated with transduction of visual stimuli [205]. Cholesterol has been reported to modulate the function of rhodopsin, a major protein of the OS membranes, by influencing membrane lipid properties [206]. Low-density lipoproteins (LDLs) are reported to be significant suppliers of PR lipids, especially cholesteryl esters [207,208]. The OSs of PRs are particularly rich in very-long-chain polyunsaturated fatty acids (PUFA), such as docasohexaenoic acid (DHA), which is considered to be essential for visual function [209], and phospholipid-containing DHA is suggested to help in isomerization of 11-cis-retinal to the all-trans form, which is further reduced for its entry into the visual cycle [210]. Recently, DHA has also been implicated in the maintenance of OS homeostasis [211] and mediating PR cell survival [212,213].

Thus, it is not surprising that disorders of lipid metabolism cause inherited PR degeneration. For example, mouse models for mutations in the elongation of very-long-chain fatty acids-like 4 (Elovl4) gene are reported to show features resembling Stargardt-like macular dystrophy in humans with cone degeneration preceding that of rods [214,215]. Mutations in genes involved in phospholipid metabolism such as Lpcat1 cause rapid PR degeneration (90% and 75% degeneration in Lpcat1^{rd11} and Lpcat1$^{rd11-2J}$ alleles, respectively by 47 days) [216]. Similarly, mutations in genes involved in cholesterol biosynthesis such as Nsdhl [217] or in the biosynthesis and regulation of DHA-containing phospholipids, such as Agpat3 and Adipor1, respectively [210], also cause PR degeneration, confirming the importance of lipids in preserving PR integrity. Since membrane phospholipid asymmetry is critical to performing various biological functions, mutations in genes important for its generation and maintenance, also lead to PR degeneration. For example, mutations in Atp8a2, a type of P4-ATPase that translocates and maintains phospholipid asymmetry show a 30–40% PR degeneration by two months of age [218]. Similarly, conditional inactivation of Tmem30a, known to be required for folding and transport of several P4-ATPases to their plasma membrane destination [219,220], also results in severe PR degeneration [221]. Tmem30a knockout mice exhibit a more severe phenotype compared to Atp8a2 knockout mice, possibly because Tmem30a binds multiple P4-ATPases [221].

Biomolecular metabolism: carbohydrate and nucleotide energy metabolism. The retina, and in particular PRs, have a high metabolic rate [222,223] to support functions that are energetically demanding, such as phototransduction during constant illumination, maintenance of ion gradients in darkness, and performing anabolic metabolism to replace the approximately 10% of OSs that are lost every day to phagocytosis by RPE cells [223]. RPE cells also perform many energy demanding functions, such as maintenance of appropriate ionic and fluid composition in the subretinal space, uptake and conversion of all-trans-retinol to 11-cis-retinal and its transport back to photoreceptor cells, and OS phagocytosis. This high energy requirement makes the retina and RPE particularly vulnerable to functional deficits induced by deficits in energy metabolism [222]. The retina relies on blood-derived glucose and oxygen for its energy requirements. Additionally, PR cells use excess lactate obtained from Müller glial cells and convert it to pyruvate to provide energy via oxidative phosphorylation [222]. In addition to carbohydrates, the retina uses fatty acids [224] and nucleotides for its energy requirements [223].

Thus, neuronal activity and energy metabolism are tightly coupled and any mutations at the level of glucose, fatty acid or nucleotide biosynthesis can lead to PR degeneration. For example, mice lacking *Hkdc1*, which encodes a kinase found in the IS that phosphorylates glucose to glucose-6-phosphate, show 40% PR degeneration by 17 months [225]. Mice mutant for *Vldlr*, which encodes the receptor facilitating the uptake of triglyceride-derived fatty acids, show reduced cellular uptake and availability of fatty acids for energy production [224]. For some alleles of *Vldlr* (*Vldlr^{m1Btlr}* and *Vldlr^{tm1Her}*), more than 50% of PRs are lost by 12–14 months [226,227], with cones being affected more significantly than rods [228]. The decrease in net available energy may lead to greater cone loss, as cones have been reported to require three times more energy than rods [222]. Similarly, while in some cases, mutations in genes involved in nucleotide metabolism such as *Nampt*, show embryonic lethality [229], others such as mutation in *Nmnat1*, show severe PR degeneration by 4–6 months [230].

Biomolecular metabolism: hormones. The physiology of eye is also dependent on the action of several hormones [231]. Mouse models mutant for thyroid hormone metabolizing genes, such as *Dio3*, which is important for local amplification of triiodothyronine (T3), show selectively detrimental effects on cone cells [232]. This confirms the proposed role of thyroid hormone signaling in regulating cone viability and cone opsin expression [232,233]. Melatonin, a hormone that plays a role in sleep patterns, is known to have protective role against oxidative stress and apoptosis, and regulates retinal circadian rhythms [234]. A mouse model, mutant for the melatonin hormone receptor *Mtnr1a*, shows very slow PR degeneration (25% in 18 months) [235].

Biomolecular metabolism: oxidative stress. The eye is constantly subjected to oxidative stress due to daily exposure to light, atmospheric oxygen, and high metabolic activities [236]. Reactive oxygen species (ROS) are derived from diatomic oxygen and processes such as mitochondrial respiration that form superoxide anion radicals, toxic bis-retinoids that undergo photo-oxidation, and lipids, such as PUFAs, that undergo peroxidation [237]. Having unpaired electrons confers a great degree of ROS reactivity that can damage biomolecules such as DNA, lipids and proteins, and organelles including mitochondria and lysosomes [238,239], thereby impairing their biological functions [203,236]. Compared to other cells, non-proliferative postmitotic cells such as PRs and RPE cells are particularly sensitive to oxidative damage due to the apparent absence of a DNA damage detection system [240–242].

Under physiological conditions, cellular redox homeostasis is maintained by a balance between ROS generation and antioxidant systems [236]. Antioxidant enzymes such as *Sod1*, *Sod2*, and *Gpx4* are known to play a major role in ROS scavenging and changes in their expression or activity or both are reported to cause increased oxidative stress and are associated with diseases such as age-related macular degeneration (AMD) [243]. For example, mutations in the *Sod1* gene, encoding a cytosolic Cu-Zn superoxide dismutase that catalyzes the conversion of superoxide to hydrogen peroxide, are known to cause PR degeneration [244]. *Sod2*, which encodes a mitochondrial Mn superoxide dismutase, is required for survival and mutations in this gene lead to embryonic lethality [244,245]. Genes such as *Nxnl1* and *Nxnl2*, known as rod-derived cone viability factors are also suggested to have antioxidant function and show cone degeneration when mutated [246,247], with *Nxnl1* also showing a progressive rod cell loss [246]. Similarly, a mouse model for loss of *Ttpa*, coding for a protein that transports vitamin E, which is known to have antioxidant function, also shows 40% PR degeneration by 20 months [248].

Organellar metabolism: lysosomes. The lysosome, a subcellular organelle is critical for performing several vital functions such as degradation of extracellular and intracellular material, nutrient sensing, energy metabolism, and maintaining cellular homeostasis [249]. Lysosomes contain a wide variety of hydrolytic enzymes that enzymatically degrade biomolecules such as polysaccharides, lipids, etc. [250]. Defects in lysosomal function results in lysosomal storage disorders, a group of inherited metabolic disorders sharing a common biochemical feature of accumulating incompletely degraded metabolites within the lysosomes. Lysosomal storage disorders are generally classified by the composition of the material accumulated within them and often differ depending on the lysosomal proteins affected, which reflect different cell biological processes that are affected but terminating in a similar pathology of reduced clearance of metabolic aggregates.

RD is an early consequence of lysosomal storage diseases, especially in neuronal ceroid lipofuscinoses (NCL) [251], also called Batten disease, an early-onset neurodegenerative disease with other systemic features such as dementia and epilepsy [252]. NCL may be caused by disruption of genes encoding lysosomal enzymes (*Ppt1* and *Cln5*) and membrane proteins (*Mfsd8*) as well as ER membrane (*Cln6* and *Cln8*) and secretory pathway (*Grn*) proteins, and is characterized by a common lysosomal accumulation of ceroid. Similar to the early retinal phenotype reported for most human NCLs, most mouse models for NCL disease show an early onset of PR degeneration, beginning at 1 month of age and showing greater than 60% degeneration by 6–9 months [253–256]. Additionally, similar to the adult-onset reported for mutations in human GRN, the mouse model for loss of *Grn* also shows a late onset PR degeneration by 12 months [257].

Mouse models for other lysosomal disorders, namely, mucopolysaccharidosis and mucolipidosis due to mutations in lysosomal proteins required for the breakdown of glycosaminoglycans and enzymes required for phosphorylation of glycoproteins, respectively, also develop PR degeneration. For example, mouse models for mucopolysaccharidosis with a mutation in *Naglu* present with a slowly progressive rod-cone degeneration [258], and for mucolipidosis with a mutation in *Gnptab* develop a severe PR degeneration with complete PR loss by 10 months [259].

The lysosome receives materials for degradation via two major pathways, autophagy and phagocytosis. Phagocytosis has an important function in maintaining retinal health since 10% of the OSs are phagocytosed daily by the RPE cells to dispose of waste such as photo-oxidative products while retaining and recycling useful contents back to the PR cells [260]. Phagocytosis by RPE requires its own machinery for processes such as recognition (e.g., *Cd36*), engulfment (e.g., *Mertk*), and degradation (lysosomal enzymes) of the extracellular material. Disruption of the phagocytic machinery due to absence/mutations in proteins involved in the phagocytic pathway, therefore, have severe consequences for PRs and can lead to PR cell death. Mouse models for mutations in genes involved in phagocytosis such as *Mertk*, *Cd36*, and *Rab28* show PR degeneration with the loss of *Mertk* showing a more severe phenotype (>80% degeneration by 60 days for *Mertk*[tm1Grl] and *Mertk*[tm1Gkm]) [261,262] than loss of *Cd36* (17% degeneration at 12 month) [263], and the model for *Rab28* loss showing a more cone-specific response [264].

Autophagy is another lysosome-mediated degradation process essential for maintaining cellular homeostasis [265]. Autophagic flux, the complete dynamic process of autophagy, includes multiple steps involving the formation of phagosomes and autophagosomes, autophagosome fusion with lysosomes, the degradation of the intra-autophagosomal contents, and recycling [266]. Thus, both lysosomal function and autophagy are interconnected wherein disruption of the hydrolytic functions of lysosomes impairs autophagic flux and, conversely, lysosomal function requires normal flux through autophagy [267,268]. In the retina, autophagy plays a dual role: promoting cell survival against harmful stress, and cell death. High basal autophagic levels are maintained in RPE and PR cells. RPE cells being post-mitotic phagocytes are not self-renewing; the autophagy of intracellular components is therefore essential for a normal cellular function of the RPE [265]. In PR cells, autophagy occurs during various cellular activities such as OS degeneration [269], rhodopsin protein expression [270], visual cycle function, and PR apoptosis [271]. Mouse models of conditional inactivation of autophagy genes such as *Atg5*, *Atg7*, and *Rb1cc1* in RPE cells show that these genes are indeed important for survival of the animal and show PR degeneration.

Organellar metabolism: mitochondria. Mitochondria, often referred to as "the powerhouse of the cell", are the major site for cellular energy production in the form of ATP via oxidative phosphorylation. They also perform other important functions such as ROS generation and scavenging, calcium regulation, steroid, and nucleotide metabolism, regulation of intermediary metabolism, and initiation of apoptosis [272]. Oxidative phosphorylation is carried out by the mitochondrial respiratory chain, which consists of five complexes located along the inner mitochondrial membrane. These complexes, in an intricately organized series of biochemical events, synthesize ATP from ADP in response to cellular energy demands. A large number of mitochondria are present in the rod and cone IS and in RPE cells. The total surface area of the inner mitochondrial membrane in cones is 3-fold greater than in rods, presumably accommodating more respiratory chain enzymes to generate more ATP. Cones require more ATP than rods as they do not saturate in bright light and use more ATP/sec for light transduction and phosphorylation [222].

Defective cellular energy production due to abnormal oxidative phosphorylation in mitochondria can therefore lead to PR degeneration. A mouse model for the Leu122Pro mutation of OPA3, a protein hypothesized to be important for maintaining the inner mitochondrial membrane, is reported to cause a multisystemic disease characterized by severely reduced vision, loss of ganglion cells and PR degeneration (by 50%) at 3–4 months of age, a much more severe progression than observed in humans [273]. Similarly, a mouse model for a mutation in the gene for NAD-specific mitochondrial enzyme isocitrate dehydrogenase 3 (*Idh3a*), catalyzing the rate limiting step of TCA cycle, also causes an early and severe PR degeneration (more than 90%) by 90 days [274].

Extra-mitochondrial components of the tricarboxylic acid cycle and oxidative phosphorylation machinery have been localized to the rod OS [275]. It has been hypothesized that perturbation of this machinery results in excess ROS production, leading to PR cell death due to oxidative stress [275–277]. Mutations in a subset of mouse RD models in Table S1 alter genes (*Mpc1, Opa3, Idh3a, Impdh1,* and *Oat*) that encode mouse homologs of mitochondria-associated proteins identified in bovine rod OS [275]. Of these, only IDH3A is directly involved in cellular energy production [274]; the others may influence oxidative phosphorylation or the TCA cycle indirectly, possibly altering the generation of ROS. It may be of interest to determine whether PR cell loss in these mouse models correlates with an altered distribution of extra-mitochondrial oxidative phosphorylation proteins in the rod OS [278], or an increased ROS production, which can be measured in retinal explants [279].

Organellar metabolism: peroxisomes. Peroxisomes are subcellular organelles with various catabolic and anabolic functions such as catabolism of long chain fatty acids and biosynthesis of DHA and bile acids [280]. Several childhood multisystem disorders with prominent ophthalmological manifestations have been ascribed to the malfunction of the peroxisomes, either at the level of peroxisomal biogenesis (PBD) or single enzyme deficiencies [281]. While little is known about the metabolic role of these organelles in retina, studies have shown the presence of peroxisomes in nearly all layers of retina and RPE, albeit with differential expression of lipid metabolizing enzymes, suggesting different functions in different cell types [282]. For example, Zellweger spectrum disorder (ZSD) is a disease continuum known to result from inherited defects in *Pex* genes essential for normal peroxisome assembly. Mice homozygous for the G844D point mutation in *Pex1* show a decreased ERG response and loss of cone PRs (up to 80%) by 22 weeks, recapitulating the abnormal retinal function phenotype in ZSD patients with mild disease [283]. The retinal pathology in such disorders suggests the importance of peroxisomes in maintaining retinal homeostasis and function.

5.2.4. Category 04: Visual Cycle and Retinoids

The visual cycle reisomerizes vitamin A retinal that has been released from visual pigments in PR cells, allowing regeneration of the bleached pigments and the subsequent detection of additional light stimuli. The process is catalyzed by enzymes located in PR and RPE cells, so the retinoid intermediates in the process must be transported between them. Mutation of genes involved in the visual cycle pathway cause PR degeneration, in most instances with a moderate to slow progression depending on the allele and the genetic background. Most *Rpe65* mutant alleles show moderately slow PR cell loss (D_{50} = 7–11 months) [284–288]. Allelic effects are observed in models bearing missense mutations, *Rpe65^{tm1Lrcb}* [289] or *Rpe65$^{tm1.1Kpal}$* [290], which cause slower progression than observed in *Rpe65^{tm1Tmr}* knockout mice [285–288]. *Abca4^{tm1Ght}* on the BALB/c strain, which also carries a homozygous *Rpe65* Leu450Met mutation, show a late-onset PR degeneration with 40% loss by 11 months of age [291].

By contrast, the same *Abca4*^{tm1Ght} mutation on a 129S4/SvJae background results in abnormal thickening of Bruch's membrane but normal ONL nuclei count and thickness [292]. Several visual cycle mutant alleles have other retinal abnormalities but normal ONL nuclei/thickness. For example, *Abca4*$^{tm1.1Rsmy}$ causes only autofluorescence and A2E accumulation [293] and *Abca4*$^{tm2.1Kpal}$ on C57BL/6*129Sv leads to a RPE defect but normal ONL nuclei count and thickness [294]. In addition, PR degeneration in *Abca4* mutants can be induced by light exposure [295] or through interaction with other genes such as *Rdh8* [296–298]. The *Lrat*^{tm1Kpal} mutation on a 129S6/SvEvTac*C57BL/6J background results in mild PR degeneration, with <10% loss at 4–5 months [299]. However, a 35% decrease in rod OS length was also reported in this model, indicating the importance of the visual cycle for OS maintenance. Another allele, *Lrat*$^{tm1.1Bok}$, showed a similar loss of rod OS length and 18% PR degeneration at 6 months of age [300]. The *Rbp3*^{tmGil} mutation results in the most rapid PR cell loss in this category (D_{50} = 0.79 months), possibly attributable to an early developmental role of the protein [301]. The *Rbp4*^{tm2Zhel} congenic mutation on C57BL/6J showed 20% PR cell loss in some peripheral areas and 10% in the central retina an age of 40 weeks [302]. Mutations in two genes that play a role in retinoid uptake in the eye also result in PR cell loss. The *Rtbdn*$^{tm1.1Itl}$ allele causes a slow degeneration with a 20% and 37% loss of PR nuclei at 240 days of age in heterozygotes and homozygotes, respectively. *Stra6*^{tm1Nbg} mice exhibit a normal number of rod PR nuclei but significant cone PR cell loss as detected by the cone-specific marker peanut agglutinin [303]. PR cell loss in *Stra6*$^{tm1.1Jvil}$ mice was more pronounced with vitamin A restriction [304].

5.2.5. Category 05: Synapse

PRs absorb light that passes through the anterior portion of the eye and convert the light to electrochemical signals that are transmitted through the neuroretina via synaptic connections to the optic nerve and visual cortex [305]. Thus, synapses, necessary for proper cell-to-cell communication, are critical for vision. Discussion of the complexity of PR synaptic development and function is reviewed in [306–308], and is beyond the scope of this review. Suffice to say that mutations in many of the components of synapses, such as presynaptic exocytotic proteins, endocytic proteins, calcium channels, postsynaptic receptors, and associated elements, must be properly organized to mediate transmission of signals, or can lead to visual problems [307]. It is interesting to note that disruption of some synaptic components of the secondary neurons (e.g., GRM6, GPR179, TRPM1, NYX, GNAO1, GNB5, and GNB3), while affecting function as assessed by ERG response, does not normally lead to PR degeneration [309]. This is also true of some presynaptic proteins, such as dystrophin [310] or dystroglycan [311]. However, disruption of some synaptic genes such as *Ache*, *Cabp4*, *Cacna1f*, *Cacna2d4*, and *Unc119* does lead to PR degeneration. For example, a null allele of *Ache* [312], causes a 50% loss of PR nuclei between 1.5 and 2 months and >80% by 6–8 months. Although it was initially determined that the ACHE protein played an important role in hydrolyzing acetylcholine at synapses, its isoforms are now recognized to have far reaching structural functions [313]. Additionally, it has been shown that the loss of secondary neurons in the null allele model is likely to cause secondary PR cell loss [312]. Null or spontaneous alleles of synaptic genes that encode subunits of calcium channels that regulate the release of neurotransmitters, and the development and maturation of exocytic function of PR ribbon synapses, *Cacna1f* [314] and *Cacna2d4* [315,316], respectively, show a slower rate of degeneration. By two months, there are approximately 10–25% of PR nuclei that have degenerated. CABP4, a protein that regulates calcium levels and neurotransmitter release at PR synapses, and modulates CACNA1F and other calcium channel activity shows a similar rate of PR degeneration of 10–25% loss at 2 months [317]. UNC119, which localizes to PR synapses (and IS) and is hypothesized to play a role in neurotransmitter release, also leads to a relatively late onset, slower rate of PR degeneration [318]. Interestingly, Haeseleer has described an interaction between synaptic genes *Cabp4* and *Unc119* [319]. It is likely that other synaptic proteins will also lead to PR degeneration through either a primary or secondary effect and that the interactions among the synaptic proteins will play a significant role in determining the relative rate of the degenerative process.

5.2.6. Category 06: Channels and Transporters

Ions such as sodium, potassium, and chloride, play important roles in the visual circuitry [320]. Their intracellular concentrations and movements within the cell, and between cells and the environment are exquisitely regulated by channels and transporters. Due to the importance of maintaining appropriate levels of these ions for proper function and maintenance of PRs, it is not surprising that disruption of these genes can lead to PR degeneration. Members of the ClC family of chloride channels, such as *Clcn2*, *Clcn3*, and *Clcn7*, show particularly early and significant PR degeneration. Compared to other channels in this section, they appear to have an enriched expression in the RPE. A 50% PR cell loss can be seen as early as 14–16 days in certain models with disruptions in these genes [231,321–323]. Indeed, rapid progression of PR cell loss is observed in mice carrying any of the following alleles: $Clcn2^{nmf240}$, $Clcn2^{tm1Tjj}$, $Clcn3^{tm1Lamb}$, $Clcn3^{tm1Tjj}$, $Clcn7^{tm1Tjj}$, $Clcn7^{tm2Tjj}$, and $Clcn7^{tm4.1Tjj}$ [231,321,322,324–327]. A similar rapid and complete loss of PRs is seen when *Atp1b2*, a Na^+/K^+-ATPase thought to play a role in cell adhesion, is inactivated [328]. A targeted mutation in *Slc6a6*, which encodes a taurine/beta-alanine transporter, also leads to rapid, complete degeneration [329]. In contrast, inactivation of the bicarbonate, amino acid transporters, and Na^+/H^+ exchangers, *Slc4a7*, *Slc7a14*, and *Slc9a8* results in a later onset, but still severe PR degeneration [330–332]. Mouse models bearing mutations affecting BSG, a protein that has a role in targeting monocarboxylate transporters such as SLC16A1 to the plasma membrane, or REEP6, which mediates trafficking of clathrin-coated vesicles from the ER to the plasma membrane at outer plexiform layer sites enriched for synaptic ribbon protein STX3, also fall in this latter late onset/severe category [333,334]. *Asic3*, an acid sensing Na^+ channel, *Clcc1*, an intracellular chloride channel, and *Slc7a14*, an intracellular arginine transporter, all cause moderately slow degeneration when mutated [331,335,336]. Slowly progressive PR cell loss is also caused by mutation of *Mfsd2a*, which encodes a sodium-dependent lipid transporter responsible for maintaining a high DHA concentration in the retina is important for OS homeostasis, as discussed in Category 03 [337]. More data are needed to see if sensing and intracellular channels/transporters generally have milder phenotypes.

5.2.7. Category 07: Adhesion and Cytoskeletal

Proper structure of the retina is developed through protein interactions between cells and within cells. The spatial and laminar organization of the retina is maintained through junctional interactions between cells that impart mechanical support to maintain retinal architecture, a means for bidirectional communication (e.g., extracellular changes to the cell and from the cell to its environment), and together can form diffusion barriers. Within cells, cytoskeletal architecture is maintained through interactions of proteins with actin, intermediate filaments, and microtubules that serve to maintain cell morphology and polarity, and as discussed elsewhere, intracellular trafficking, contractility, motility, and cell division. Examples of disrupted proteins that lead to gaps between cell layers, presumably through aberrant adhesion, are mutations in *Adam9* and *Rs1*. The null allele of *Adam9*, a single pass transmembrane protein with disintegrin and metalloprotease domains that has been shown to interact with a number of integrins [338], leads to aberrant adhesion between the apical processes of the RPE and OS and to late onset PR degeneration [339]. Likewise, mutations in RS1, a protein with a discoid domain, which has been implicated in cell adhesion and cell–cell interactions [340] lead to a splitting of the inner retinal layer and progressive PR loss [341–343]. RS1 binding to phospholipids on the membrane surface, together with other proteins [340] may provide a stabilizing scaffold that is important in cell–matrix, cell–cell, and cytoskeletal organization.

CRB1 and its interacting partners, such MPP3, MPP5, and PARD6A, have been shown to be important in establishing proper retinal lamination presumably through their essential roles in establishing cellular apical basal polarity [344]. A primary defect of a disruption in CRB1 is the fragmentation of the outer limiting membrane [345,346]. As reviewed previously [344,347], the outer limiting membrane consists of adherens/tight junctions formed in part by the CRB1 complexes between Müller glia and the rod or cone IS that form a diffusion barrier. Loss of components of the CRB1 complexes (CRB1-MPP5-PATJ, CRB1-MPP5-MPDZ, and CRB1-PARD6A-MPP5-MPP3/MPP4) leads to lamination defects with formation of rosettes and a progressive loss of PRs. Although yet to be reported, it is likely that mutations in PATJ, PARD3, MPDZ, and MPP4 will lead to similar disease phenotypes, as a reduction in ERG response in MPDZ mutants [348] and a reduced ERG with abnormal retinal morphology have been indicated for PARD3 mutants [41,43].

Equally important to the function and maintenance of the retina are the intracellular components that make up the cytoskeletal cell structure. Disruption of proteins that interact with actin intracellularly have been shown to lead to PR degeneration. For example, CDC42, a small GTPase that is a key regulator of actin dynamics [349] leads to an early onset, progressive PR degeneration when disrupted. Models caused by mutations in FSCN2, an actin crosslinking protein [350,351], and by a hypomorphic variant of CTNNA1, a protein that coordinates cell surface cadherins with the intracellular actin filament network [352], show slow-paced PR cell loss. The proper localization of organelles within the cell is also mediated by the cytoskeletal architecture and can have an untoward effect when disrupted. For example, SYNE2, a nuclear outer membrane protein that binds to F-actin, tethers the nucleus to the cytoskeleton and is necessary for the structural integrity of the nucleus [353,354]. Without it, early onset, moderately paced PR cell loss occurs.

5.2.8. Category 08: Signaling

Molecules such as growth factors/cytokines, hormones, neurotransmitters, and extracellular matrix proteins, or alternatively, mechanical stimuli, are examples of signals used to communicate environmental changes to the cell. Surface or intracellular (e.g., nuclear) receptors recognize the signals and effect changes within the cell, often setting in motion amplifying transduction cascades that mediate responses such as activation or inhibition of protein activity or migration to different cellular localizations. Further, signals can also be transmitted from the cell to other cells, for example, through neurotransmitters. Since intra- and intercellular communication is crucial for the proper development or function of cells, it is not surprising that a large number of mutations in cellular signaling lead to defects in retinal development, which in turn affects PR survival. For example, vascular development is affected in mutants bearing disruptions in *Fzd5*, *Lrp5*, *Ndp*, and *Tspan12*—all components of the Wnt signaling pathway. Integral membrane frizzled receptors, of which they are 10, together with coreceptors, LRP5 and LRP6, mediate canonical Wnt signaling [355]. Thus, conditional *Fzd5* null mutants develop microphthalmia, coloboma and persistent fetal vasculature, and late-onset progressive RD [356] and *Lrp5* mutants exhibit similar vascular and retinal phenotypes [357]. Mice that are null for NDP, a ligand for FZD4, exhibit delayed retinal vasculature development, retrolental masses, disorganization of the ganglion cell layer, and occasionally focal areas of ONL absence at later stages of the disease [358]. TSPAN12, mediates NDP-FZD4-LRP5 signaling in the retinal vasculature, where it localizes, and a mutation leads to vascular defects that phenocopies disruptions in *Ndp*, *Fzd4*, and *Lrp5*, and at 3 months exhibits a 50% loss of PRs [359]. In all of these models, it is likely that the loss of PRs is caused by the aberrant retinal vasculature having secondary effects on PRs. A review by Hackam suggests that Wnt signaling may affect the apoptotic pathway and neurotrophin release, dysregulation of which may affect PR survival [360]. MFRP, which bears a CRD domain shared by all frizzled proteins, also leads to PR degeneration when disrupted [361,362], as does the human knock-in allele, p.S163R, of its bicistronic partner, CTRP5 [363]. The exact role or function of either protein has yet to be fully elucidated.

Like the frizzled-associated proteins whose pathological effects on PRs are likely to be mediated through an aberrant retinal vasculature, other signaling molecules, *Ptpn11* and *Fyn*, appear to mediate their effects on PRs through another cell type as well, in this case, Müller glia cells, and PRKQ through the RPE. A *Six3-cre* mediated conditional knockout of *Ptpn11* [364] leads to altered ERK and MAPK signaling in Müller glia and alteration in their adhesive capabilities. FYN, a Src-kinase membrane associated tyrosine kinase, localizes to Müller glia cells, and FYN deficiency leads to altered adhesion properties of Müller cells and retinal dysmorphology [365]. PRKCQ, a serine threonine protein kinase, which localizes to the lateral surface of the RPE cells, causes a reduction in adhesion between the apical processes of the RPE and OSs when it is disrupted. The reduction in adhesion may be responsible for the retinal detachment and subsequent PR loss observed in this model [366].

The family of PI3Ks or phosphoinositide 3-kinases, made up of catalytic and regulatory subunits, function to phosphorylate the inositol ring of phosphatidylinositol and thereby regulate growth, proliferation, differentiation, motility, survival, and intracellular trafficking. For example, it mediates insulin-stimulated increase in glucose uptake and glycogen synthesis and responds to signals such as FGFRs and PDGFRs. Conditional knockouts of *Pik3cb*, encoding a catalytic subunit [367] and *Pik3r1*, encoding a regulatory subunit [368], using the cone-specific CRE, Tg(OPN1LW-cre)4Yzl, lead to progressive cone PR loss. IRS2, necessary for the integration of signals from insulin and IGF1 receptors, causes an early-onset, moderately paced PR loss [369]. Additionally, a targeted conditional allele of PDGFRB developed diabetic retinopathy like features with angiogenesis, proliferative DR-like lesions, pericyte drop out, and eventual PR loss [370]. Disruption of MAP3K1, a serine/threonine kinase, which participates in the ERK, JNK, and NF-κB signaling pathways, leads to retinal laminar and vascular defects, aberrant RPE, and PR cell death [371]. SEMA4A, a transmembrane protein, also causes PR loss, most probably through its effects on endosomal sorting [372].

5.3. Category 09: Transcription Factors

In mice, cone and rod PRs are born and develop between approximately E12 and P0, and approximately E13.5 and P7, respectively, from the same multipotent retinal progenitor cell (RPC) pool [373]. PR development, orchestrated by a network of transcription factors, is divided into five phases: proliferation of multipotent RPCs, restriction of RPC competence, cell fate specification, expression of genes important for PR function, and finally, PR structural maturation [374,375]. RB1 and E2F1 function by controlling the G1 to S phase transition in the cell cycle; RB1 plays an inhibitory role until activated by phosphorylation, balancing cell proliferation and cell fate specification [376]. OTX2 is critical for fate determination, while CRX is necessary for terminal PR differentiation and acts at different steps in PR development. Transcriptional factors important for rod PR subtype specification include RORβ, NRL, and NR2E3, and for generation of the cone subtypes, TRβ2 and RXRγ [374,375]. Further, transcription factors regulate the expression of other transcription factors in the network (e.g., CRX interacts with *Nrl*, *Rorb*, and *Mef2d*, to name a few, to mediate rod differentiation, cone differentiation, and proteins necessary for the maturation of the PR, respectively).

The importance of transcription factors in retinal development has been explored in many studies resulting in a number of mouse models with different disease phenotypes (MGI JAX). In many cases, disruption of transcription factors, especially those affecting earlier phases of PR development lead to a reduction in the total number of retinal cells generated. We have only included within this category those disrupted transcription factors that eventually lead to PR degeneration. Interestingly, the onset of degeneration of the PR transcription factor models is highly variable—14 days to 2 months of age—and appears to be dependent upon the method used to generate the model and possibly background strain, as variation of severity and onset differs among different models of the same gene. Interestingly, the *Crx* models provide a series that recapitulate the clinical diagnoses of autosomal dominant cone-rod dystrophy, Leber congenital amaurosis, and late-onset dominant retinitis pigmentosa. *Crx*^{Rip} heterozygotes showed 34% degeneration at five weeks, compared to mice homozygous for the mutation, which reached 55% degeneration at the same age [377]. *Crx*$^{tm1.1Smgc}$ was also noted to have a heterozygous disease presentation more similar to a cone-rod dystrophy, while the homozygous mutant presented with a disease phenotype similar to Leber congenital amaurosis with 70% loss of PRs at one month of age [378].

Other transcriptional factors necessary for the proper maturation of the PRs, such as, MEF2D, shown to be important in regulating transcription of OS and synaptic proteins [379], or NRF1 [380], important in mitochondrial biogenesis also develop PR degeneration when disrupted. Finally, there are transcriptional factors that are important in the development or function of supporting cells such as

ONECUT1 for horizontal cells [381] and MITF for RPE and/or choroidal melanocytes [382], which affect PR survival when disrupted.

5.4. Category 10: DNA Repair, RNA Biogenesis, and Protein Modification

Among the many disrupted genes that lead to PR degeneration, several instances have been documented in genes necessary for producing fully functional proteins, from transcription through post-translational modification. Defects in these genes are likely to impact the function of many other genes that they act upon, and hence, have a greater effect. Since they play a central and basic role, when disrupted they often lead to prenatal lethality in mice, and the adult phenotype is unknown unless a conditional knockout or hypomorphic allele is generated. For example, disruption of DNA repair genes such as *Ercc1*, RNA splicing genes such as *Prpf3, Prpf6, Prpf8, Prpf31*, and *Bnc2*, and miRNA processing genes, *Dicer1* and *Dgcr8* are prenatal lethal in a homozygous state [34,383]. In contrast, homozygous null alleles of *Bmi1* [384] and *Msi1* [385], both involved in repression of regulatory genes in embryonic development, are viable, suggesting potential compensatory mechanisms for the functional loss of these genes. Thus, germline, conditional or hypomorphic models were considered in this category.

Review of genes in this category suggested that a DNA damage response network to ensure transcription in the face of DNA lesions might be required for PR cell maintenance. DNA lesions, such as pyrimidine dimers, interstrand crosslinks, or double-strand breaks (DSBs), are induced by many mechanisms that include UV radiation or free radicals. Repair of such damage is essential for DNA replication and, of particular importance for long-lived post-mitotic neuronal cells, transcription [386–388]. Proteins encoded by *Bmi1, Dgcr8, Dicer1, Elp1, Ercc1, Ercc6, Msi1, Sirt6, Top2b, Ubb*, and *Uchl3* are known to participate in the DNA damage response [387,389–398], some in transcription-coupled DNA repair. For example, BMI1 represses transcription at sites of UV-induced DNA damage to allow repair [389]; ELP1 is a required component of the Elongator complex [399], which couples RNA polymerase II to an alkyladenine glycosylase that initiates base excision repair [392]; ERCC6 promotes DSB repair in actively transcribed regions by displacing RNA polymerase from the lesion site [387], and DGCR8 interacts with both RNA polymerase II and ERCC6 to mediate transcription-coupled nucleotide excision repair of UV-induced DNA lesions [390]. Intriguingly, topoisomerase TOP2B, which creates DSBs during transcriptional activation [396], has been identified as a key regulator of transcription during the last stages of postnatal PR development [400]. Thus, DSBs in PR cells may arise in part from transcriptional activation of genes that encode components destined for the OS. Additionally supporting the importance of DNA repair to PR maintenance, Category 01 gene *Atr* encodes a master regulator of the DNA damage response that has surprisingly been linked to retinal degenerative disease and localized to the cilium [401]. Further, Category 03 gene *Nmnat1* encodes an enzyme that synthesizes nicotinamide adenine dinucleotide in the nucleus, which may regulate the large-scale polyADP-ribosylation of protein targets at sites of DNA damage [402]. Mutations in the genes encoding these proteins all result in PR cell loss [230,384,385,400,401,403–411]. Mutations in five of these genes as included in Figure 6 (*Cwc27, Ercc1, Ercc6, Sirt6*, and *Ubb*) caused moderate to slow progression of PR cell loss ($D_{50} \geq 2$ months), consistent with a steady accumulation of unresolved DNA damage with age. The rapid PR cell loss observed in *Atr^{tm1Ofc}* mice ($D_{50} = 13$ days) may reflect its direct involvement in OS development [401] in addition to the DNA damage response.

Due to the high percentage of alternatively spliced genes in the human retina [412,413], it is not surprising that mutations in mRNA splicing genes: *PRPF3, PRPF4, PRPF6, PRPF8, PRPF31, PDAP1*, and *BNC2* have been shown to lead to PR degeneration in humans [3]. In fact, in human retinal disease, 14% of disease genes are categorized as playing a role in RNA metabolism [383]. Interestingly, heterozygous humanized alleles of *PRPF3* and *PRPF8* and the null allele of *Prpf31* in mice do not recapitulate PR degeneration observed in humans but rather exhibit late-onset RPE degeneration [414]. In contrast, a hypomorphic allele of the mRNA splicing gene, *Cwc27*, with reduced viability, does lead to moderate onset PR degeneration [415]. The differences observed among species require additional studies to unravel the complexities that govern genetic interactions.

Post-translational modification, which occurs by adding modifying molecules to amino acids or removing or altering these modified amino acids, is important for proper folding, transport/trafficking, localization, function, regulation, and/or degradation of proteins. Examples of post-translational modifications include phosphorylation, glycosylation, acetylation, ubiquitination, sumoylation, methylation, and lipidation [416]. Kinases that affect activity by mediating phosphorylation states are described elsewhere, however, post-translational modification genes affecting glycosylation and lipidation/prenylation are prominent among those that lead to PR degeneration. For example, the encoded proteins of *Fkrp*, *Large1*, *Pomt1*, and *PomgnT1*, necessary for the glycosylation of alpha-dystroglycan, essential for formation of the dystroglycan complex and for proper retinal lamination, lead to moderate rates of PR degeneration when disrupted. Prenylation is critical for proper trafficking and localization of retinal proteins. Of the three genes important in the prenylation and postprenylation processes, conditional loss of *Rce1* leads to an absence of phosphodiesterase subunits PDE6A, PDE6B, and PDE6C from the rod OS, probably due to a failure to prenylate one or more of these proteins [417]. By contrast, ablation of *Icmt* does not appear to affect phosphodiesterase transport but rather results in lowered levels of prenylated proteins GNAT1, PDE6G, and GRK1 [418], which are essential PR proteins. The null mutation of farnesyl-diphosphate farnesyltransferase 1, which adds a farnesyl group to the cysteine of the CAAX amino acid motif is prenatal lethal, but as a conditional tissue specific knockout may result in the same PR effects.

Two additional types of post-translational modification involve glycylation and glutamylation of proteins essential for normal connecting cilia function. Disruption of *Ttll3*, encoding a protein-glycine ligase necessary for glycylation of tubulin, results in an absence of glycylation in PR cells, shortening of the connecting cilia, and slow PR cell loss [419]. Interestingly, PR tubulin glutamylation increased in *Ttll3* mutant mice. TTLL5, tubulin tyrosine ligase like 5, adds glutamate residues on proteins. Sun et al. [420] reported that *Ttll5* disruption leads to late onset, slowly progressive PR cell loss that phenocopied retinal disease observed in *Rpgr* mutants. Perhaps this is not surprising as these investigators determined that TTLL5 glutamylates RPGR, a modification that is necessary for normal RPGR function in the PR cilium. *Agtpbp1* encodes a metallocarboxypeptidase that deglutamylates target proteins. Its disruption in *pcd* mutants leads to abnormal tubulin glutamylation [419] and an accumulation of vesicles in the interphotoreceptor space [421], indicating the importance of proper post-translational modification for PR survival.

5.5. Category 11: Immune Response

As resident immune cells, microglia survey the retina constantly, presumably with the goal of removing unwanted debris and responding to damage arising from environmental and/or genetic stressors. They respond to damage by eliciting various responses that can range from regenerative to inflammatory depending on the type of injury. Thus, although microglia are unlikely to be instigators in RD, it may well be the case that microglia influence the severity of responses to ocular damage depending on mutations. Mutations in several genes central to the immune system lead to PR degeneration in mouse models. *Aire*[tm1.1Doi] show early onset PR degeneration with 20% of ONL thickness loss at 10 weeks with rapid progression to 60% ONL thickness loss by 18 weeks [422]. *C3ar1*[tm1Cge] mutants show very slow PR degeneration with about 20% loss at 14 months [423]. *Cd46*[tm1Atk] show different rates of PR nuclei loss in male and female mice with 23% and 31% at 12 months of age, respectively [424]. Mutations in *Cx3cr1*, normally expressed in immune cells including microglia, were associated with PR cell loss. Homozygous *Cx3cr1*[tm1Litt] [425] and *Cx3cr1*[tm1Zm] [426] mice on the same C57BL/6J background showed similar rates of PR degeneration with 30% and 40% loss, respectively, at 16–18 months of age. However, *Cx3cr1*[tm1Zm] mice on the BALB/cJ background show complete nuclei loss at 4 months of age [426]. *Cxcr5*[tm1Lipp] causes late onset PR degeneration with 20% loss of ONL thickness at 17 months of age and RPE disorganization [427], whereas ablation of *Irf3* and *Igfbp3* showed mild PR degeneration at 2–4 months of age, about 10–14% [428,429]. *Ccl2* and *Ccr2* mutations also led to PR degeneration and fundus lesions, ONL loss in some areas and development of neovascular lesions, resembling phenotypes of AMD [430]. *Cfh^{tm1Mbo}* was shown to have an impairment of rod and cone function by ERG and 29% decreased thickness of Bruch's membrane; however, rod opsin was distributed normally and no significant reduction in the number of PR cells was observed [431]. *Cfh^{tm1.1Song}* demonstrated retinal whitening and cotton wool spots by fundus imaging [432]. Other genes involved in immune function that also showed PR degeneration as conditional knockouts encode transforming growth factor beta receptor II (*Tgfbr2*) [433] and aryl hydrocarbon receptor (*Ahr*) [434].

5.6. Omitted Models with PR Abnormalities that May be of Interest

Based on the exclusion criteria described in the Methods section, a number of models with PR abnormalities caused by single gene mutations were not included in our final Table S1. Since we narrowly defined PR degeneration models as post-developmental loss of PR nuclei, some models, which were described with only OS alterations or ERG differences, were not included. For example, mice bearing a spontaneous point mutation in the *Ttc26^{hop}* [435] that leads to the generation of a stop codon, Tyr430Ter, were reported to show OS shortening at one year of age with no PR loss. Likewise, ectopic expression of cone opsins in rod OSs led to scotopic ERG abnormalities but not PR degeneration in *Samd7^{tm1TFur}* mice at 12 months of age [436]. The many allelic variants that cause ERG abnormalities without PR cell loss are listed in the MGI database and can be accessed through a phenotype query.

5.7. Factors Leading to Phenotypic Variability

5.7.1. Effects of Allelic Heterogeneity

Allelic heterogeneity is frequently a cause of phenotypic variability. For mouse models, this is often encountered when comparing a knockout model with spontaneous or induced mutations that still allow a protein to be produced. The latter would primarily be hypomorphic alleles due to amino acid substitutions, some splicing mutations that leave alternate splice forms intact and some C-terminal truncating mutations, which may retain some protein function. Often the knockout allele will be the more severe, presumably because in addition to the loss of protein function, the loss of the protein itself may cause secondary defects such as the failure to form a molecular complex that normally needs the native protein to form.

Mutations in the voltage gated calcium channel, *Cacna1f*, cause congenital stationary night blindness in humans due to abnormal neurotransmitter release in PR synapses. A null mutation in the *Cacna1f* gene (ΔEx14–17) leads to an absent b-wave, abnormal PR synapses, lack of Ca^{2+} response in PR terminals and PR degeneration to 8 rows in the ONL at 8 months [314]. In contrast, an Ile756Thr amino acid substitution found in human patients and introduced into mouse, led to a different phenotype with reduced b-wave, some intact ribbon synapses, a strong abnormal Ca^{2+} response, and a more severe degeneration (3–4 rows at 8 months of age [314]). Here the human allele represents a gain-of-function mutation that in addition to the loss of the original enzyme activity results in a new activity, or causes cell stress, which then induces additional phenotypes and makes the disease presentation more severe.

Within an allelic series of amino acid substitutions there are also frequently gradations of phenotypic severity. If a protein has several functional domains, mutations in different domains may lead to distinct phenotypes. In addition, some mutations can lead to an abnormal tertiary structure of the protein. Such structural changes can lead to a failure to interact with binding partners or substrates/ligands or change the nature of such interactions [437]. Structural changes can also affect export of the protein from the endoplasmic reticulum (ER) and result in ER stress and eventually apoptosis of the cell [438].

One of the larger allelic series available is for human PRPH2 with more than 150 disease causing mutations reported [439]. Although only the secondary structure of the protein is available, some clustering of disease phenotypes is apparent. For example, the area around amino acids 190–220 on the intradiscal loop 2 is enriched for mutations causing autosomal dominant retinitis pigmentosa. This area is thought to interact with ROM1. Mutations leading to macular degeneration are more frequently present between amino acids 142 and 172. However, some macular degeneration and autosomal dominant retinitis pigmentosa mutations are also found elsewhere in the protein [439,440]. Once a 3D structure is available, we may find that the disease specific mutations may well be in spatial proximity and a clearer picture of the genotype-phenotype relation may be revealed.

Allelic heterogeneity can also arise from the intron/exon structure of the gene itself. Many genes produce several distinct transcripts through alternative splicing of their exons [441]. These differing transcripts can each produce proteins, which possess unique functions. For example, the *Rpgrip1* gene produces two splice variants that code for proteins that differ at their C-terminus, a full-length transcript and a shorter transcript encompassing exons 1–13 plus three additional C-terminal amino acids. An insertion between exons 14 and 15 of the full-length transcript leads to PRs with vertically stacked OS discs [442], whereas, a chemically induced mutation in the splice acceptor site in intron 6 that leads to a loss of both splice variant forms results in a failure to develop OSs altogether [443].

Despite the promise of genotype–phenotype correlation analyses to aid in the functional annotation of retinal proteins as well as in the diagnosis and prognosis of retinal degenerative diseases, few allelic series are yet available. In humans the analysis is complicated by the fact that environment and genetic background effects can confound the allelic effect. In animal models, large allelic series are not yet available.

Until recently allelic heterogeneity posed a problem for the generation of mouse models for human retinal diseases because only transgenesis and the generation of knockout models by homologous recombination were available. The removal of the gene products using knockouts can only model recessive or haploinsufficiency diseases, and often the complete lack of the protein will lead to embryonic lethality.

Transgenic models are associated with their own set of problems. Depending on the transgene integration site, the expression of the transgene can be reduced or cellularly restricted. Integration into an unrelated gene can disrupt expression of that gene and cause a phenotype that is not related to the transgene. The use of directed transgene insertion into safe sites, such as the Rosa26 locus (*Gt(ROSA)26Sor*) provides a workaround for some of these problems, although the choice of a promoter that faithfully mimics the native expression is still a difficult process. For these reasons, transgenic mouse models were not included in this review.

With the advent of CRISPR/Cas9 technology to produce precise cuts in genomic DNA, and the ability to perform gene editing through homology directed repair, it is now feasible to recreate human mutations in the mouse and directly probe for the phenotypic effects of allelic heterogeneity [444]. Comitato et al. present an interesting phenotype comparison of transgenic and knock-in rhodopsin P23H models [445].

5.7.2. Effects of Genetic Interactions

Gene interaction, or epistasis, is frequently observed during genetic analysis when two or more alleles at different loci combine to alter the onset, type, or severity of disease phenotypes. Such phenotype altering interactions arise from the organization of proteins and RNAs into macromolecular complexes and/or biochemical and regulatory pathways and networks. For example, consider hypomorphic mutations in two proteins that are components of a linear enzymatic pathway. Individually the reduced activity may not greatly impact the flux through the pathway, but combined in the same cell, the pathway flux may be reduced and become severe enough to induce a disease phenotype due to a lack of sufficient pathway product. Alternatively, a mutation may impair Pathway A, so that a disease phenotype arises. A second mutation may arise in a Pathway B that allows it to compensate for the malfunction in Pathway A and thus reduce the severity of the original disease phenotype. Mutations of this latter type of interacting mutations are called suppressor mutations and are extremely useful because they directly identify potential drug targets whose manipulation may be used to treat disease.

In general, identification of genetic interactors can be useful for placing the primary mutated gene in a biological context and help to define its cellular and organismal function. Often, the known function of a gene and its biology can suggest candidate interacting genes. Similar to the first hypothetical interaction case above, mutations in two proteins involved in iron homeostasis, ceruloplasmin (CP), a ferroxidase associated with transferrin transport across the plasma membrane, and hephaestin (HEPH), implicated in iron transport across cells, individually do not show obvious PR degeneration. Combined in a double mutant mouse model, however, they lead to iron overload in the retina and subsequent RPE abnormalities and PR degeneration [446]. Another example involves two proteins necessary for retinoid recycling, ABCA4 and RDH8. Mutations in each alone do not show any phenotype; combined they cause all-*trans*-retinoid accumulation and PR degeneration [296]. Since previous studies had suggested that activation of TLR3 may lead to inflammation and mediating apoptosis [447], the authors explored the role of *Tlr3* in their *Abca4/Rdh8* double mutant model. Importantly, adding a targeted mutation of *Tlr3* to make a triple mutant mouse resulted in rescue of PR cells [448]. Here then the *Tlr3* mutation acts as a suppressor of the degenerative phenotype of the *Abca4/Rdh8* double mutant.

Additional interacting gene pairs have been found that affect PR degeneration, among them *Mertk*^{tm1Grl}; *Tyro3*^{tm1Grl} [449], *Cep290*^{rd16}; *Bbs4*^{tm1Vcs} [450], *Cep290*^{rd16}; *Mkks*^{tm1Vcs} [451], *Rpgr*^{tm1Tili}; *Cep290*^{rd16} [452], *Cngb1*$^{tm1.1Biel}$; *Cnga3*^{tm1Biel}; *Hcn1*^{tm2Kndl} [453], *Crb1*$^{tm1.1Wij}$; *Crb2*$^{tm1.1Wij}$ [454], *Dio3*^{tm1Stg}; *Dio2*^{tm1Vag} [455], and *Ercc6*^{tm1Gvh}; and *Xpa*^{tm1Hvs} [456].

In addition to testing candidate interacting genes, methods have been developed to identify such interactors in an unbiased fashion that is illustrated below.

Effects of genetic background. For the calcium channel gene *Cacna1f* mentioned above, there is a third allele available. Chang et al. [457] reported the phenotype of the *nob2* mutation, an out-of-frame insertion of a transposable element into the *Cacna1f* gene, which is predicted to cause a truncation after 32 amino acids. The authors demonstrated by western blot that this is a null mutation and no protein is detected. Compared to the ΔEx14–17 null mutation, however, the phenotype of *nob2* is much milder with no apparent PR degradation [457]. The most likely explanation for this discrepancy can be deduced from the fact that the *nob2* mutation arose on the AxB6 recombinant inbred strain, a strain whose DNA is composed of alternate segments derived from C57BL/6J and A/J. It is likely that the A/J strain carries one or more modifier loci that suppress the PR degeneration induced by a *Cacna1f* null mutation.

Upon outcrossing an inbred strain carrying a mutation that leads to a particular phenotype with a different inbred strain, it is frequently observed that the phenotype of the offspring differs from that of the parents. This was often encountered in the past when knockout alleles were created in embryonic stem cells derived from strain 129/Sv and the founder animals were then made congenic on the C57BL/6 background. An early example is a study of a homozygous *Rho* knockout that was shown to lose PR nuclei significantly faster on the 129Sv background than on the C57BL/6 background [458]. Corresponding differences were also found in the number of apoptotic nuclei and in ERG responses. It was concluded that the B6 strain carries protective alleles of modifier genes that lead to a slower rate of PR degeneration [458]. Alternatively, it is also possible that 129Sv carries modifier alleles that accelerate degeneration.

Other inbred strains have also been reported to modify retinal phenotypes. For example, a targeted mutation of *Rp1* (*Rp1*^{tm1Eap}) only showed moderate PR degeneration as an incipient congenic (N6) on the A/J strain background, but not on C57BL/6J or DBA/1J backgrounds [459]. ONL dysplasia and excess blue cone formation caused by loss of *Nr2e3* in C57BL/6J are suppressed by the genetic backgrounds of CAST/EiJ, AKR/J, and NOD.NON-*H2*^{nb1} strains [460].

In principle, all inbred strains will carry modifier alleles. However, which strain modifies a particular mutation will depend on the primary mutation. It should be emphasized that an inbred strain represents a single genotype. In order to model the phenotypic spectrum of a human disease-causing mutation, many inbred strain backgrounds would have to be examined. Recently, advanced genetically diverse mouse populations have become available, such as the collaborative cross (CC) or the diversity outcross (DO) populations, that allow for more efficient modeling of human populations compared to the classical inbred strains [461,462].

Modifier screens. Modifier screens are a tool to identify genes that modify phenotypic traits caused by a particular mutation. The disease modifying properties of inbred strains have been used for many decades to identify the underlying modifier genes by using genetic crosses, marker assisted genetic mapping of modifying loci, and positional cloning or more recently high throughput whole exome or whole genome sequencing approaches. For example, when B6.Cg-$Nr2e3^{rd7}$ homozygotes are outcrossed to CAST/EiJ, AKR/J, or NOD.NON-$H2^{nb1}$ and then the F1 mice intercrossed, homozygous $Nr2e3^{rd7}$ mice of the F2 generation are found that unlike the parental B6.Cg-$Nr2e3^{rd7}$ homozygotes have fewer spots on fundus examination and no PR layer dysplasia in histological sections [460]. This phenotypic variability is caused by the genetic interaction between the $Nr2e3^{rd7}$ disease allele and variants of so-called modifier genes that are specific to the outcross partner strain. Several quantitative trait loci (QTL) on chromosomes 7, 8, 11, and 19 were mapped [460]. Generation of a congenic line carrying the Chr11 modifier, along with further fine mapping, reduced the critical genomic interval to 3.3 cM. Several candidate genes were sequenced and a single nucleotide polymorphism was found in a nuclear receptor gene, Nr1d1, that is predicted to lead to an Arg409Gln amino acid change. Causality was confirmed by phenotypic rescue of the rd7-associated phenotypes by in vivo electroporation of a wild-type Nr1d1 expression construct [463].

Several other modifiers have been mapped and identified based on inbred strain differences. For example, mapping crosses have been carried out for rd3 (BALB/cJ and C57BL/6J, [464]), rd1 (C3H/HeOu and FVB/N, [465]), Crb1 (C57BL/6N and C57BL/6JOlaHsd, Chr15, [466]), Mfrp (B6.C3Ga and CAST/EiJ, Chr 1, 6, and 11 [467]), and Tub and Tulp1 (C57BL/6J and AKR/J, Mtap1a, [468]).

Although not yet widely used as a means to explore retinal biology, a very efficient way to identify modifier genes is the use of a sensitized mutagenesis screen in which a male mouse carrying a mutation of interest is given a chemical mutagen and its offspring are examined for any change in the original phenotype. Offspring carrying a potential mutation is backcrossed to the unmutagenized parental inbred strain to test for heritability and to reduce the mutational load. Mutations are identified using whole exome sequencing of the pheno-deviant mouse. This approach avoids the limited genetic diversity of inbred strains since in principle all genes can be mutated. An example of the utility of mutagenesis to search for modifier genes is the identification of a suppressor mutation in Frmd4b that prevents the PR dysplasia and external limiting membrane fragmentation observed in $Nr2e3^{rd7}$ mutant mice [469].

5.7.3. Effects of Environment on PR Degeneration

PR cell loss has been shown to be induced by a number of environmental factors such as light, diet, and smoking in combination with particular genotypes. Perhaps not surprisingly, light exposure in some models bearing mutations in genes that function directly or in an ancillary fashion in the visual transduction pathway trend toward hastening PR degeneration [470,471]. For example, transgenic mice bearing the rhodopsin VPP mutation, widely used in visual transduction studies, is susceptible to light-exacerbated PR degeneration [472]. Likewise, mice carrying a homozygous Prom1 null mutation are particularly susceptible to light-induced degeneration. At eye opening, with exposure to light, degeneration initiates at P14, and all PRs are gone by P20, whereas dark rearing from P8 to P30 leads to significant preservation of PRs [471]. Dark-rearing has also been demonstrated to delay PR degeneration in $Slc6a6^{tm1Dhau}$ (10% loss vs. 90% loss in normal vivarium lighting at three weeks of age) [473] or have no effect in C57BL/6-$Mitf^{mi-vit}$/J homozygotes [474]. In some situations, light may actually trigger the disease phenotype, as is the case in Sag knockout mice [198,199], with three Class B1 Rhodopsin missense mutations, Tvrm1 and Tvrm4 [157] or Tvrm144 [18], and in null mutation models of Rdh12 [475], Asic2 [476], Myo7a [477], Whrn [478], or Akt2 [479]. Sag mutants must be reared in the dark to observe any PR cells. Under normal vivarium lighting conditions, the other light-sensitive mouse models do not show PR degeneration or only a slight shortening of OS at one year of age, as in the those carrying *Rho* alleles *Tvrm1*, *Tvrm4*, or *Tvrm144*, and in retinol dehydrogenase (*Rdh12*) mutant mice. However, exposure to bright light or rearing under cyclic moderate-lighting, even subjecting mice to fundus examination, leads to PR degeneration. A comprehensive list of animal models and the effects of dark-rearing or light exposure can be found in reference [470].

Like light exposure, smoking and high fat intake have been proposed to have a negative impact on retinal function by increasing oxidative stress and inflammation in PR and RPE cells [480]. Smoking has been implicated as a major risk factor in the development of age-related macular degeneration in humans [481,482], and the results have been replicated in mouse models as well. Smoking leads to increased oxidative stress and inflammation in B6 mice [483] and in the presence of *Nfe2l2* deficiency [484]. Likewise, combinations of smoking and high fat intake in the presence of an *ApoB* mutation that promotes production of the APOB100 isoform [485] leads to significant loss of PRs [484]. Further, high-fat diet intake for certain genotypes, such as mutations of *Ldlr* [486] or certain alleles of *Apoe* [487], has been shown to compromise PR integrity in mice.

The majority of pharmacological or dietary interventions that have been reported in the relationship to PR degeneration in mouse models are associated with the goal of increasing vitamin A derivative availability [488–490] or reducing oxidative stress [491,492] in the retina. Heritable mutations in enzymes, such as LRAT or RPE65, required for processing of vitamin A within the retina are known to cause early onset RD due a deficiency of the 11-*cis*-retinal chromophore. Efficacy of treatment with 9-*cis*-retinal derivatives of mice with null mutations in *Lrat* and *Rpe65* mice is thoroughly discussed in a review by Perusek and Maeda [488,489]. Administration of antioxidants has in some cases improved PR survival. *Rs1*[tm1Web] homozygous females or hemizygous males fed a diet high in DHA [493] or *Pde6b*[rd10] mice fed lutein and zeaxanthin [494] showed a significant PR preservation. Further, injections of a mixture of antioxidants—alpha tocopheral, ascorbic acid, alpha-lipoic acid, and/or Mn(III)tetrakis porphyrin—were able to slow the loss of cone/rod PRs in *Pde6b*[rd1] [495], and *Pde6b*[rd10] mice and in mice with a rhodopsin Q344ter mutation [492]. Environmental enhancement of *Pde6b*[rd10] mice was able to significantly reduce PR loss presumably by reducing retinal oxidative stress [496].

5.8. Relationship to Human Disease Genes

Of the 273 retinal degenerative disease genes in RetNet [3] for which mouse homologs exist, mouse models are available for 110 or 40% of them, including both germline and conditional mutants (Figure 7). Through our survey, we found 120 additional genes, in which mutations lead to PR degeneration. These genes could serve as candidates for yet to be identified human retinal diseases. The available mouse models, for the most part, recapitulate the human disease phenotype well and permit mechanistic and therapeutic studies. However, apparent failures of mouse models do occur. When mutations in *MFRP* were first identified in humans [497], mice were thought to be a poor model because unlike humans [498], mice were previously reported to develop PR degeneration [499], and the microphthalmia and hyperopia found in human patients had not been reported in homozygous *Mfrp*[rd6] mice. In subsequent years, numerous human patients have been identified that do show a degenerative phenotype [500] and hyperopia was detected both in a mouse model carrying a human *MFRP* c.498_499insC allele [501] and the original *Mfrp*[rd6] mouse (our unpublished observations). An important family of deaf–blindness diseases, Usher syndrome, was also thought to be poorly recapitulated in mice, because early models like the shaker-1 mouse had only the characteristic hearing loss, but no retinal degeneration [502]. Later, however, it was found that moderate light exposure does result in photoreceptor degeneration in shaker-1 mice [477]. In addition, a knock-in of the Acadian *USH1C* c.216G>A mutation into the mouse *Ush1c* gene recapitulates both deafness and retinal degeneration phenotypes [503]. In many cases, discordance between the human and mouse phenotypes can be attributed to insufficient information about variation in the human disease, or to allelic effects (knockout vs. hypomorph or gain of function, expression of alternatively splice isoforms), or strain background (modifier genes) in the mouse models. Such shortcomings in mouse models can often be addressed by testing multiple models, including human disease alleles, and by using multiple genetic backgrounds.

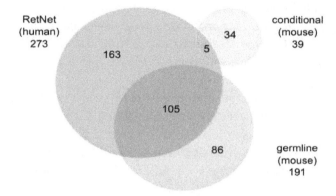

Figure 7. Comparison of the number of RD genes identified in human (RetNet) and mouse as listed in Table S1 and summarized in Figure 3. The total number of genes in the RetNet database that cause monogenic disease and have mouse homologs is indicated, as is the total for which conditional or germline mutations have been associated with PR cell loss in mice, as described in this review. Numbers within the overlapping areas of the diagram represent genes present in both RetNet and Table S1; the remaining numbers represent genes that are unique to the indicated category.

Although humans and mice share about 98% of their genes, species differences do exist and need to be considered when selecting a model. Examples of vision-related genes that mice lack are *EYS*, *ARMS2*, and *CETP*. Species differences are the result of different evolutionary histories; humans and mice have encountered different pathogens, resulting in adaptations of our respective immune systems. Mice have different nutritional requirements, resulting in differences in lipid metabolism. Additionally, mouse eyes are adapted to a nocturnal life, resulting in a rod dominated retina with no macula. Nevertheless, mice possess all of the same retinal cell types necessary for vision and the vast majority of the same genes, and even when missing genes are introduced into mice they result in relevant phenotypes. For example, in a transgenic mouse model for Stargardt-like macular degeneration 3 due to a mutation in *Elovl4*, PR cell loss occurs in the central retina in a pattern that resembles the human disease [504]. For the many retinal diseases still in need of models, including complex diseases such as AMD or diabetic retinopathy, it remains the case that valuable new insights into disease mechanism and basic eye biology can still be obtained from mouse studies.

6. Discussion

6.1. Variability in Measuring PR Cell Loss

We noted an extremely large variability in PR cell loss data presented in the various reports, which were based on several different types of measures, such as ONL thickness obtained from toluidine-stained plastic sections, hematoxylin and eosin-stained paraffin sections, or DAPI-stained cryosections; counts of rows of ONL nuclei in the same preparations; counts of the total number of ONL nuclei in a fixed retinal area; spider plots assessing ONL thickness over the full perimeter; ONL thickness from OCT B-scans. Cone numbers were assessed in sections or whole mounts stained with cone opsins, peanut agglutinin lectin, or cone arrestin. Methods to count cone cell nuclei efficiently might benefit from studies that examine the effect of mutations in genes that specifically affect cones. Perhaps more challenging is that many studies provided insufficient sample sizes or number of time points to assess the progression of PR cell loss. Some of this variability reflects the evolution of methods and quantitative approaches over several decades, and some may be attributed to the different choices each laboratory makes depending on what works best given resources and interests. However, to aid future efforts to compare PR cell loss between studies, we recommend that at least three ages be assessed, one prior to the onset of PR cell loss, and at least two within the age range where PR cells are declining exponentially (that is, between 95% and 5% of wild-type values), and that the data be quantified relative to gender-matched controls at these same ages.

Although a decrease in PR cell numbers as estimated above is widely accepted as evidence for RD, an alternative explanation may apply in some instances. $Mcoln1^{tm1Sasl}$ homozygotes exhibit an apparent decrease in PR cells to 54% of wild-type at one month of age, a value that remained unchanged at two and six months [505]. TUNEL analysis revealed no increase in apoptosis at any age compared to controls, and both histology and OCT indicated a decrease in total retinal thickness. It is possible that the rapid initial decrease to a stable value may result from retinal thinning as the eye enlarges due to myopia during postnatal development, an occasionally observed feature of $MCOLN1$-associated disease in humans [506]. Methods are available to measure axial length in mice [507], which might be used to determine whether the observed change in nuclear layer thickness is due to ocular enlargement. Models in Table S1 with a similar phenotype include $Guca1a^{tm1.1Hunt}$ and $Ctnna1^{Tvrm5}$.

6.2. Correlation of PR Cell Loss with Gene Function

As a fortuitous consequence of our inquiry, in some cases, the progress of PR cell loss could be correlated with gene function within categories. For example, in the ciliary function and trafficking section we see trends in the onset and progression of RD depending on the role and location of gene products within the PR. Mice with mutations in genes involved in ciliogenesis or in transition zone protein complexes, typically result in a PR degeneration that begins at 2 weeks during OS biogenesis and progresses rapidly through OS maturation. Null mutations in genes that encode components of the IFT machinery tend to result in premature death or embryonic lethality, and conditional ablation of these genes in the retina typically leads to early and rapid PR loss. Models with disruptions in protein complexes with roles in BBSome assembly or regulation, protein/lipid trafficking, axoneme extension, or disc morphogenesis tend to have a moderate to slow degeneration. Lastly, mice with mutations that disturb basal body and pericentriolar anchoring and integrity such as the Usher periciliary membrane complex undergo a very slow form of RD, which results in partial PR function throughout the life of the mouse. It remains possible that the slower progression of PR cell loss, especially when associated with members of protein complexes, may be the result of genetic redundancy where multiple genes encode proteins that have similar biochemical functions.

It was also interesting to note that disruption of chloride channels appeared to be particularly deleterious to PR survival. Many of the models we identified with early and rapid progression of PR cell loss, including those affecting a subset of the ciliary genes discussed above or the OS components $Prom1$, $Prph2$, and Rho, appear to be required for OS assembly. Chloride channel defects resulted in similar progression, raising the possibility that chloride homeostasis is important for OS development. This idea is supported by evidence that chloride transport by the chloride channel ANO1 is required for ciliogenesis [508] and that control of intracellular chloride ion levels by this channel regulates the membrane organization of phosphatidylinositol 4,5-bisphosphate [509], a prominent lipid that regulates ciliary development [131,510]. Characterization of early OS development in mouse models defective in chloride channels CLCN2, CLCN3, or CLCN7 may provide mechanistic clues on the role of intracellular chloride in ciliogenesis.

Finally, our analysis revealed links between PR cell loss and a network of 13 genes known to participate in the cellular response to DNA damage, four of which have been directly associated with transcription-coupled DNA repair. Based on canonical indicators of DNA repair, such as the colocalization of phosphorylated histone H2AX and TRP53BP1 (also known as 53BP1) at DSBs, it has been reported that rod PR cells in mice lack a robust canonical DNA damage response, [241,511]. An attenuated response may reflect an adaptation to improve rod cell survival [241,511]. Nevertheless, mechanisms are present in rod cells to repair DNA damage, as evidenced by the robust levels of DNA repair factors [241] and by our results indicating that a network of DNA damage response genes is required for maintaining PR cell viability. Together, these results support the idea that a non-canonical

DNA damage response pathway exists in rod PR cells [512]. Further study of the DNA damage response genes linked to PR cell loss in mice may be useful for elucidating this pathway.

7. Conclusions

This review highlights mouse models of monogenic retinal degenerative diseases that cause rod or cone PR cell loss. The models include germline mutations and conditional alleles, in which characterization of retinal phenotypes in germline mutations was not possible due to embryonic or perinatal lethality. By providing an extensive list of these models as well as a means of comparing their progression, we hope to benefit researchers who seek to optimize their experimental approaches.

Author Contributions: Conceptualization, P.M.N., M.P.K.; methodology, M.P.K., B.C., P.M.N.; software, M.P.K.; formal analysis, M.P.K.; investigation, G.B.C., N.G., N.D., J.P., L.F.H., L.S., J.K.N., M.P.K., P.M.N.; resources, B.C., J.K.N., P.M.N.; data curation, G.B.C., N.G., N.D., J.P., L.F.H., L.S., J.K.N., M.P.K., P.M.N.; writing—original draft preparation, G.B.C., N.G., N.D., J.P., L.H., J.K.N., M.P.K., P.M.N.; writing—review and editing, G.B.C., N.G., J.K.N., M.P.K., P.M.N.; visualization, B.C., M.P.K.; supervision, J.K.N., P.M.N.; project administration, P.M.N.; funding acquisition, M.P.K., B.C., J.K.N., P.M.N. All authors have read and agree to the published version of the manuscript.

Acknowledgments: The authors thank James Kadin and Grace Stafford for help with scripts to filter PubMed data, Cynthia Smith for her contributions to Table S1 and for coordinating our efforts with those at MGI, Melissa Berry for assistance with nomenclature, Bernard Fitzmaurice and Wanda Hicks for fundus and/or OCT imaging, and Jane Cha for drawing Figure 1.

References

1. Cremers, F.P.M.; Boon, C.J.F.; Bujakowska, K.; Zeitz, C. Special Issue Introduction: Inherited Retinal Disease: Novel Candidate Genes, Genotype-Phenotype Correlations, and Inheritance Models. *Genes (Basel)* **2018**, *9*, 215. [CrossRef] [PubMed]
2. Hanany, M.; Rivolta, C.; Sharon, D. Worldwide carrier frequency and genetic prevalence of autosomal recessive inherited retinal diseases. *Proc. Natl. Acad. Sci. USA* **2020**, *117*, 2710–2716. [CrossRef] [PubMed]
3. RetNet—Retinal Information Network. Available online: https://sph.uth.edu/retnet/home.htm (accessed on 8 December 2019).
4. Picaud, S.; Dalkara, D.; Marazova, K.; Goureau, O.; Roska, B.; Sahel, J.A. The primate model for understanding and restoring vision. *Proc. Natl. Acad. Sci. USA* **2019**, *116*, 26280–26287. [CrossRef] [PubMed]
5. Bunel, M.; Chaudieu, G.; Hamel, C.; Lagoutte, L.; Manes, G.; Botherel, N.; Brabet, P.; Pilorge, P.; Andre, C.; Quignon, P. Natural models for retinitis pigmentosa: Progressive retinal atrophy in dog breeds. *Hum. Genet.* **2019**, *138*, 441–453. [CrossRef] [PubMed]
6. Fletcher, E.L.; Jobling, A.I.; Vessey, K.A.; Luu, C.; Guymer, R.H.; Baird, P.N. Animal models of retinal disease. *Prog. Mol. Biol. Transl. Sci.* **2011**, *100*, 211–286. [CrossRef]
7. Veleri, S.; Lazar, C.H.; Chang, B.; Sieving, P.A.; Banin, E.; Swaroop, A. Biology and therapy of inherited retinal degenerative disease: Insights from mouse models. *Dis. Model. Mech.* **2015**, *8*, 109–129. [CrossRef]
8. Angueyra, J.M.; Kindt, K.S. Leveraging Zebrafish to Study Retinal Degenerations. *Front. Cell Dev. Biol.* **2018**, *6*, 110. [CrossRef]
9. Lehmann, M.; Knust, E.; Hebbar, S. Drosophila melanogaster: A Valuable Genetic Model Organism to Elucidate the Biology of Retinitis Pigmentosa. *Methods Mol. Biol.* **2019**, *1834*, 221–249. [CrossRef]
10. Travis, G.H.; Brennan, M.B.; Danielson, P.E.; Kozak, C.A.; Sutcliffe, J.G. Identification of a photoreceptor-specific mRNA encoded by the gene responsible for retinal degeneration slow (rds). *Nature* **1989**, *338*, 70–73. [CrossRef]

11. Dryja, T.P.; McGee, T.L.; Reichel, E.; Hahn, L.B.; Cowley, G.S.; Yandell, D.W.; Sandberg, M.A.; Berson, E.L. A point mutation of the rhodopsin gene in one form of retinitis pigmentosa. *Nature* **1990**, *343*, 364–366. [CrossRef]

12. Bowes, C.; Li, T.; Danciger, M.; Baxter, L.C.; Applebury, M.L.; Farber, D.B. Retinal degeneration in the rd mouse is caused by a defect in the beta subunit of rod cGMP-phosphodiesterase. *Nature* **1990**, *347*, 677–680. [CrossRef] [PubMed]

13. Wheway, G.; Parry, D.A.; Johnson, C.A. The role of primary cilia in the development and disease of the retina. *Organogenesis* **2014**, *10*, 69–85. [CrossRef] [PubMed]

14. Baehr, W.; Hanke-Gogokhia, C.; Sharif, A.; Reed, M.; Dahl, T.; Frederick, J.M.; Ying, G. Insights into photoreceptor ciliogenesis revealed by animal models. *Prog. Retin. Eye Res.* **2019**, *71*, 26–56. [CrossRef] [PubMed]

15. Chang, B.; Hawes, N.L.; Hurd, R.E.; Davisson, M.T.; Nusinowitz, S.; Heckenlively, J.R. Retinal degeneration mutants in the mouse. *Vis. Res.* **2002**, *42*, 517–525. [CrossRef]

16. Chang, B.; Hawes, N.L.; Hurd, R.E.; Wang, J.; Howell, D.; Davisson, M.T.; Roderick, T.H.; Nusinowitz, S.; Heckenlively, J.R. Mouse models of ocular diseases. *Vis. NeuroSci.* **2005**, *22*, 587–593. [CrossRef] [PubMed]

17. Won, J.; Shi, L.Y.; Hicks, W.; Wang, J.; Hurd, R.; Naggert, J.K.; Chang, B.; Nishina, P.M. Mouse model resources for vision research. *J. Ophthalmol.* **2011**, *2011*, 391384. [CrossRef]

18. Won, J.; Shi, L.Y.; Hicks, W.; Wang, J.; Naggert, J.K.; Nishina, P.M. Translational vision research models program. *Adv. Exp. Med. Biol.* **2012**, *723*, 391–397. [CrossRef]

19. Chang, B. Mouse models for studies of retinal degeneration and diseases. *Methods Mol. Biol.* **2013**, *935*, 27–39. [CrossRef]

20. Chang, B. Mouse Models as Tools to Identify Genetic Pathways for Retinal Degeneration, as Exemplified by Leber's Congenital Amaurosis. *Methods Mol. Biol.* **2016**, *1438*, 417–430. [CrossRef]

21. Krebs, M.P.; Collin, G.B.; Hicks, W.L.; Yu, M.; Charette, J.R.; Shi, L.Y.; Wang, J.; Naggert, J.K.; Peachey, N.S.; Nishina, P.M. Mouse models of human ocular disease for translational research. *PLoS ONE* **2017**, *12*, e0183837. [CrossRef]

22. Do, M.T.; Yau, K.W. Intrinsically photosensitive retinal ganglion cells. *Physiol. Rev.* **2010**, *90*, 1547–1581. [CrossRef] [PubMed]

23. Goldberg, A.F.; Moritz, O.L.; Williams, D.S. Molecular basis for photoreceptor outer segment architecture. *Prog. Retin. Eye Res.* **2016**, *55*, 52–81. [CrossRef] [PubMed]

24. Rachel, R.A.; Li, T.; Swaroop, A. Photoreceptor sensory cilia and ciliopathies: Focus on CEP290, RPGR and their interacting proteins. *Cilia* **2012**, *1*, 22. [CrossRef] [PubMed]

25. Wang, J.; O'Sullivan, M.L.; Mukherjee, D.; Punal, V.M.; Farsiu, S.; Kay, J.N. Anatomy and spatial organization of Muller glia in mouse retina. *J. Comp. Neurol.* **2017**, *525*, 1759–1777. [CrossRef]

26. Reichenbach, A.; Bringmann, A. Glia of the human retina. *Glia* **2019**, *68*, 768–796. [CrossRef]

27. Strauss, O. The retinal pigment epithelium in visual function. *Physiol. Rev.* **2005**, *85*, 845–881. [CrossRef]

28. Verbakel, S.K.; van Huet, R.A.C.; Boon, C.J.F.; den Hollander, A.I.; Collin, R.W.J.; Klaver, C.C.W.; Hoyng, C.B.; Roepman, R.; Klevering, B.J. Non-syndromic retinitis pigmentosa. *Prog. Retin. Eye Res.* **2018**, *66*, 157–186. [CrossRef]

29. Kumaran, N.; Moore, A.T.; Weleber, R.G.; Michaelides, M. Leber congenital amaurosis/early-onset severe retinal dystrophy: Clinical features, molecular genetics and therapeutic interventions. *Br. J. Ophthalmol.* **2017**, *101*, 1147–1154. [CrossRef]

30. Parisi, M.A. The molecular genetics of Joubert syndrome and related ciliopathies: The challenges of genetic and phenotypic heterogeneity. *Transl. Sci. Rare Dis.* **2019**, *4*, 25–49. [CrossRef]

31. Suspitsin, E.N.; Imyanitov, E.N. Bardet-Biedl Syndrome. *Mol. Syndromol.* **2016**, *7*, 62–71. [CrossRef]

32. Mathur, P.; Yang, J. Usher syndrome: Hearing loss, retinal degeneration and associated abnormalities. *Biochim. Biophys. Acta* **2015**, *1852*, 406–420. [CrossRef] [PubMed]

33. Kumaran, N.; Michaelides, M.; Smith, A.J.; Ali, R.R.; Bainbridge, J.W.B. Retinal gene therapy. *Br. Med. Bull.* **2018**, *126*, 13–25. [CrossRef] [PubMed]

34. Mouse Genome Database (MGD) at the Mouse Genome Informatics website, The Jackson Laboratory, Bar Harbor, Maine. Available online: http://www.informatics.jax.org (accessed on 18 October 2019).

35. PubMed [Internet]. Bethesda (MD): National Library of Medicine (US), National Center for Biotechnology Information. Available online: https://www.ncbi.nlm.nih.gov/pubmed/ (accessed on 15 October 2019).

36. Clarke, G.; Collins, R.A.; Leavitt, B.R.; Andrews, D.F.; Hayden, M.R.; Lumsden, C.J.; McInnes, R.R. A one-hit model of cell death in inherited neuronal degenerations. *Nature* **2000**, *406*, 195–199. [CrossRef] [PubMed]

37. Krebs, M.P.; Xiao, M.; Sheppard, K.; Hicks, W.; Nishina, P.M. Bright-Field Imaging and Optical Coherence Tomography of the Mouse Posterior Eye. *Methods Mol. Biol.* **2016**, *1438*, 395–415. [CrossRef] [PubMed]

38. Krebs, M.P. Using Vascular Landmarks to Orient 3D Optical Coherence Tomography Images of the Mouse Eye. *Curr. Protoc. Mouse Biol.* **2017**, *7*, 176–190. [CrossRef]

39. Dyer, M.A.; Donovan, S.L.; Zhang, J.; Gray, J.; Ortiz, A.; Tenney, R.; Kong, J.; Allikmets, R.; Sohocki, M.M. Retinal degeneration in Aipl1-deficient mice: A new genetic model of Leber congenital amaurosis. *Brain Res. Mol. Brain Res.* **2004**, *132*, 208–220. [CrossRef]

40. Liu, X.; Bulgakov, O.V.; Wen, X.H.; Woodruff, M.L.; Pawlyk, B.; Yang, J.; Fain, G.L.; Sandberg, M.A.; Makino, C.L.; Li, T. AIPL1, the protein that is defective in Leber congenital amaurosis, is essential for the biosynthesis of retinal rod cGMP phosphodiesterase. *Proc. Natl. Acad. Sci. USA* **2004**, *101*, 13903–13908. [CrossRef]

41. Dickinson, M.E.; Flenniken, A.M.; Ji, X.; Teboul, L.; Wong, M.D.; White, J.K.; Meehan, T.F.; Weninger, W.J.; Westerberg, H.; Adissu, H.; et al. High-throughput discovery of novel developmental phenotypes. *Nature* **2016**, *537*, 508–514. [CrossRef]

42. Hanke-Gogokhia, C.; Wu, Z.; Gerstner, C.D.; Frederick, J.M.; Zhang, H.; Baehr, W. Arf-like Protein 3 (ARL3) Regulates Protein Trafficking and Ciliogenesis in Mouse Photoreceptors. *J. Biol. Chem.* **2016**, *291*, 7142–7155. [CrossRef]

43. International Mouse Phenotyping Consortium: Home—IMPC. Available online: https://www.mousephenotype.org/ (accessed on 22 December 2019).

44. Bujakowska, K.M.; Liu, Q.; Pierce, E.A. Photoreceptor Cilia and Retinal Ciliopathies. *Cold Spring Harb. Perspect. Biol.* **2017**, *9*, a028274. [CrossRef]

45. Gilliam, J.C.; Chang, J.T.; Sandoval, I.M.; Zhang, Y.; Li, T.; Pittler, S.J.; Chiu, W.; Wensel, T.G. Three-dimensional architecture of the rod sensory cilium and its disruption in retinal neurodegeneration. *Cell* **2012**, *151*, 1029–1041. [CrossRef] [PubMed]

46. Rohlich, P. The sensory cilium of retinal rods is analogous to the transitional zone of motile cilia. *Cell Tiss. Res.* **1975**, *161*, 421–430. [CrossRef] [PubMed]

47. Goncalves, J.; Pelletier, L. The Ciliary Transition Zone: Finding the Pieces and Assembling the Gate. *Mol. Cells* **2017**, *40*, 243–253. [CrossRef] [PubMed]

48. Seo, S.; Datta, P. Photoreceptor outer segment as a sink for membrane proteins: Hypothesis and implications in retinal ciliopathies. *Hum. Mol. Genet.* **2017**, *26*, R75–R82. [CrossRef]

49. Khanna, H. Photoreceptor Sensory Cilium: Traversing the Ciliary Gate. *Cells* **2015**, *4*, 674–686. [CrossRef]

50. Garcia-Gonzalo, F.R.; Corbit, K.C.; Sirerol-Piquer, M.S.; Ramaswami, G.; Otto, E.A.; Noriega, T.R.; Seol, A.D.; Robinson, J.F.; Bennett, C.L.; Josifova, D.J.; et al. A transition zone complex regulates mammalian ciliogenesis and ciliary membrane composition. *Nat. Genet.* **2011**, *43*, 776–784. [CrossRef]

51. Sedmak, T.; Wolfrum, U. Intraflagellar transport proteins in ciliogenesis of photoreceptor cells. *Biol. Cell* **2011**, *103*, 449–466. [CrossRef]

52. Salinas, R.Y.; Pearring, J.N.; Ding, J.D.; Spencer, W.J.; Hao, Y.; Arshavsky, V.Y. Photoreceptor discs form through peripherin-dependent suppression of ciliary ectosome release. *J. Cell Biol.* **2017**, *216*, 1489–1499. [CrossRef]

53. LaVail, M.M. Kinetics of rod outer segment renewal in the developing mouse retina. *J. Cell Biol.* **1973**, *58*, 650–661. [CrossRef]

54. De Robertis, E. Morphogenesis of the retinal rods; an electron microscope study. *J. Biophys. Biochem. Cytol.* **1956**, *2*, 209–218. [CrossRef]

55. Insinna, C.; Besharse, J.C. Intraflagellar transport and the sensory outer segment of vertebrate photoreceptors. *Dev. Dyn.* **2008**, *237*, 1982–1992. [CrossRef] [PubMed]

56. Rosenbaum, J.L.; Cole, D.G.; Diener, D.R. Intraflagellar transport: The eyes have it. *J. Cell Biol.* **1999**, *144*, 385–388. [CrossRef]

57. Chuang, J.Z.; Zhao, Y.; Sung, C.H. SARA-regulated vesicular targeting underlies formation of the light-sensing organelle in mammalian rods. *Cell* **2007**, *130*, 535–547. [CrossRef] [PubMed]

58. Chuang, J.Z.; Hsu, Y.C.; Sung, C.H. Ultrastructural visualization of trans-ciliary rhodopsin cargoes in mammalian rods. *Cilia* **2015**, *4*, 4. [CrossRef] [PubMed]

59. Steinberg, R.H.; Fisher, S.K.; Anderson, D.H. Disc morphogenesis in vertebrate photoreceptors. *J. Comp. Neurol.* **1980**, *190*, 501–508. [CrossRef]

60. Ding, J.D.; Salinas, R.Y.; Arshavsky, V.Y. Discs of mammalian rod photoreceptors form through the membrane evagination mechanism. *J. Cell Biol.* **2015**, *211*, 495–502. [CrossRef]

61. Burgoyne, T.; Meschede, I.P.; Burden, J.J.; Bailly, M.; Seabra, M.C.; Futter, C.E. Rod disc renewal occurs by evagination of the ciliary plasma membrane that makes cadherin-based contacts with the inner segment. *Proc. Natl. Acad. Sci. USA* **2015**, *112*, 15922–15927. [CrossRef]

62. Young, R.W. The renewal of photoreceptor cell outer segments. *J. Cell Biol.* **1967**, *33*, 61–72. [CrossRef]

63. Jin, H.; White, S.R.; Shida, T.; Schulz, S.; Aguiar, M.; Gygi, S.P.; Bazan, J.F.; Nachury, M.V. The conserved Bardet-Biedl syndrome proteins assemble a coat that traffics membrane proteins to cilia. *Cell* **2010**, *141*, 1208–1219. [CrossRef]

64. Liew, G.M.; Ye, F.; Nager, A.R.; Murphy, J.P.; Lee, J.S.; Aguiar, M.; Breslow, D.K.; Gygi, S.P.; Nachury, M.V. The intraflagellar transport protein IFT27 promotes BBSome exit from cilia through the GTPase ARL6/BBS3. *Dev. Cell* **2014**, *31*, 265–278. [CrossRef]

65. Taub, D.G.; Liu, Q. The Role of Intraflagellar Transport in the Photoreceptor Sensory Cilium. *Adv. Exp. Med. Biol.* **2016**, *854*, 627–633. [CrossRef] [PubMed]

66. Pazour, G.J.; Baker, S.A.; Deane, J.A.; Cole, D.G.; Dickert, B.L.; Rosenbaum, J.L.; Witman, G.B.; Besharse, J.C. The intraflagellar transport protein, IFT88, is essential for vertebrate photoreceptor assembly and maintenance. *J. Cell Biol.* **2002**, *157*, 103–113. [CrossRef] [PubMed]

67. Jensen, V.L.; Leroux, M.R. Gates for soluble and membrane proteins, and two trafficking systems (IFT and LIFT), establish a dynamic ciliary signaling compartment. *Curr. Opin. Cell Biol.* **2017**, *47*, 83–91. [CrossRef] [PubMed]

68. Baehr, W. Membrane protein transport in photoreceptors: The function of PDEdelta: The Proctor lecture. *Investig. Ophthalmol. Vis. Sci.* **2014**, *55*, 8653–8666. [CrossRef]

69. Hsu, Y.; Garrison, J.E.; Kim, G.; Schmitz, A.R.; Searby, C.C.; Zhang, Q.; Datta, P.; Nishimura, D.Y.; Seo, S.; Sheffield, V.C. BBSome function is required for both the morphogenesis and maintenance of the photoreceptor outer segment. *PLoS Genet.* **2017**, *13*, e1007057. [CrossRef]

70. Jiang, L.; Wei, Y.; Ronquillo, C.C.; Marc, R.E.; Yoder, B.K.; Frederick, J.M.; Baehr, W. Heterotrimeric kinesin-2 (KIF3) mediates transition zone and axoneme formation of mouse photoreceptors. *J. Biol. Chem.* **2015**, *290*, 12765–12778. [CrossRef]

71. Ronquillo, C.C.; Hanke-Gogokhia, C.; Revelo, M.P.; Frederick, J.M.; Jiang, L.; Baehr, W. Ciliopathy-associated IQCB1/NPHP5 protein is required for mouse photoreceptor outer segment formation. *FASEB J.* **2016**, *30*, 3400–3412. [CrossRef]

72. Hanke-Gogokhia, C.; Wu, Z.; Sharif, A.; Yazigi, H.; Frederick, J.M.; Baehr, W. The guanine nucleotide exchange factor Arf-like protein 13b is essential for assembly of the mouse photoreceptor transition zone and outer segment. *J. Biol. Chem.* **2017**, *292*, 21442–21456. [CrossRef]

73. Cantagrel, V.; Silhavy, J.L.; Bielas, S.L.; Swistun, D.; Marsh, S.E.; Bertrand, J.Y.; Audollent, S.; Attie-Bitach, T.; Holden, K.R.; Dobyns, W.B.; et al. Mutations in the cilia gene ARL13B lead to the classical form of Joubert syndrome. *Am. J. Hum. Genet.* **2008**, *83*, 170–179. [CrossRef]

74. Caspary, T.; Larkins, C.E.; Anderson, K.V. The graded response to Sonic Hedgehog depends on cilia architecture. *Dev. Cell* **2007**, *12*, 767–778. [CrossRef]

75. Eblimit, A.; Agrawal, S.A.; Thomas, K.; Anastassov, I.A.; Abulikemu, T.; Moayedi, Y.; Mardon, G.; Chen, R. Conditional loss of Spata7 in photoreceptors causes progressive retinal degeneration in mice. *Exp. Eye Res.* **2018**, *166*, 120–130. [CrossRef] [PubMed]

76. Singla, V.; Reiter, J.F. The primary cilium as the cell's antenna: Signaling at a sensory organelle. *Science* **2006**, *313*, 629–633. [CrossRef]

77. Garcia-Gonzalo, F.R.; Reiter, J.F. Open Sesame: How Transition Fibers and the Transition Zone Control Ciliary Composition. *Cold Spring Harb. Perspect. Biol.* **2017**, *9*, a028134. [CrossRef]

78. Shi, X.; Garcia, G., 3rd; Van De Weghe, J.C.; McGorty, R.; Pazour, G.J.; Doherty, D.; Huang, B.; Reiter, J.F. Super-resolution microscopy reveals that disruption of ciliary transition-zone architecture causes Joubert syndrome. *Nat. Cell Biol.* **2017**, *19*, 1178–1188. [CrossRef] [PubMed]

79. Williams, C.L.; Li, C.; Kida, K.; Inglis, P.N.; Mohan, S.; Semenec, L.; Bialas, N.J.; Stupay, R.M.; Chen, N.; Blacque, O.E.; et al. MKS and NPHP modules cooperate to establish basal body/transition zone membrane associations and ciliary gate function during ciliogenesis. *J. Cell Biol.* **2011**, *192*, 1023–1041. [CrossRef] [PubMed]

80. Knorz, V.J.; Spalluto, C.; Lessard, M.; Purvis, T.L.; Adigun, F.F.; Collin, G.B.; Hanley, N.A.; Wilson, D.I.; Hearn, T. Centriolar association of ALMS1 and likely centrosomal functions of the ALMS motif-containing proteins C10orf90 and KIAA1731. *Mol. Biol. Cell* **2010**, *21*, 3617–3629. [CrossRef] [PubMed]

81. Hearn, T.; Renforth, G.L.; Spalluto, C.; Hanley, N.A.; Piper, K.; Brickwood, S.; White, C.; Connolly, V.; Taylor, J.F.; Russell-Eggitt, I.; et al. Mutation of ALMS1, a large gene with a tandem repeat encoding 47 amino acids, causes Alstrom syndrome. *Nat. Genet.* **2002**, *31*, 79–83. [CrossRef]

82. Collin, G.B.; Marshall, J.D.; Ikeda, A.; So, W.V.; Russell-Eggitt, I.; Maffei, P.; Beck, S.; Boerkoel, C.F.; Sicolo, N.; Martin, M.; et al. Mutations in ALMS1 cause obesity, type 2 diabetes and neurosensory degeneration in Alstrom syndrome. *Nat. Genet.* **2002**, *31*, 74–78. [CrossRef]

83. Collin, G.B.; Cyr, E.; Bronson, R.; Marshall, J.D.; Gifford, E.J.; Hicks, W.; Murray, S.A.; Zheng, Q.Y.; Smith, R.S.; Nishina, P.M.; et al. Alms1-disrupted mice recapitulate human Alstrom syndrome. *Hum. Mol. Genet.* **2005**, *14*, 2323–2333. [CrossRef]

84. Brun, A.; Yu, X.; Obringer, C.; Ajoy, D.; Haser, E.; Stoetzel, C.; Roux, M.J.; Messaddeq, N.; Dollfus, H.; Marion, V. In vivo phenotypic and molecular characterization of retinal degeneration in mouse models of three ciliopathies. *Exp. Eye Res.* **2019**, *186*, 107721. [CrossRef]

85. May-Simera, H.L.; Gumerson, J.D.; Gao, C.; Campos, M.; Cologna, S.M.; Beyer, T.; Boldt, K.; Kaya, K.D.; Patel, N.; Kretschmer, F.; et al. Loss of MACF1 Abolishes Ciliogenesis and Disrupts Apicobasal Polarity Establishment in the Retina. *Cell Rep.* **2016**, *17*, 1399–1413. [CrossRef] [PubMed]

86. Gerding, W.M.; Schreiber, S.; Schulte-Middelmann, T.; de Castro Marques, A.; Atorf, J.; Akkad, D.A.; Dekomien, G.; Kremers, J.; Dermietzel, R.; Gal, A.; et al. Ccdc66 null mutation causes retinal degeneration and dysfunction. *Hum. Mol. Genet.* **2011**, *20*, 3620–3631. [CrossRef] [PubMed]

87. Insolera, R.; Shao, W.; Airik, R.; Hildebrandt, F.; Shi, S.H. SDCCAG8 regulates pericentriolar material recruitment and neuronal migration in the developing cortex. *Neuron* **2014**, *83*, 805–822. [CrossRef] [PubMed]

88. Veleri, S.; Manjunath, S.H.; Fariss, R.N.; May-Simera, H.; Brooks, M.; Foskett, T.A.; Gao, C.; Longo, T.A.; Liu, P.; Nagashima, K.; et al. Ciliopathy-associated gene Cc2d2a promotes assembly of subdistal appendages on the mother centriole during cilia biogenesis. *Nat. Commun.* **2014**, *5*, 4207. [CrossRef]

89. Tallila, J.; Jakkula, E.; Peltonen, L.; Salonen, R.; Kestila, M. Identification of CC2D2A as a Meckel syndrome gene adds an important piece to the ciliopathy puzzle. *Am. J. Hum. Genet.* **2008**, *82*, 1361–1367. [CrossRef]

90. Gorden, N.T.; Arts, H.H.; Parisi, M.A.; Coene, K.L.; Letteboer, S.J.; van Beersum, S.E.; Mans, D.A.; Hikida, A.; Eckert, M.; Knutzen, D.; et al. CC2D2A is mutated in Joubert syndrome and interacts with the ciliopathy-associated basal body protein CEP290. *Am. J. Hum. Genet.* **2008**, *83*, 559–571. [CrossRef]

91. Mejecase, C.; Hummel, A.; Mohand-Said, S.; Andrieu, C.; El Shamieh, S.; Antonio, A.; Condroyer, C.; Boyard, F.; Foussard, M.; Blanchard, S.; et al. Whole exome sequencing resolves complex phenotype and identifies CC2D2A mutations underlying non-syndromic rod-cone dystrophy. *Clin. Genet.* **2019**, *95*, 329–333. [CrossRef]

92. Lewis, W.R.; Bales, K.L.; Revell, D.Z.; Croyle, M.J.; Engle, S.E.; Song, C.J.; Malarkey, E.B.; Uytingco, C.R.; Shan, D.; Antonellis, P.J.; et al. Mks6 mutations reveal tissue- and cell type-specific roles for the cilia transition zone. *FASEB J.* **2019**, *33*, 1440–1455. [CrossRef]

93. Sorusch, N.; Bauss, K.; Plutniok, J.; Samanta, A.; Knapp, B.; Nagel-Wolfrum, K.; Wolfrum, U. Characterization of the ternary Usher syndrome SANS/ush2a/whirlin protein complex. *Hum. Mol. Genet.* **2017**, *26*, 1157–1172. [CrossRef]

94. Liu, X.; Bulgakov, O.V.; Darrow, K.N.; Pawlyk, B.; Adamian, M.; Liberman, M.C.; Li, T. Usherin is required for maintenance of retinal photoreceptors and normal development of cochlear hair cells. *Proc. Natl. Acad. Sci. USA* **2007**, *104*, 4413–4418. [CrossRef]

95.   Yang, J.; Liu, X.; Zhao, Y.; Adamian, M.; Pawlyk, B.; Sun, X.; McMillan, D.R.; Liberman, M.C.; Li, T. Ablation of whirlin long isoform disrupts the USH2 protein complex and causes vision and hearing loss. *PLoS Genet.* **2010**, *6*, e1000955. [CrossRef] [PubMed]

96.   Khattree, N.; Ritter, L.M.; Goldberg, A.F. Membrane curvature generation by a C-terminal amphipathic helix in peripherin-2/rds, a tetraspanin required for photoreceptor sensory cilium morphogenesis. *J. Cell Sci.* **2013**, *126*, 4659–4670. [CrossRef] [PubMed]

97.   Molday, R.S.; Hicks, D.; Molday, L. Peripherin. A rim-specific membrane protein of rod outer segment discs. *Investig. Ophthalmol. Vis. Sci.* **1987**, *28*, 50–61. [PubMed]

98.   Wood, C.R.; Huang, K.; Diener, D.R.; Rosenbaum, J.L. The cilium secretes bioactive ectosomes. *Curr. Biol.* **2013**, *23*, 906–911. [CrossRef]

99.   Wood, C.R.; Rosenbaum, J.L. Ciliary ectosomes: Transmissions from the cell's antenna. *Trends Cell Biol.* **2015**, *25*, 276–285. [CrossRef] [PubMed]

100. Stuck, M.W.; Conley, S.M.; Naash, M.I. The Y141C knockin mutation in RDS leads to complex phenotypes in the mouse. *Hum. Mol. Genet.* **2014**, *23*, 6260–6274. [CrossRef]

101. Chakraborty, D.; Conley, S.M.; Zulliger, R.; Naash, M.I. The K153Del PRPH2 mutation differentially impacts photoreceptor structure and function. *Hum. Mol. Genet.* **2016**, *25*, 3500–3514. [CrossRef]

102. Sanyal, S.; De Ruiter, A.; Hawkins, R.K. Development and degeneration of retina in rds mutant mice: Light microscopy. *J. Comp. Neurol.* **1980**, *194*, 193–207. [CrossRef]

103. Sanyal, S.; Hawkins, R.K. Development and degeneration of retina in rds mutant mice: Effects of light on the rate of degeneration in albino and pigmented homozygous and heterozygous mutant and normal mice. *Vis. Res.* **1986**, *26*, 1177–1185. [CrossRef]

104. McNally, N.; Kenna, P.F.; Rancourt, D.; Ahmed, T.; Stitt, A.; Colledge, W.H.; Lloyd, D.G.; Palfi, A.; O'Neill, B.; Humphries, M.M.; et al. Murine model of autosomal dominant retinitis pigmentosa generated by targeted deletion at codon 307 of the rds-peripherin gene. *Hum. Mol. Genet.* **2002**, *11*, 1005–1016. [CrossRef]

105. Chakraborty, D.; Conley, S.M.; Al-Ubaidi, M.R.; Naash, M.I. Initiation of rod outer segment disc formation requires RDS. *PLoS ONE* **2014**, *9*, e98939. [CrossRef] [PubMed]

106. Kajiwara, K.; Berson, E.L.; Dryja, T.P. Digenic retinitis pigmentosa due to mutations at the unlinked peripherin/RDS and ROM1 loci. *Science* **1994**, *264*, 1604–1608. [CrossRef] [PubMed]

107. Clarke, G.; Goldberg, A.F.; Vidgen, D.; Collins, L.; Ploder, L.; Schwarz, L.; Molday, L.L.; Rossant, J.; Szel, A.; Molday, R.S.; et al. Rom-1 is required for rod photoreceptor viability and the regulation of disk morphogenesis. *Nat. Genet.* **2000**, *25*, 67–73. [CrossRef] [PubMed]

108. Sato, H.; Suzuki, T.; Ikeda, K.; Masuya, H.; Sezutsu, H.; Kaneda, H.; Kobayashi, K.; Miura, I.; Kurihara, Y.; Yokokura, S.; et al. A monogenic dominant mutation in Rom1 generated by N-ethyl-N-nitrosourea mutagenesis causes retinal degeneration in mice. *Mol. Vis.* **2010**, *16*, 378–391.

109. Spencer, W.J.; Pearring, J.N.; Salinas, R.Y.; Loiselle, D.R.; Skiba, N.P.; Arshavsky, V.Y. Progressive Rod-Cone Degeneration (PRCD) Protein Requires N-Terminal S-Acylation and Rhodopsin Binding for Photoreceptor Outer Segment Localization and Maintaining Intracellular Stability. *Biochemistry* **2016**, *55*, 5028–5037. [CrossRef]

110. Allon, G.; Mann, I.; Remez, L.; Sehn, E.; Rizel, L.; Nevet, M.J.; Perlman, I.; Wolfrum, U.; Ben-Yosef, T. PRCD is Concentrated at the Base of Photoreceptor Outer Segments and is Involved in Outer Segment Disc Formation. *Hum. Mol. Genet.* **2019**, *28*, 4078–4088. [CrossRef]

111. Zangerl, B.; Goldstein, O.; Philp, A.R.; Lindauer, S.J.; Pearce-Kelling, S.E.; Mullins, R.F.; Graphodatsky, A.S.; Ripoll, D.; Felix, J.S.; Stone, E.M.; et al. Identical mutation in a novel retinal gene causes progressive rod-cone degeneration in dogs and retinitis pigmentosa in humans. *Genomics* **2006**, *88*, 551–563. [CrossRef]

112. Spencer, W.J.; Ding, J.D.; Lewis, T.R.; Yu, C.; Phan, S.; Pearring, J.N.; Kim, K.Y.; Thor, A.; Mathew, R.; Kalnitsky, J.; et al. PRCD is essential for high-fidelity photoreceptor disc formation. *Proc. Natl. Acad. Sci. USA* **2019**, *116*, 13087–13096. [CrossRef]

113. Pedersen, L.B.; Rosenbaum, J.L. Intraflagellar transport (IFT) role in ciliary assembly, resorption and signalling. *Curr. Top. Dev. Biol.* **2008**, *85*, 23–61. [CrossRef]

114. Cortellino, S.; Wang, C.; Wang, B.; Bassi, M.R.; Caretti, E.; Champeval, D.; Calmont, A.; Jarnik, M.; Burch, J.; Zaret, K.S.; et al. Defective ciliogenesis, embryonic lethality and severe impairment of the Sonic Hedgehog pathway caused by inactivation of the mouse complex A intraflagellar transport gene Ift122/Wdr10, partially overlapping with the DNA repair gene Med1/Mbd4. *Dev. Biol.* **2009**, *325*, 225–237. [CrossRef]

115. Murcia, N.S.; Richards, W.G.; Yoder, B.K.; Mucenski, M.L.; Dunlap, J.R.; Woychik, R.P. The Oak Ridge Polycystic Kidney (orpk) disease gene is required for left-right axis determination. *Development* **2000**, *127*, 2347–2355. [PubMed]

116. Stottmann, R.W.; Tran, P.V.; Turbe-Doan, A.; Beier, D.R. Ttc21b is required to restrict sonic hedgehog activity in the developing mouse forebrain. *Dev. Biol.* **2009**, *335*, 166–178. [CrossRef] [PubMed]

117. Gorivodsky, M.; Mukhopadhyay, M.; Wilsch-Braeuninger, M.; Phillips, M.; Teufel, A.; Kim, C.; Malik, N.; Huttner, W.; Westphal, H. Intraflagellar transport protein 172 is essential for primary cilia formation and plays a vital role in patterning the mammalian brain. *Dev. Biol.* **2009**, *325*, 24–32. [CrossRef] [PubMed]

118. Rix, S.; Calmont, A.; Scambler, P.J.; Beales, P.L. An Ift80 mouse model of short rib polydactyly syndromes shows defects in hedgehog signalling without loss or malformation of cilia. *Hum. Mol. Genet.* **2011**, *20*, 1306–1314. [CrossRef]

119. Berbari, N.F.; Kin, N.W.; Sharma, N.; Michaud, E.J.; Kesterson, R.A.; Yoder, B.K. Mutations in Traf3ip1 reveal defects in ciliogenesis, embryonic development, and altered cell size regulation. *Dev. Biol.* **2011**, *360*, 66–76. [CrossRef]

120. Bangs, F.; Anderson, K.V. Primary Cilia and Mammalian Hedgehog Signaling. *Cold Spring Harb. Perspect. Biol.* **2017**, *9*, a028175. [CrossRef]

121. Ko, H.W.; Liu, A.; Eggenschwiler, J.T. Analysis of hedgehog signaling in mouse intraflagellar transport mutants. *Methods Cell Biol.* **2009**, *93*, 347–369. [CrossRef]

122. Gupta, P.R.; Pendse, N.; Greenwald, S.H.; Leon, M.; Liu, Q.; Pierce, E.A.; Bujakowska, K.M. Ift172 conditional knock-out mice exhibit rapid retinal degeneration and protein trafficking defects. *Hum. Mol. Genet.* **2018**, *27*, 2012–2024. [CrossRef]

123. Keady, B.T.; Le, Y.Z.; Pazour, G.J. IFT20 is required for opsin trafficking and photoreceptor outer segment development. *Mol. Biol. Cell* **2011**, *22*, 921–930. [CrossRef]

124. Resh, M.D. Trafficking and signaling by fatty-acylated and prenylated proteins. *Nat. Chem. Biol.* **2006**, *2*, 584–590. [CrossRef]

125. Schwarz, N.; Hardcastle, A.J.; Cheetham, M.E. Arl3 and RP2 mediated assembly and traffic of membrane associated cilia proteins. *Vis. Res.* **2012**, *75*, 2–4. [CrossRef] [PubMed]

126. Li, L.; Khan, N.; Hurd, T.; Ghosh, A.K.; Cheng, C.; Molday, R.; Heckenlively, J.R.; Swaroop, A.; Khanna, H. Ablation of the X-linked retinitis pigmentosa 2 (Rp2) gene in mice results in opsin mislocalization and photoreceptor degeneration. *Investig. Ophthalmol. Vis. Sci.* **2013**, *54*, 4503–4511. [CrossRef] [PubMed]

127. Zhang, H.; Hanke-Gogokhia, C.; Jiang, L.; Li, X.; Wang, P.; Gerstner, C.D.; Frederick, J.M.; Yang, Z.; Baehr, W. Mistrafficking of prenylated proteins causes retinitis pigmentosa 2. *FASEB J.* **2015**, *29*, 932–942. [CrossRef] [PubMed]

128. Wright, Z.C.; Singh, R.K.; Alpino, R.; Goldberg, A.F.; Sokolov, M.; Ramamurthy, V. ARL3 regulates trafficking of prenylated phototransduction proteins to the rod outer segment. *Hum. Mol. Genet.* **2016**, *25*, 2031–2044. [CrossRef]

129. Schrick, J.J.; Vogel, P.; Abuin, A.; Hampton, B.; Rice, D.S. ADP-ribosylation factor-like 3 is involved in kidney and photoreceptor development. *Am. J. Pathol.* **2006**, *168*, 1288–1298. [CrossRef]

130. Rao, K.N.; Zhang, W.; Li, L.; Anand, M.; Khanna, H. Prenylated retinal ciliopathy protein RPGR interacts with PDE6delta and regulates ciliary localization of Joubert syndrome-associated protein INPP5E. *Hum. Mol. Genet.* **2016**, *25*, 4533–4545. [CrossRef]

131. Xu, W.; Jin, M.; Hu, R.; Wang, H.; Zhang, F.; Yuan, S.; Cao, Y. The Joubert Syndrome Protein Inpp5e Controls Ciliogenesis by Regulating Phosphoinositides at the Apical Membrane. *J. Am. Soc. Nephrol.* **2017**, *28*, 118–129. [CrossRef]

132. Gillespie, P.G.; Prusti, R.K.; Apel, E.D.; Beavo, J.A. A soluble form of bovine rod photoreceptor phosphodiesterase has a novel 15-kDa subunit. *J. Biol. Chem.* **1989**, *264*, 12187–12193.

133. Thompson, D.A.; Khan, N.W.; Othman, M.I.; Chang, B.; Jia, L.; Grahek, G.; Wu, Z.; Hiriyanna, S.; Nellissery, J.; Li, T.; et al. Rd9 is a naturally occurring mouse model of a common form of retinitis pigmentosa caused by mutations in RPGR-ORF15. *PLoS ONE* **2012**, *7*, e35865. [CrossRef]

134. Hong, D.H.; Pawlyk, B.S.; Shang, J.; Sandberg, M.A.; Berson, E.L.; Li, T. A retinitis pigmentosa GTPase regulator (RPGR)-deficient mouse model for X-linked retinitis pigmentosa (RP3). *Proc. Natl. Acad. Sci. USA* **2000**, *97*, 3649–3654. [CrossRef]

135. Zhang, H.; Li, S.; Doan, T.; Rieke, F.; Detwiler, P.B.; Frederick, J.M.; Baehr, W. Deletion of PrBP/delta impedes transport of GRK1 and PDE6 catalytic subunits to photoreceptor outer segments. *Proc. Natl. Acad. Sci. USA* **2007**, *104*, 8857–8862. [CrossRef] [PubMed]

136. Ramamurthy, V.; Niemi, G.A.; Reh, T.A.; Hurley, J.B. Leber congenital amaurosis linked to AIPL1: A mouse model reveals destabilization of cGMP phosphodiesterase. *Proc. Natl. Acad. Sci. USA* **2004**, *101*, 13897–13902. [CrossRef] [PubMed]

137. Yadav, R.P.; Artemyev, N.O. AIPL1: A specialized chaperone for the phototransduction effector. *Cell Signal.* **2017**, *40*, 183–189. [CrossRef] [PubMed]

138. Scheidecker, S.; Etard, C.; Pierce, N.W.; Geoffroy, V.; Schaefer, E.; Muller, J.; Chennen, K.; Flori, E.; Pelletier, V.; Poch, O.; et al. Exome sequencing of Bardet-Biedl syndrome patient identifies a null mutation in the BBSome subunit BBIP1 (BBS18). *J. Med. Genet.* **2014**, *51*, 132–136. [CrossRef] [PubMed]

139. Eichers, E.R.; Abd-El-Barr, M.M.; Paylor, R.; Lewis, R.A.; Bi, W.; Lin, X.; Meehan, T.P.; Stockton, D.W.; Wu, S.M.; Lindsay, E.; et al. Phenotypic characterization of Bbs4 null mice reveals age-dependent penetrance and variable expressivity. *Hum. Genet.* **2006**, *120*, 211–226. [CrossRef] [PubMed]

140. Mykytyn, K.; Mullins, R.F.; Andrews, M.; Chiang, A.P.; Swiderski, R.E.; Yang, B.; Braun, T.; Casavant, T.; Stone, E.M.; Sheffield, V.C. Bardet-Biedl syndrome type 4 (BBS4)-null mice implicate Bbs4 in flagella formation but not global cilia assembly. *Proc. Natl. Acad. Sci. USA* **2004**, *101*, 8664–8669. [CrossRef] [PubMed]

141. Koch, K.W.; Dell'Orco, D. Protein and Signaling Networks in Vertebrate Photoreceptor Cells. *Front. Mol. Neurosci.* **2015**, *8*, 67. [CrossRef]

142. Pinto, L.H.; Vitaterna, M.H.; Shimomura, K.; Siepka, S.M.; McDearmon, E.L.; Fenner, D.; Lumayag, S.L.; Omura, C.; Andrews, A.W.; Baker, M.; et al. Generation, characterization, and molecular cloning of the Noerg-1 mutation of rhodopsin in the mouse. *Vis. Neurosci.* **2005**, *22*, 619–629. [CrossRef]

143. Liu, H.; Wang, M.; Xia, C.H.; Du, X.; Flannery, J.G.; Ridge, K.D.; Beutler, B.; Gong, X. Severe retinal degeneration caused by a novel rhodopsin mutation. *Investig. Ophthalmol. Vis. Sci.* **2010**, *51*, 1059–1065. [CrossRef]

144. Sakami, S.; Maeda, T.; Bereta, G.; Okano, K.; Golczak, M.; Sumaroka, A.; Roman, A.J.; Cideciyan, A.V.; Jacobson, S.G.; Palczewski, K. Probing mechanisms of photoreceptor degeneration in a new mouse model of the common form of autosomal dominant retinitis pigmentosa due to P23H opsin mutations. *J. Biol. Chem.* **2011**, *286*, 10551–10567. [CrossRef]

145. Chiang, W.C.; Kroeger, H.; Sakami, S.; Messah, C.; Yasumura, D.; Matthes, M.T.; Coppinger, J.A.; Palczewski, K.; LaVail, M.M.; Lin, J.H. Robust Endoplasmic Reticulum-Associated Degradation of Rhodopsin Precedes Retinal Degeneration. *Mol. Neurobiol.* **2015**, *52*, 679–695. [CrossRef] [PubMed]

146. Comitato, A.; Schiroli, D.; Montanari, M.; Marigo, V. Calpain Activation Is the Major Cause of Cell Death in Photoreceptors Expressing a Rhodopsin Misfolding Mutation. *Mol. Neurobiol.* **2020**, *57*, 589–599. [CrossRef] [PubMed]

147. Athanasiou, D.; Aguila, M.; Bevilacqua, D.; Novoselov, S.S.; Parfitt, D.A.; Cheetham, M.E. The cell stress machinery and retinal degeneration. *FEBS Lett.* **2013**, *587*, 2008–2017. [CrossRef] [PubMed]

148. Athanasiou, D.; Aguila, M.; Bellingham, J.; Kanuga, N.; Adamson, P.; Cheetham, M.E. The role of the ER stress-response protein PERK in rhodopsin retinitis pigmentosa. *Hum. Mol. Genet.* **2017**, *26*, 4896–4905. [CrossRef]

149. Zhang, N.; Kolesnikov, A.V.; Jastrzebska, B.; Mustafi, D.; Sawada, O.; Maeda, T.; Genoud, C.; Engel, A.; Kefalov, V.J.; Palczewski, K. Autosomal recessive retinitis pigmentosa E150K opsin mice exhibit photoreceptor disorganization. *J. Clin. Investig.* **2013**, *123*, 121–137. [CrossRef]

150. Sakami, S.; Kolesnikov, A.V.; Kefalov, V.J.; Palczewski, K. P23H opsin knock-in mice reveal a novel step in retinal rod disc morphogenesis. *Hum. Mol. Genet.* **2014**, *23*, 1723–1741. [CrossRef]

151. Hollingsworth, T.J.; Gross, A.K. The severe autosomal dominant retinitis pigmentosa rhodopsin mutant Ter349Glu mislocalizes and induces rapid rod cell death. *J. Biol. Chem.* **2013**, *288*, 29047–29055. [CrossRef]

152. Humphries, M.M.; Rancourt, D.; Farrar, G.J.; Kenna, P.; Hazel, M.; Bush, R.A.; Sieving, P.A.; Sheils, D.M.; McNally, N.; Creighton, P.; et al. Retinopathy induced in mice by targeted disruption of the rhodopsin gene. *Nat. Genet.* **1997**, *15*, 216–219. [CrossRef]

153. Lem, J.; Krasnoperova, N.V.; Calvert, P.D.; Kosaras, B.; Cameron, D.A.; Nicolo, M.; Makino, C.L.; Sidman, R.L. Morphological, physiological, and biochemical changes in rhodopsin knockout mice. *Proc. Natl. Acad. Sci. USA* **1999**, *96*, 736–741. [CrossRef]

154. Faber, S.; Roepman, R. Balancing the Photoreceptor Proteome: Proteostasis Network Therapeutics for Inherited Retinal Disease. *Genes* **2019**, *10*, 557. [CrossRef]

155. Sancho-Pelluz, J.; Cui, X.; Lee, W.; Tsai, Y.T.; Wu, W.H.; Justus, S.; Washington, I.; Hsu, C.W.; Park, K.S.; Koch, S.; et al. Mechanisms of neurodegeneration in a preclinical autosomal dominant retinitis pigmentosa knock-in model with a Rho(D190N) mutation. *Cell Mol. Life Sci.* **2019**, *76*, 3657–3665. [CrossRef] [PubMed]

156. Park, P.S. Constitutively active rhodopsin and retinal disease. *Adv. Pharmacol.* **2014**, *70*, 1–36. [CrossRef] [PubMed]

157. Budzynski, E.; Gross, A.K.; McAlear, S.D.; Peachey, N.S.; Shukla, M.; He, F.; Edwards, M.; Won, J.; Hicks, W.L.; Wensel, T.G.; et al. Mutations of the opsin gene (Y102H and I307N) lead to light-induced degeneration of photoreceptors and constitutive activation of phototransduction in mice. *J. Biol. Chem.* **2010**, *285*, 14521–14533. [CrossRef] [PubMed]

158. Daniele, L.L.; Insinna, C.; Chance, R.; Wang, J.; Nikonov, S.S.; Pugh, E.N., Jr. A mouse M-opsin monochromat: Retinal cone photoreceptors have increased M-opsin expression when S-opsin is knocked out. *Vis. Res.* **2011**, *51*, 447–458. [CrossRef] [PubMed]

159. Zhang, Y.; Deng, W.T.; Du, W.; Zhu, P.; Li, J.; Xu, F.; Sun, J.; Gerstner, C.D.; Baehr, W.; Boye, S.L.; et al. Gene-based Therapy in a Mouse Model of Blue Cone Monochromacy. *Sci. Rep.* **2017**, *7*, 6690. [CrossRef] [PubMed]

160. Carter-Dawson, L.D.; LaVail, M.M.; Sidman, R.L. Differential effect of the rd mutation on rods and cones in the mouse retina. *Investig. Ophthalmol. Vis. Sci.* **1978**, *17*, 489–498. [PubMed]

161. Calvert, P.D.; Krasnoperova, N.V.; Lyubarsky, A.L.; Isayama, T.; Nicolo, M.; Kosaras, B.; Wong, G.; Gannon, K.S.; Margolskee, R.F.; Sidman, R.L.; et al. Phototransduction in transgenic mice after targeted deletion of the rod transducin alpha -subunit. *Proc. Natl. Acad. Sci. USA* **2000**, *97*, 13913–13918. [CrossRef]

162. Barber, A.C.; Hippert, C.; Duran, Y.; West, E.L.; Bainbridge, J.W.; Warre-Cornish, K.; Luhmann, U.F.; Lakowski, J.; Sowden, J.C.; Ali, R.R.; et al. Repair of the degenerate retina by photoreceptor transplantation. *Proc. Natl. Acad. Sci. USA* **2013**, *110*, 354–359. [CrossRef]

163. Miyamoto, M.; Aoki, M.; Sugimoto, S.; Kawasaki, K.; Imai, R. IRD1 and IRD2 mice, naturally occurring models of hereditary retinal dysfunction, show late-onset and progressive retinal degeneration. *Curr. Eye Res.* **2010**, *35*, 137–145. [CrossRef]

164. Mejecase, C.; Laurent-Coriat, C.; Mayer, C.; Poch, O.; Mohand-Said, S.; Prevot, C.; Antonio, A.; Boyard, F.; Condroyer, C.; Michiels, C.; et al. Identification of a Novel Homozygous Nonsense Mutation Confirms the Implication of GNAT1 in Rod-Cone Dystrophy. *PLoS ONE* **2016**, *11*, e0168271. [CrossRef]

165. Carrigan, M.; Duignan, E.; Humphries, P.; Palfi, A.; Kenna, P.F.; Farrar, G.J. A novel homozygous truncating GNAT1 mutation implicated in retinal degeneration. *Br. J. Ophthalmol.* **2016**, *100*, 495–500. [CrossRef] [PubMed]

166. Zenteno, J.C.; Garcia-Montano, L.A.; Cruz-Aguilar, M.; Ronquillo, J.; Rodas-Serrano, A.; Aguilar-Castul, L.; Matsui, R.; Vencedor-Meraz, C.I.; Arce-Gonzalez, R.; Graue-Wiechers, F.; et al. Extensive genic and allelic heterogeneity underlying inherited retinal dystrophies in Mexican patients molecularly analyzed by next-generation sequencing. *Mol. Genet. Genomic Med.* **2020**, *8*. [CrossRef] [PubMed]

167. Deng, W.T.; Sakurai, K.; Liu, J.; Dinculescu, A.; Li, J.; Pang, J.; Min, S.H.; Chiodo, V.A.; Boye, S.L.; Chang, B.; et al. Functional interchangeability of rod and cone transducin alpha-subunits. *Proc. Natl. Acad. Sci. USA* **2009**, *106*, 17681–17686. [CrossRef] [PubMed]

168. Chang, B.; Hawes, N.L.; Hurd, R.E.; Wang, J.; Davisson, M.T.; Nusinowitz, S.; Heckenlively, J.R. A New Mouse Model of Retinal Degeneration (rd17). Proceedings of ARVO Annual Meeting Abstract, Fort Lauderdale, FL, USA, 6–10 May 2007.

169. Lobanova, E.S.; Finkelstein, S.; Herrmann, R.; Chen, Y.M.; Kessler, C.; Michaud, N.A.; Trieu, L.H.; Strissel, K.J.; Burns, M.E.; Arshavsky, V.Y. Transducin gamma-subunit sets expression levels of alpha- and beta-subunits and is crucial for rod viability. *J. Neurosci.* **2008**, *28*, 3510–3520. [CrossRef] [PubMed]

170. Kolesnikov, A.V.; Rikimaru, L.; Hennig, A.K.; Lukasiewicz, P.D.; Fliesler, S.J.; Govardovskii, V.I.; Kefalov, V.J.; Kisselev, O.G. G-protein betagamma-complex is crucial for efficient signal amplification in vision. *J. Neurosci.* **2011**, *31*, 8067–8077. [CrossRef]

171. Lobanova, E.S.; Finkelstein, S.; Skiba, N.P.; Arshavsky, V.Y. Proteasome overload is a common stress factor in multiple forms of inherited retinal degeneration. *Proc. Natl. Acad. Sci. USA* **2013**, *110*, 9986–9991. [CrossRef]

172. Jobling, A.I.; Vessey, K.A.; Waugh, M.; Mills, S.A.; Fletcher, E.L. A naturally occurring mouse model of achromatopsia: Characterization of the mutation in cone transducin and subsequent retinal phenotype. *Investig. Ophthalmol. Vis. Sci.* **2013**, *54*, 3350–3359. [CrossRef]

173. Chang, B.; Dacey, M.S.; Hawes, N.L.; Hitchcock, P.F.; Milam, A.H.; Atmaca-Sonmez, P.; Nusinowitz, S.; Heckenlively, J.R. Cone photoreceptor function loss-3, a novel mouse model of achromatopsia due to a mutation in Gnat2. *Investig. Ophthalmol. Vis. Sci.* **2006**, *47*, 5017–5021. [CrossRef]

174. Ronning, K.E.; Allina, G.P.; Miller, E.B.; Zawadzki, R.J.; Pugh, E.N., Jr.; Herrmann, R.; Burns, M.E. Loss of cone function without degeneration in a novel Gnat2 knock-out mouse. *Exp. Eye Res.* **2018**, *171*, 111–118. [CrossRef]

175. Hirji, N.; Aboshiha, J.; Georgiou, M.; Bainbridge, J.; Michaelides, M. Achromatopsia: Clinical features, molecular genetics, animal models and therapeutic options. *Ophthalmic Genet.* **2018**, *39*, 149–157. [CrossRef]

176. Michaelides, M.; Aligianis, I.A.; Holder, G.E.; Simunovic, M.; Mollon, J.D.; Maher, E.R.; Hunt, D.M.; Moore, A.T. Cone dystrophy phenotype associated with a frameshift mutation (M280fsX291) in the alpha-subunit of cone specific transducin (GNAT2). *Br. J. Ophthalmol.* **2003**, *87*, 1317–1320. [CrossRef]

177. Du, J.; An, J.; Linton, J.D.; Wang, Y.; Hurley, J.B. How Excessive cGMP Impacts Metabolic Proteins in Retinas at the Onset of Degeneration. *Adv. Exp. Med. Biol.* **2018**, *1074*, 289–295. [CrossRef]

178. Tolone, A.; Belhadj, S.; Rentsch, A.; Schwede, F.; Paquet-Durand, F. The cGMP Pathway and Inherited Photoreceptor Degeneration: Targets, Compounds, and Biomarkers. *Genes* **2019**, *10*, 453. [CrossRef] [PubMed]

179. Sothilingam, V.; Garcia Garrido, M.; Jiao, K.; Buena-Atienza, E.; Sahaboglu, A.; Trifunovic, D.; Balendran, S.; Koepfli, T.; Muhlfriedel, R.; Schon, C.; et al. Retinitis pigmentosa: Impact of different Pde6a point mutations on the disease phenotype. *Hum. Mol. Genet.* **2015**, *24*, 5486–5499. [CrossRef]

180. Sakamoto, K.; McCluskey, M.; Wensel, T.G.; Naggert, J.K.; Nishina, P.M. New mouse models for recessive retinitis pigmentosa caused by mutations in the Pde6a gene. *Hum. Mol. Genet.* **2009**, *18*, 178–192. [CrossRef]

181. Power, M.; Das, S.; Schutze, K.; Marigo, V.; Ekstrom, P.; Paquet-Durand, F. Cellular mechanisms of hereditary photoreceptor degeneration—Focus on cGMP. *Prog. Retin. Eye Res.* **2020**, *74*, 100772. [CrossRef] [PubMed]

182. Tsang, S.H.; Gouras, P.; Yamashita, C.K.; Kjeldbye, H.; Fisher, J.; Farber, D.B.; Goff, S.P. Retinal degeneration in mice lacking the gamma subunit of the rod cGMP phosphodiesterase. *Science* **1996**, *272*, 1026–1029. [CrossRef] [PubMed]

183. Thiadens, A.A.; Somervuo, V.; van den Born, L.I.; Roosing, S.; van Schooneveld, M.J.; Kuijpers, R.W.; van Moll-Ramirez, N.; Cremers, F.P.; Hoyng, C.B.; Klaver, C.C. Progressive loss of cones in achromatopsia: An imaging study using spectral-domain optical coherence tomography. *Investig. Ophthalmol. Vis. Sci.* **2010**, *51*, 5952–5957. [CrossRef] [PubMed]

184. Brennenstuhl, C.; Tanimoto, N.; Burkard, M.; Wagner, R.; Bolz, S.; Trifunovic, D.; Kabagema-Bilan, C.; Paquet-Durand, F.; Beck, S.C.; Huber, G.; et al. Targeted ablation of the Pde6h gene in mice reveals cross-species differences in cone and rod phototransduction protein isoform inventory. *J. Biol. Chem.* **2015**, *290*, 10242–10255. [CrossRef]

185. Kohl, S.; Coppieters, F.; Meire, F.; Schaich, S.; Roosing, S.; Brennenstuhl, C.; Bolz, S.; van Genderen, M.M.; Riemslag, F.C.; European Retinal Disease, C.; et al. A nonsense mutation in PDE6H causes autosomal-recessive incomplete achromatopsia. *Am. J. Hum. Genet.* **2012**, *91*, 527–532. [CrossRef]

186. Pedurupillay, C.R.; Landsend, E.C.; Vigeland, M.D.; Ansar, M.; Frengen, E.; Misceo, D.; Stromme, P. Segregation of Incomplete Achromatopsia and Alopecia Due to PDE6H and LPAR6 Variants in a Consanguineous Family from Pakistan. *Genes* **2016**, *7*, 41. [CrossRef]

187. Weitz, D.; Ficek, N.; Kremmer, E.; Bauer, P.J.; Kaupp, U.B. Subunit stoichiometry of the CNG channel of rod photoreceptors. *Neuron* **2002**, *36*, 881–889. [CrossRef]

188. Zheng, J.; Trudeau, M.C.; Zagotta, W.N. Rod cyclic nucleotide-gated channels have a stoichiometry of three CNGA1 subunits and one CNGB1 subunit. *Neuron* **2002**, *36*, 891–896. [CrossRef]

189. Huttl, S.; Michalakis, S.; Seeliger, M.; Luo, D.G.; Acar, N.; Geiger, H.; Hudl, K.; Mader, R.; Haverkamp, S.; Moser, M.; et al. Impaired channel targeting and retinal degeneration in mice lacking the cyclic nucleotide-gated channel subunit CNGB1. *J. Neurosci.* **2005**, *25*, 130–138. [CrossRef] [PubMed]

190. Vinberg, F.; Wang, T.; Molday, R.S.; Chen, J.; Kefalov, V.J. A new mouse model for stationary night blindness with mutant Slc24a1 explains the pathophysiology of the associated human disease. *Hum. Mol. Genet.* **2015**, *24*, 5915–5929. [CrossRef] [PubMed]

191. Yang, R.B.; Robinson, S.W.; Xiong, W.H.; Yau, K.W.; Birch, D.G.; Garbers, D.L. Disruption of a retinal guanylyl cyclase gene leads to cone-specific dystrophy and paradoxical rod behavior. *J. Neurosci.* **1999**, *19*, 5889–5897. [CrossRef] [PubMed]

192. Bouzia, Z.; Georgiou, M.; Hull, S.; Robson, A.G.; Fujinami, K.; Rotsos, T.; Pontikos, N.; Arno, G.; Webster, A.R.; Hardcastle, A.J.; et al. GUCY2D-Associated Leber Congenital Amaurosis: A Retrospective Natural History Study in Preparation for Trials of Novel Therapies. *Am. J. Ophthalmol.* **2020**, *210*, 59–70. [CrossRef]

193. Baehr, W.; Karan, S.; Maeda, T.; Luo, D.G.; Li, S.; Bronson, J.D.; Watt, C.B.; Yau, K.W.; Frederick, J.M.; Palczewski, K. The function of guanylate cyclase 1 and guanylate cyclase 2 in rod and cone photoreceptors. *J. Biol. Chem.* **2007**, *282*, 8837–8847. [CrossRef]

194. Mendez, A.; Burns, M.E.; Sokal, I.; Dizhoor, A.M.; Baehr, W.; Palczewski, K.; Baylor, D.A.; Chen, J. Role of guanylate cyclase-activating proteins (GCAPs) in setting the flash sensitivity of rod photoreceptors. *Proc. Natl. Acad. Sci. USA* **2001**, *98*, 9948–9953. [CrossRef]

195. Buch, P.K.; Mihelec, M.; Cottrill, P.; Wilkie, S.E.; Pearson, R.A.; Duran, Y.; West, E.L.; Michaelides, M.; Ali, R.R.; Hunt, D.M. Dominant cone-rod dystrophy: A mouse model generated by gene targeting of the GCAP1/Guca1a gene. *PLoS ONE* **2011**, *6*, e18089. [CrossRef]

196. Marino, V.; Dal Cortivo, G.; Oppici, E.; Maltese, P.E.; D'Esposito, F.; Manara, E.; Ziccardi, L.; Falsini, B.; Magli, A.; Bertelli, M.; et al. A novel p.(Glu111Val) missense mutation in GUCA1A associated with cone-rod dystrophy leads to impaired calcium sensing and perturbed second messenger homeostasis in photoreceptors. *Hum. Mol. Genet.* **2018**, *27*, 4204–4217. [CrossRef] [PubMed]

197. Chen, C.K.; Burns, M.E.; Spencer, M.; Niemi, G.A.; Chen, J.; Hurley, J.B.; Baylor, D.A.; Simon, M.I. Abnormal photoresponses and light-induced apoptosis in rods lacking rhodopsin kinase. *Proc. Natl. Acad. Sci. USA* **1999**, *96*, 3718–3722. [CrossRef] [PubMed]

198. Xu, J.; Dodd, R.L.; Makino, C.L.; Simon, M.I.; Baylor, D.A.; Chen, J. Prolonged photoresponses in transgenic mouse rods lacking arrestin. *Nature* **1997**, *389*, 505–509. [CrossRef] [PubMed]

199. Chen, J.; Simon, M.I.; Matthes, M.T.; Yasumura, D.; LaVail, M.M. Increased susceptibility to light damage in an arrestin knockout mouse model of Oguchi disease (stationary night blindness). *Investig. Ophthalmol. Vis. Sci.* **1999**, *40*, 2978–2982. [PubMed]

200. Charette, J.R.; Samuels, I.S.; Yu, M.; Stone, L.; Hicks, W.; Shi, L.Y.; Krebs, M.P.; Naggert, J.K.; Nishina, P.M.; Peachey, N.S. A Chemical Mutagenesis Screen Identifies Mouse Models with ERG Defects. *Adv. Exp. Med. Biol.* **2016**, *854*, 177–183. [CrossRef] [PubMed]

201. Rajappa, M.; Goyal, A.; Kaur, J. Inherited metabolic disorders involving the eye: A clinico-biochemical perspective. *Eye* **2010**, *24*, 507–518. [CrossRef] [PubMed]

202. Poll-The, B.T.; Maillette de Buy Wenniger-Prick, C.J. The eye in metabolic diseases: Clues to diagnosis. *Eur. J. Paediatr. Neurol.* **2011**, *15*, 197–204. [CrossRef]

203. Wright, A.F.; Chakarova, C.F.; Abd El-Aziz, M.M.; Bhattacharya, S.S. Photoreceptor degeneration: Genetic and mechanistic dissection of a complex trait. *Nat. Rev. Genet.* **2010**, *11*, 273–284. [CrossRef]

204. Fliesler, S.J.; Anderson, R.E. Chemistry and metabolism of lipids in the vertebrate retina. *Prog. Lipid Res.* **1983**, *22*, 79–131. [CrossRef]

205. Giusto, N.M.; Pasquare, S.J.; Salvador, G.A.; Ilincheta de Boschero, M.G. Lipid second messengers and related enzymes in vertebrate rod outer segments. *J. Lipid Res.* **2010**, *51*, 685–700. [CrossRef]

206. Niu, S.L.; Mitchell, D.C.; Litman, B.J. Manipulation of cholesterol levels in rod disk membranes by methyl-beta-cyclodextrin: Effects on receptor activation. *J. Biol. Chem.* **2002**, *277*, 20139–20145. [CrossRef] [PubMed]

207. Bretillon, L.; Thuret, G.; Gregoire, S.; Acar, N.; Joffre, C.; Bron, A.M.; Gain, P.; Creuzot-Garcher, C.P. Lipid and fatty acid profile of the retina, retinal pigment epithelium/choroid, and the lacrimal gland, and associations with adipose tissue fatty acids in human subjects. *Exp. Eye Res.* **2008**, *87*, 521–528. [CrossRef]

208. Fliesler, S.J.; Bretillon, L. The ins and outs of cholesterol in the vertebrate retina. *J. Lipid Res.* **2010**, *51*, 3399–3413. [CrossRef]

209. German, O.L.; Agnolazza, D.L.; Politi, L.E.; Rotstein, N.P. Light, lipids and photoreceptor survival: Live or let die? *Photochem. Photobiol. Sci.* **2015**, *14*, 1737–1753. [CrossRef] [PubMed]

210. Shindou, H.; Koso, H.; Sasaki, J.; Nakanishi, H.; Sagara, H.; Nakagawa, K.M.; Takahashi, Y.; Hishikawa, D.; Iizuka-Hishikawa, Y.; Tokumasu, F.; et al. Docosahexaenoic acid preserves visual function by maintaining correct disc morphology in retinal photoreceptor cells. *J. Biol. Chem.* **2017**, *292*, 12054–12064. [CrossRef] [PubMed]

211. Lobanova, E.S.; Schuhmann, K.; Finkelstein, S.; Lewis, T.R.; Cady, M.A.; Hao, Y.; Keuthan, C.; Ash, J.D.; Burns, M.E.; Shevchenko, A.; et al. Disrupted Blood-Retina Lysophosphatidylcholine Transport Impairs Photoreceptor Health But Not Visual Signal Transduction. *J. Neurosci.* **2019**, *39*, 9689–9701. [CrossRef] [PubMed]

212. Pham, T.L.; He, J.; Kakazu, A.H.; Jun, B.; Bazan, N.G.; Bazan, H.E.P. Defining a mechanistic link between pigment epithelium-derived factor, docosahexaenoic acid, and corneal nerve regeneration. *J. Biol. Chem.* **2017**, *292*, 18486–18499. [CrossRef]

213. Comitato, A.; Subramanian, P.; Turchiano, G.; Montanari, M.; Becerra, S.P.; Marigo, V. Pigment epithelium-derived factor hinders photoreceptor cell death by reducing intracellular calcium in the degenerating retina. *Cell Death Dis.* **2018**, *9*, 560. [CrossRef]

214. Bernstein, P.S.; Tammur, J.; Singh, N.; Hutchinson, A.; Dixon, M.; Pappas, C.M.; Zabriskie, N.A.; Zhang, K.; Petrukhin, K.; Leppert, M.; et al. Diverse macular dystrophy phenotype caused by a novel complex mutation in the ELOVL4 gene. *Investig. Ophthalmol. Vis. Sci.* **2001**, *42*, 3331–3336.

215. Vasireddy, V.; Jablonski, M.M.; Mandal, M.N.; Raz-Prag, D.; Wang, X.F.; Nizol, L.; Iannaccone, A.; Musch, D.C.; Bush, R.A.; Salem, N., Jr.; et al. Elovl4 5-bp-deletion knock-in mice develop progressive photoreceptor degeneration. *Investig. Ophthalmol. Vis. Sci.* **2006**, *47*, 4558–4568. [CrossRef]

216. Friedman, J.S.; Chang, B.; Krauth, D.S.; Lopez, I.; Waseem, N.H.; Hurd, R.E.; Feathers, K.L.; Branham, K.E.; Shaw, M.; Thomas, G.E.; et al. Loss of lysophosphatidylcholine acyltransferase 1 leads to photoreceptor degeneration in rd11 mice. *Proc. Natl. Acad. Sci. USA* **2010**, *107*, 15523–15528. [CrossRef] [PubMed]

217. Perkovic, T.; Duh, D.; Peterlin, B.; Gregoric, J. The Str mouse as a model for incontinentia pigmenti. *Pflugers Arch.* **2000**, *440*, R53–R54. [CrossRef] [PubMed]

218. Coleman, J.A.; Zhu, X.; Djajadi, H.R.; Molday, L.L.; Smith, R.S.; Libby, R.T.; John, S.W.; Molday, R.S. Phospholipid flippase ATP8A2 is required for normal visual and auditory function and photoreceptor and spiral ganglion cell survival. *J. Cell Sci.* **2014**, *127*, 1138–1149. [CrossRef] [PubMed]

219. Bryde, S.; Hennrich, H.; Verhulst, P.M.; Devaux, P.F.; Lenoir, G.; Holthuis, J.C. CDC50 proteins are critical components of the human class-1 P4-ATPase transport machinery. *J. Biol. Chem.* **2010**, *285*, 40562–40572. [CrossRef]

220. van der Velden, L.M.; Wichers, C.G.; van Breevoort, A.E.; Coleman, J.A.; Molday, R.S.; Berger, R.; Klomp, L.W.; van de Graaf, S.F. Heteromeric interactions required for abundance and subcellular localization of human CDC50 proteins and class 1 P4-ATPases. *J. Biol. Chem.* **2010**, *285*, 40088–40096. [CrossRef]

221. Zhang, L.; Yang, Y.; Li, S.; Zhang, S.; Zhu, X.; Tai, Z.; Yang, M.; Liu, Y.; Guo, X.; Chen, B.; et al. Loss of Tmem30a leads to photoreceptor degeneration. *Sci. Rep.* **2017**, *7*, 9296. [CrossRef]

222. Wong-Riley, M.T. Energy metabolism of the visual system. *Eye Brain* **2010**, *2*, 99–116. [CrossRef] [PubMed]

223. Du, J.; Rountree, A.; Cleghorn, W.M.; Contreras, L.; Lindsay, K.J.; Sadilek, M.; Gu, H.; Djukovic, D.; Raftery, D.; Satrustegui, J.; et al. Phototransduction Influences Metabolic Flux and Nucleotide Metabolism in Mouse Retina. *J. Biol. Chem.* **2016**, *291*, 4698–4710. [CrossRef]

224. Joyal, J.S.; Sun, Y.; Gantner, M.L.; Shao, Z.; Evans, L.P.; Saba, N.; Fredrick, T.; Burnim, S.; Kim, J.S.; Patel, G.; et al. Retinal lipid and glucose metabolism dictates angiogenesis through the lipid sensor Ffar1. *Nat. Med.* **2016**, *22*, 439–445. [CrossRef]

225. Zhang, L.; Sun, Z.; Zhao, P.; Huang, L.; Xu, M.; Yang, Y.; Chen, X.; Lu, F.; Zhang, X.; Wang, H.; et al. Whole-exome sequencing revealed HKDC1 as a candidate gene associated with autosomal-recessive retinitis pigmentosa. *Hum. Mol. Genet.* **2018**, *27*, 4157–4168. [CrossRef]

226. Xia, C.H.; Lu, E.; Liu, H.; Du, X.; Beutler, B.; Gong, X. The role of Vldlr in intraretinal angiogenesis in mice. *Investig. Ophthalmol. Vis. Sci.* **2011**, *52*, 6572–6579. [CrossRef] [PubMed]

227. Hu, W.; Jiang, A.; Liang, J.; Meng, H.; Chang, B.; Gao, H.; Qiao, X. Expression of VLDLR in the retina and evolution of subretinal neovascularization in the knockout mouse model's retinal angiomatous proliferation. *Investig. Ophthalmol. Vis. Sci.* **2008**, *49*, 407–415. [CrossRef] [PubMed]

228. Chen, Y.; Hu, Y.; Moiseyev, G.; Zhou, K.K.; Chen, D.; Ma, J.X. Photoreceptor degeneration and retinal inflammation induced by very low-density lipoprotein receptor deficiency. *Microvasc. Res.* **2009**, *78*, 119–127. [CrossRef] [PubMed]

229. Lin, J.B.; Kubota, S.; Ban, N.; Yoshida, M.; Santeford, A.; Sene, A.; Nakamura, R.; Zapata, N.; Kubota, M.; Tsubota, K.; et al. NAMPT-Mediated NAD(+) Biosynthesis Is Essential for Vision In Mice. *Cell Rep.* **2016**, *17*, 69–85. [CrossRef]

230. Greenwald, S.H.; Charette, J.R.; Staniszewska, M.; Shi, L.Y.; Brown, S.D.M.; Stone, L.; Liu, Q.; Hicks, W.L.; Collin, G.B.; Bowl, M.R.; et al. Mouse Models of NMNAT1-Leber Congenital Amaurosis (LCA9) Recapitulate Key Features of the Human Disease. *Am. J. Pathol.* **2016**, *186*, 1925–1938. [CrossRef]

231. Bosl, M.R.; Stein, V.; Hubner, C.; Zdebik, A.A.; Jordt, S.E.; Mukhopadhyay, A.K.; Davidoff, M.S.; Holstein, A.F.; Jentsch, T.J. Male germ cells and photoreceptors, both dependent on close cell-cell interactions, degenerate upon ClC-2 Cl(-) channel disruption. *EMBO J.* **2001**, *20*, 1289–1299. [CrossRef]

232. Ng, L.; Lyubarsky, A.; Nikonov, S.S.; Ma, M.; Srinivas, M.; Kefas, B.; St Germain, D.L.; Hernandez, A.; Pugh, E.N., Jr.; Forrest, D. Type 3 deiodinase, a thyroid-hormone-inactivating enzyme, controls survival and maturation of cone photoreceptors. *J. Neurosci.* **2010**, *30*, 3347–3357. [CrossRef]

233. Ng, L.; Hurley, J.B.; Dierks, B.; Srinivas, M.; Salto, C.; Vennstrom, B.; Reh, T.A.; Forrest, D. A thyroid hormone receptor that is required for the development of green cone photoreceptors. *Nat. Genet.* **2001**, *27*, 94–98. [CrossRef]

234. Gianesini, C.; Hiragaki, S.; Laurent, V.; Hicks, D.; Tosini, G. Cone Viability Is Affected by Disruption of Melatonin Receptors Signaling. *Investig. Ophthalmol. Vis. Sci.* **2016**, *57*, 94–104. [CrossRef]

235. Baba, K.; Pozdeyev, N.; Mazzoni, F.; Contreras-Alcantara, S.; Liu, C.; Kasamatsu, M.; Martinez-Merlos, T.; Strettoi, E.; Iuvone, P.M.; Tosini, G. Melatonin modulates visual function and cell viability in the mouse retina via the MT1 melatonin receptor. *Proc. Natl. Acad. Sci. USA* **2009**, *106*, 15043–15048. [CrossRef]

236. Chen, Y.; Mehta, G.; Vasiliou, V. Antioxidant defenses in the ocular surface. *Ocul. Surf.* **2009**, *7*, 176–185. [CrossRef]

237. Nita, M.; Grzybowski, A. The Role of the Reactive Oxygen Species and Oxidative Stress in the Pathomechanism of the Age-Related Ocular Diseases and Other Pathologies of the Anterior and Posterior Eye Segments in Adults. *Oxid. Med. Cell Longev.* **2016**, *2016*, 3164734. [CrossRef] [PubMed]

238. Chen, H.; Lukas, T.J.; Du, N.; Suyeoka, G.; Neufeld, A.H. Dysfunction of the retinal pigment epithelium with age: Increased iron decreases phagocytosis and lysosomal activity. *Investig. Ophthalmol. Vis. Sci.* **2009**, *50*, 1895–1902. [CrossRef] [PubMed]

239. Blasiak, J.; Glowacki, S.; Kauppinen, A.; Kaarniranta, K. Mitochondrial and nuclear DNA damage and repair in age-related macular degeneration. *Int. J. Mol. Sci.* **2013**, *14*, 2996–3010. [CrossRef]

240. Tan, B.L.; Norhaizan, M.E.; Liew, W.P.; Sulaiman Rahman, H. Antioxidant and Oxidative Stress: A Mutual Interplay in Age-Related Diseases. *Front. Pharmacol.* **2018**, *9*, 1162. [CrossRef]

241. Frohns, A.; Frohns, F.; Naumann, S.C.; Layer, P.G.; Lobrich, M. Inefficient double-strand break repair in murine rod photoreceptors with inverted heterochromatin organization. *Curr. Biol.* **2014**, *24*, 1080–1090. [CrossRef]

242. Blasiak, J.; Petrovski, G.; Vereb, Z.; Facsko, A.; Kaarniranta, K. Oxidative stress, hypoxia, and autophagy in the neovascular processes of age-related macular degeneration. *Biomed. Res. Int.* **2014**, *2014*, 768026. [CrossRef]

243. Tokarz, P.; Kaarniranta, K.; Blasiak, J. Role of antioxidant enzymes and small molecular weight antioxidants in the pathogenesis of age-related macular degeneration (AMD). *Biogerontology* **2013**, *14*, 461–482. [CrossRef]

244. Hashizume, K.; Hirasawa, M.; Imamura, Y.; Noda, S.; Shimizu, T.; Shinoda, K.; Kurihara, T.; Noda, K.; Ozawa, Y.; Ishida, S.; et al. Retinal dysfunction and progressive retinal cell death in SOD1-deficient mice. *Am. J. Pathol.* **2008**, *172*, 1325–1331. [CrossRef]

245. Biswal, M.R.; Ildefonso, C.J.; Mao, H.; Seo, S.J.; Wang, Z.; Li, H.; Le, Y.Z.; Lewin, A.S. Conditional Induction of Oxidative Stress in RPE: A Mouse Model of Progressive Retinal Degeneration. *Adv. Exp. Med. Biol.* **2016**, *854*, 31–37. [CrossRef]

246. Cronin, T.; Raffelsberger, W.; Lee-Rivera, I.; Jaillard, C.; Niepon, M.L.; Kinzel, B.; Clerin, E.; Petrosian, A.; Picaud, S.; Poch, O.; et al. The disruption of the rod-derived cone viability gene leads to photoreceptor dysfunction and susceptibility to oxidative stress. *Cell Death Differ.* **2010**, *17*, 1199–1210. [CrossRef] [PubMed]

247. Jaillard, C.; Mouret, A.; Niepon, M.L.; Clerin, E.; Yang, Y.; Lee-Rivera, I.; Ait-Ali, N.; Millet-Puel, G.; Cronin, T.; Sedmak, T.; et al. Nxnl2 splicing results in dual functions in neuronal cell survival and maintenance of cell integrity. *Hum. Mol. Genet.* **2012**, *21*, 2298–2311. [CrossRef] [PubMed]

248. Yokota, T.; Igarashi, K.; Uchihara, T.; Jishage, K.; Tomita, H.; Inaba, A.; Li, Y.; Arita, M.; Suzuki, H.; Mizusawa, H.; et al. Delayed-onset ataxia in mice lacking alpha -tocopherol transfer protein: Model for neuronal degeneration caused by chronic oxidative stress. *Proc. Natl. Acad. Sci. USA* **2001**, *98*, 15185–15190. [CrossRef] [PubMed]

249. Mukherjee, A.B.; Appu, A.P.; Sadhukhan, T.; Casey, S.; Mondal, A.; Zhang, Z.; Bagh, M.B. Emerging new roles of the lysosome and neuronal ceroid lipofuscinoses. *Mol. Neurodegener.* **2019**, *14*, 4. [CrossRef] [PubMed]

250. Schulze, H.; Kolter, T.; Sandhoff, K. Principles of lysosomal membrane degradation: Cellular topology and biochemistry of lysosomal lipid degradation. *Biochim. Biophys. Acta* **2009**, *1793*, 674–683. [CrossRef] [PubMed]

251. Birch, D.G. Retinal degeneration in retinitis pigmentosa and neuronal ceroid lipofuscinosis: An overview. *Mol. Genet. Metab.* **1999**, *66*, 356–366. [CrossRef]

252. Ostergaard, J.R. Juvenile neuronal ceroid lipofuscinosis (Batten disease): Current insights. *Degener. Neurol. Neuromuscul. Dis.* **2016**, *6*, 73–83. [CrossRef]

253. Leinonen, H.; Keksa-Goldsteine, V.; Ragauskas, S.; Kohlmann, P.; Singh, Y.; Savchenko, E.; Puranen, J.; Malm, T.; Kalesnykas, G.; Koistinaho, J.; et al. Retinal Degeneration In A Mouse Model Of CLN5 Disease Is Associated With Compromised Autophagy. *Sci. Rep.* **2017**, *7*, 1597. [CrossRef]

254. Bartsch, U.; Galliciotti, G.; Jofre, G.F.; Jankowiak, W.; Hagel, C.; Braulke, T. Apoptotic photoreceptor loss and altered expression of lysosomal proteins in the nclf mouse model of neuronal ceroid lipofuscinosis. *Investig. Ophthalmol. Vis. Sci.* **2013**, *54*, 6952–6959. [CrossRef]

255. Jankowiak, W.; Brandenstein, L.; Dulz, S.; Hagel, C.; Storch, S.; Bartsch, U. Retinal Degeneration in Mice Deficient in the Lysosomal Membrane Protein CLN7. *Investig. Ophthalmol. Vis. Sci.* **2016**, *57*, 4989–4998. [CrossRef]

256. Chang, B.; Bronson, R.T.; Hawes, N.L.; Roderick, T.H.; Peng, C.; Hageman, G.S.; Heckenlively, J.R. Retinal degeneration in motor neuron degeneration: A mouse model of ceroid lipofuscinosis. *Investig. Ophthalmol. Vis. Sci.* **1994**, *35*, 1071–1076. [PubMed]

257. Hafler, B.P.; Klein, Z.A.; Jimmy Zhou, Z.; Strittmatter, S.M. Progressive retinal degeneration and accumulation of autofluorescent lipopigments in Progranulin deficient mice. *Brain Res.* **2014**, *1588*, 168–174. [CrossRef] [PubMed]

258. Heldermon, C.D.; Hennig, A.K.; Ohlemiller, K.K.; Ogilvie, J.M.; Herzog, E.D.; Breidenbach, A.; Vogler, C.; Wozniak, D.F.; Sands, M.S. Development of sensory, motor and behavioral deficits in the murine model of Sanfilippo syndrome type B. *PLoS ONE* **2007**, *2*, e772. [CrossRef] [PubMed]

259. Gelfman, C.M.; Vogel, P.; Issa, T.M.; Turner, C.A.; Lee, W.S.; Kornfeld, S.; Rice, D.S. Mice lacking alpha/beta subunits of GlcNAc-1-phosphotransferase exhibit growth retardation, retinal degeneration, and secretory cell lesions. *Investig. Ophthalmol. Vis. Sci.* **2007**, *48*, 5221–5228. [CrossRef] [PubMed]

260. Kevany, B.M.; Palczewski, K. Phagocytosis of retinal rod and cone photoreceptors. *Physiology* **2010**, *25*, 8–15. [CrossRef] [PubMed]

261. Prasad, D.; Rothlin, C.V.; Burrola, P.; Burstyn-Cohen, T.; Lu, Q.; Garcia de Frutos, P.; Lemke, G. TAM receptor function in the retinal pigment epithelium. *Mol. Cell Neurosci.* **2006**, *33*, 96–108. [CrossRef] [PubMed]

262. Duncan, J.L.; LaVail, M.M.; Yasumura, D.; Matthes, M.T.; Yang, H.; Trautmann, N.; Chappelow, A.V.; Feng, W.; Earp, H.S.; Matsushima, G.K.; et al. An RCS-like retinal dystrophy phenotype in mer knockout mice. *Investig. Ophthalmol. Vis. Sci.* **2003**, *44*, 826–838. [CrossRef]

263. Houssier, M.; Raoul, W.; Lavalette, S.; Keller, N.; Guillonneau, X.; Baragatti, B.; Jonet, L.; Jeanny, J.C.; Behar-Cohen, F.; Coceani, F.; et al. CD36 deficiency leads to choroidal involution via COX2 down-regulation in rodents. *PLoS Med.* **2008**, *5*, e39. [CrossRef]

264. Ying, G.; Boldt, K.; Ueffing, M.; Gerstner, C.D.; Frederick, J.M.; Baehr, W. The small GTPase RAB28 is required for phagocytosis of cone outer segments by the murine retinal pigmented epithelium. *J. Biol. Chem.* **2018**, *293*, 17546–17558. [CrossRef]

265. Lin, W.; Xu, G. Autophagy: A Role in the Apoptosis, Survival, Inflammation, and Development of the Retina. *Ophthalmic Res.* **2019**, *61*, 65–72. [CrossRef]

266. Seranova, E.; Connolly, K.J.; Zatyka, M.; Rosenstock, T.R.; Barrett, T.; Tuxworth, R.I.; Sarkar, S. Dysregulation of autophagy as a common mechanism in lysosomal storage diseases. *Essays Biochem.* **2017**, *61*, 733–749. [CrossRef] [PubMed]

267. Byrne, S.; Jansen, L.; JM, U.K.-I.; Siddiqui, A.; Lidov, H.G.; Bodi, I.; Smith, L.; Mein, R.; Cullup, T.; Dionisi-Vici, C.; et al. EPG5-related Vici syndrome: A paradigm of neurodevelopmental disorders with defective autophagy. *Brain* **2016**, *139*, 765–781. [CrossRef] [PubMed]

268. Smucker, W.D.; Kontak, J.R. Adverse drug reactions causing hospital admission in an elderly population: Experience with a decision algorithm. *J. Am. Board Fam. Pract.* **1990**, *3*, 105–109. [PubMed]

269. Kim, J.Y.; Zhao, H.; Martinez, J.; Doggett, T.A.; Kolesnikov, A.V.; Tang, P.H.; Ablonczy, Z.; Chan, C.C.; Zhou, Z.; Green, D.R.; et al. Noncanonical autophagy promotes the visual cycle. *Cell* **2013**, *154*, 365–376. [CrossRef] [PubMed]

270. Mohlin, C.; Taylor, L.; Ghosh, F.; Johansson, K. Autophagy and ER-stress contribute to photoreceptor degeneration in cultured adult porcine retina. *Brain Res.* **2014**, *1585*, 167–183. [CrossRef]

271. Chen, Y.; Sawada, O.; Kohno, H.; Le, Y.Z.; Subauste, C.; Maeda, T.; Maeda, A. Autophagy protects the retina from light-induced degeneration. *J. Biol. Chem.* **2013**, *288*, 7506–7518. [CrossRef]

272. Falk, M.J. Neurodevelopmental manifestations of mitochondrial disease. *J. Dev. Behav. Pediatr.* **2010**, *31*, 610–621. [CrossRef]

273. Davies, V.J.; Powell, K.A.; White, K.E.; Yip, W.; Hogan, V.; Hollins, A.J.; Davies, J.R.; Piechota, M.; Brownstein, D.G.; Moat, S.J.; et al. A missense mutation in the murine Opa3 gene models human Costeff syndrome. *Brain* **2008**, *131*, 368–380. [CrossRef]

274. Findlay, A.S.; Carter, R.N.; Starbuck, B.; McKie, L.; Novakova, K.; Budd, P.S.; Keighren, M.A.; Marsh, J.A.; Cross, S.H.; Simon, M.M.; et al. Mouse Idh3a mutations cause retinal degeneration and reduced mitochondrial function. *Dis. Model. Mech.* **2018**, *11*, 036426. [CrossRef]

275. Bruschi, M.; Petretto, A.; Caicci, F.; Bartolucci, M.; Calzia, D.; Santucci, L.; Manni, L.; Ramenghi, L.A.; Ghiggeri, G.; Traverso, C.E.; et al. Proteome of Bovine Mitochondria and Rod Outer Segment Disks: Commonalities and Differences. *J. Proteome Res.* **2018**, *17*, 918–925. [CrossRef]

276. Calzia, D.; Barabino, S.; Bianchini, P.; Garbarino, G.; Oneto, M.; Caicci, F.; Diaspro, A.; Tacchetti, C.; Manni, L.; Candiani, S.; et al. New findings in ATP supply in rod outer segments: Insights for retinopathies. *Biol. Cell* **2013**, *105*, 345–358. [CrossRef] [PubMed]

277. Funk, R.H.; Schumann, U.; Engelmann, K.; Becker, K.A.; Roehlecke, C. Blue light induced retinal oxidative stress: Implications for macular degeneration. *World J. Ophthalmol.* **2014**, *4*, 29–34. [CrossRef]

278. Calzia, D.; Garbarino, G.; Caicci, F.; Manni, L.; Candiani, S.; Ravera, S.; Morelli, A.; Traverso, C.E.; Panfoli, I. Functional expression of electron transport chain complexes in mouse rod outer segments. *Biochimie* **2014**, *102*, 78–82. [CrossRef] [PubMed]

279. Roehlecke, C.; Schumann, U.; Ader, M.; Brunssen, C.; Bramke, S.; Morawietz, H.; Funk, R.H. Stress reaction in outer segments of photoreceptors after blue light irradiation. *PLoS ONE* **2013**, *8*, e71570. [CrossRef] [PubMed]

280. Wanders, R.J.; Waterham, H.R.; Ferdinandusse, S. Metabolic Interplay between Peroxisomes and Other Subcellular Organelles Including Mitochondria and the Endoplasmic Reticulum. *Front. Cell Dev. Biol.* **2015**, *3*, 83. [CrossRef]

281. Folz, S.J.; Trobe, J.D. The peroxisome and the eye. *Surv. Ophthalmol.* **1991**, *35*, 353–368. [CrossRef]

282. Das, Y.; Roose, N.; De Groef, L.; Fransen, M.; Moons, L.; Van Veldhoven, P.P.; Baes, M. Differential distribution of peroxisomal proteins points to specific roles of peroxisomes in the murine retina. *Mol. Cell Biochem.* **2019**, *456*, 53–62. [CrossRef]

283. Hiebler, S.; Masuda, T.; Hacia, J.G.; Moser, A.B.; Faust, P.L.; Liu, A.; Chowdhury, N.; Huang, N.; Lauer, A.; Bennett, J.; et al. The Pex1-G844D mouse: A model for mild human Zellweger spectrum disorder. *Mol. Genet. Metab.* **2014**, *111*, 522–532. [CrossRef]

284. Pang, J.J.; Chang, B.; Hawes, N.L.; Hurd, R.E.; Davisson, M.T.; Li, J.; Noorwez, S.M.; Malhotra, R.; McDowell, J.H.; Kaushal, S.; et al. Retinal degeneration 12 (rd12): A new, spontaneously arising mouse model for human Leber congenital amaurosis (LCA). *Mol. Vis.* **2005**, *11*, 152–162.

285. Wright, C.B.; Chrenek, M.A.; Feng, W.; Getz, S.E.; Duncan, T.; Pardue, M.T.; Feng, Y.; Redmond, T.M.; Boatright, J.H.; Nickerson, J.M. The Rpe65 rd12 allele exerts a semidominant negative effect on vision in mice. *Investig. Ophthalmol. Vis. Sci.* **2014**, *55*, 2500–2515. [CrossRef]

286. Redmond, T.M.; Yu, S.; Lee, E.; Bok, D.; Hamasaki, D.; Chen, N.; Goletz, P.; Ma, J.X.; Crouch, R.K.; Pfeifer, K. Rpe65 is necessary for production of 11-cis-vitamin A in the retinal visual cycle. *Nat. Genet.* **1998**, *20*, 344–351. [CrossRef] [PubMed]

287. Tanabu, R.; Sato, K.; Monai, N.; Yamauchi, K.; Gonome, T.; Xie, Y.; Takahashi, S.; Ishiguro, S.I.; Nakazawa, M. The findings of optical coherence tomography of retinal degeneration in relation to the morphological and electroretinographic features in RPE65-/- mice. *PLoS ONE* **2019**, *14*, e0210439. [CrossRef] [PubMed]

288. Woodruff, M.L.; Wang, Z.; Chung, H.Y.; Redmond, T.M.; Fain, G.L.; Lem, J. Spontaneous activity of opsin apoprotein is a cause of Leber congenital amaurosis. *Nat. Genet.* **2003**, *35*, 158–164. [CrossRef] [PubMed]

289. Samardzija, M.; von Lintig, J.; Tanimoto, N.; Oberhauser, V.; Thiersch, M.; Reme, C.E.; Seeliger, M.; Grimm, C.; Wenzel, A. R91W mutation in Rpe65 leads to milder early-onset retinal dystrophy due to the generation of low levels of 11-cis-retinal. *Hum. Mol. Genet.* **2008**, *17*, 281–292. [CrossRef] [PubMed]

290. Choi, E.H.; Suh, S.; Sander, C.L.; Hernandez, C.J.O.; Bulman, E.R.; Khadka, N.; Dong, Z.; Shi, W.; Palczewski, K.; Kiser, P.D. Insights into the pathogenesis of dominant retinitis pigmentosa associated with a D477G mutation in RPE65. *Hum. Mol. Genet.* **2018**, *27*, 2225–2243. [CrossRef]

291. Radu, R.A.; Yuan, Q.; Hu, J.; Peng, J.H.; Lloyd, M.; Nusinowitz, S.; Bok, D.; Travis, G.H. Accelerated accumulation of lipofuscin pigments in the RPE of a mouse model for ABCA4-mediated retinal dystrophies following Vitamin A supplementation. *Investig. Ophthalmol. Vis. Sci.* **2008**, *49*, 3821–3829. [CrossRef]

292. Weng, J.; Mata, N.L.; Azarian, S.M.; Tzekov, R.T.; Birch, D.G.; Travis, G.H. Insights into the function of Rim protein in photoreceptors and etiology of Stargardt's disease from the phenotype in abcr knockout mice. *Cell* **1999**, *98*, 13–23. [CrossRef]

293. Molday, L.L.; Wahl, D.; Sarunic, M.V.; Molday, R.S. Localization and functional characterization of the p.Asn965Ser (N965S) ABCA4 variant in mice reveal pathogenic mechanisms underlying Stargardt macular degeneration. *Hum. Mol. Genet.* **2018**, *27*, 295–306. [CrossRef]

294. Zhang, N.; Tsybovsky, Y.; Kolesnikov, A.V.; Rozanowska, M.; Swider, M.; Schwartz, S.B.; Stone, E.M.; Palczewska, G.; Maeda, A.; Kefalov, V.J.; et al. Protein misfolding and the pathogenesis of ABCA4-associated retinal degenerations. *Hum. Mol. Genet.* **2015**, *24*, 3220–3237. [CrossRef]

295. Wu, L.; Ueda, K.; Nagasaki, T.; Sparrow, J.R. Light damage in Abca4 and Rpe65rd12 mice. *Investig. Ophthalmol. Vis. Sci.* **2014**, *55*, 1910–1918. [CrossRef]

296. Maeda, A.; Maeda, T.; Golczak, M.; Palczewski, K. Retinopathy in mice induced by disrupted all-trans-retinal clearance. *J. Biol. Chem.* **2008**, *283*, 26684–26693. [CrossRef]

297. Chen, Y.; Okano, K.; Maeda, T.; Chauhan, V.; Golczak, M.; Maeda, A.; Palczewski, K. Mechanism of all-trans-retinal toxicity with implications for stargardt disease and age-related macular degeneration. *J. Biol. Chem.* **2012**, *287*, 5059–5069. [CrossRef] [PubMed]

298. Okano, K.; Maeda, A.; Chen, Y.; Chauhan, V.; Tang, J.; Palczewska, G.; Sakai, T.; Tsuneoka, H.; Palczewski, K.; Maeda, T. Retinal cone and rod photoreceptor cells exhibit differential susceptibility to light-induced damage. *J. Neurochem.* **2012**, *121*, 146–156. [CrossRef] [PubMed]

299. Batten, M.L.; Imanishi, Y.; Maeda, T.; Tu, D.C.; Moise, A.R.; Bronson, D.; Possin, D.; Van Gelder, R.N.; Baehr, W.; Palczewski, K. Lecithin-retinol acyltransferase is essential for accumulation of all-trans-retinyl esters in the eye and in the liver. *J. Biol. Chem.* **2004**, *279*, 10422–10432. [CrossRef] [PubMed]

300. Ruiz, A.; Ghyselinck, N.B.; Mata, N.; Nusinowitz, S.; Lloyd, M.; Dennefeld, C.; Chambon, P.; Bok, D. Somatic ablation of the Lrat gene in the mouse retinal pigment epithelium drastically reduces its retinoid storage. *Investig. Ophthalmol. Vis. Sci.* **2007**, *48*, 5377–5387. [CrossRef]

301. Liou, G.I.; Fei, Y.; Peachey, N.S.; Matragoon, S.; Wei, S.; Blaner, W.S.; Wang, Y.; Liu, C.; Gottesman, M.E.; Ripps, H. Early onset photoreceptor abnormalities induced by targeted disruption of the interphotoreceptor retinoid-binding protein gene. *J. Neurosci.* **1998**, *18*, 4511–4520. [CrossRef]

302. Shen, J.; Shi, D.; Suzuki, T.; Xia, Z.; Zhang, H.; Araki, K.; Wakana, S.; Takeda, N.; Yamamura, K.; Jin, S.; et al. Severe ocular phenotypes in Rbp4-deficient mice in the C57BL/6 genetic background. *Lab. Investig.* **2016**, *96*, 680–691. [CrossRef]

303. Ruiz, A.; Mark, M.; Jacobs, H.; Klopfenstein, M.; Hu, J.; Lloyd, M.; Habib, S.; Tosha, C.; Radu, R.A.; Ghyselinck, N.B.; et al. Retinoid content, visual responses, and ocular morphology are compromised in the retinas of mice lacking the retinol-binding protein receptor, STRA6. *Investig. Ophthalmol. Vis. Sci.* **2012**, *53*, 3027–3039. [CrossRef]

304. Amengual, J.; Zhang, N.; Kemerer, M.; Maeda, T.; Palczewski, K.; Von Lintig, J. STRA6 is critical for cellular vitamin A uptake and homeostasis. *Hum. Mol. Genet.* **2014**, *23*, 5402–5417. [CrossRef]

305. Wu, S.M. Synaptic transmission in the outer retina. *Annu. Rev. Physiol.* **1994**, *56*, 141–168. [CrossRef]

306. Wu, S.M. Synaptic organization of the vertebrate retina: General principles and species-specific variations: The Friedenwald lecture. *Investig. Ophthalmol. Vis. Sci.* **2010**, *51*, 1263–1274. [CrossRef] [PubMed]

307. Mercer, A.J.; Thoreson, W.B. The dynamic architecture of photoreceptor ribbon synapses: Cytoskeletal, extracellular matrix, and intramembrane proteins. *Vis. Neurosci.* **2011**, *28*, 453–471. [CrossRef] [PubMed]

308. Furukawa, T.; Ueno, A.; Omori, Y. Molecular mechanisms underlying selective synapse formation of vertebrate retinal photoreceptor cells. *Cell Mol. Life Sci.* **2019**, *77*, 1251–1266. [CrossRef] [PubMed]

309. Pardue, M.T.; Peachey, N.S. Mouse b-wave mutants. *Doc. Ophthalmol.* **2014**, *128*, 77–89. [CrossRef] [PubMed]

310. Pillers, D.A.; Weleber, R.G.; Woodward, W.R.; Green, D.G.; Chapman, V.M.; Ray, P.N. mdxCv3 mouse is a model for electroretinography of Duchenne/Becker muscular dystrophy. *Investig. Ophthalmol. Vis. Sci.* **1995**, *36*, 462–466.

311. Satz, J.S.; Philp, A.R.; Nguyen, H.; Kusano, H.; Lee, J.; Turk, R.; Riker, M.J.; Hernandez, J.; Weiss, R.M.; Anderson, M.G.; et al. Visual impairment in the absence of dystroglycan. *J. Neurosci.* **2009**, *29*, 13136–13146. [CrossRef]

312. Bytyqi, A.H.; Lockridge, O.; Duysen, E.; Wang, Y.; Wolfrum, U.; Layer, P.G. Impaired formation of the inner retina in an AChE knockout mouse results in degeneration of all photoreceptors. *Eur. J. Neurosci.* **2004**, *20*, 2953–2962. [CrossRef]

313. Grisaru, D.; Sternfeld, M.; Eldor, A.; Glick, D.; Soreq, H. Structural roles of acetylcholinesterase variants in biology and pathology. *Eur. J. Biochem.* **1999**, *264*, 672–686. [CrossRef]

314. Regus-Leidig, H.; Atorf, J.; Feigenspan, A.; Kremers, J.; Maw, M.A.; Brandstatter, J.H. Photoreceptor degeneration in two mouse models for congenital stationary night blindness type 2. *PLoS ONE* **2014**, *9*, e86769. [CrossRef]

315. Kerov, V.; Laird, J.G.; Joiner, M.L.; Knecht, S.; Soh, D.; Hagen, J.; Gardner, S.H.; Gutierrez, W.; Yoshimatsu, T.; Bhattarai, S.; et al. alpha2delta-4 Is Required for the Molecular and Structural Organization of Rod and Cone Photoreceptor Synapses. *J. Neurosci.* **2018**, *38*, 6145–6160. [CrossRef]

316. Ruether, K.; Grosse, J.; Matthiessen, E.; Hoffmann, K.; Hartmann, C. Abnormalities of the photoreceptor-bipolar cell synapse in a substrain of C57BL/10 mice. *Investig. Ophthalmol. Vis. Sci.* **2000**, *41*, 4039–4047. [PubMed]

317. Haeseleer, F.; Imanishi, Y.; Maeda, T.; Possin, D.E.; Maeda, A.; Lee, A.; Rieke, F.; Palczewski, K. Essential role of Ca2+-binding protein 4, a Cav1.4 channel regulator, in photoreceptor synaptic function. *Nat. Neurosci.* **2004**, *7*, 1079–1087. [CrossRef] [PubMed]

318. Ishiba, Y.; Higashide, T.; Mori, N.; Kobayashi, A.; Kubota, S.; McLaren, M.J.; Satoh, H.; Wong, F.; Inana, G. Targeted inactivation of synaptic HRG4 (UNC119) causes dysfunction in the distal photoreceptor and slow retinal degeneration, revealing a new function. *Exp. Eye Res.* **2007**, *84*, 473–485. [CrossRef] [PubMed]

319. Haeseleer, F. Interaction and colocalization of CaBP4 and Unc119 (MRG4) in photoreceptors. *Investig. Ophthalmol. Vis. Sci.* **2008**, *49*, 2366–2375. [CrossRef]

320. Giblin, J.P.; Comes, N.; Strauss, O.; Gasull, X. Ion Channels in the Eye: Involvement in Ocular Pathologies. *Adv. Protein Chem. Struct. Biol.* **2016**, *104*, 157–231. [CrossRef]

321. Edwards, M.M.; Marin de Evsikova, C.; Collin, G.B.; Gifford, E.; Wu, J.; Hicks, W.L.; Whiting, C.; Varvel, N.H.; Maphis, N.; Lamb, B.T.; et al. Photoreceptor degeneration, azoospermia, leukoencephalopathy, and abnormal RPE cell function in mice expressing an early stop mutation in CLCN2. *Investig. Ophthalmol. Vis. Sci.* **2010**, *51*, 3264–3272. [CrossRef]

322. Stobrawa, S.M.; Breiderhoff, T.; Takamori, S.; Engel, D.; Schweizer, M.; Zdebik, A.A.; Bosl, M.R.; Ruether, K.; Jahn, H.; Draguhn, A.; et al. Disruption of ClC-3, a chloride channel expressed on synaptic vesicles, leads to a loss of the hippocampus. *Neuron* **2001**, *29*, 185–196. [CrossRef]

323. Rajan, I.; Read, R.; Small, D.L.; Perrard, J.; Vogel, P. An alternative splicing variant in Clcn7-/- mice prevents osteopetrosis but not neural and retinal degeneration. *Vet. Pathol.* **2011**, *48*, 663–675. [CrossRef]

324. Dickerson, L.W.; Bonthius, D.J.; Schutte, B.C.; Yang, B.; Barna, T.J.; Bailey, M.C.; Nehrke, K.; Williamson, R.A.; Lamb, F.S. Altered GABAergic function accompanies hippocampal degeneration in mice lacking ClC-3 voltage-gated chloride channels. *Brain Res.* **2002**, *958*, 227–250. [CrossRef]

325. Kornak, U.; Kasper, D.; Bosl, M.R.; Kaiser, E.; Schweizer, M.; Schulz, A.; Friedrich, W.; Delling, G.; Jentsch, T.J. Loss of the ClC-7 chloride channel leads to osteopetrosis in mice and man. *Cell* **2001**, *104*, 205–215. [CrossRef]

326. Kasper, D.; Planells-Cases, R.; Fuhrmann, J.C.; Scheel, O.; Zeitz, O.; Ruether, K.; Schmitt, A.; Poet, M.; Steinfeld, R.; Schweizer, M.; et al. Loss of the chloride channel ClC-7 leads to lysosomal storage disease and neurodegeneration. *EMBO J.* **2005**, *24*, 1079–1091. [CrossRef] [PubMed]

327. Weinert, S.; Jabs, S.; Hohensee, S.; Chan, W.L.; Kornak, U.; Jentsch, T.J. Transport activity and presence of ClC-7/Ostm1 complex account for different cellular functions. *EMBO Rep.* **2014**, *15*, 784–791. [CrossRef] [PubMed]

328. Weber, P.; Bartsch, U.; Schachner, M.; Montag, D. Na,K-ATPase subunit beta1 knock-in prevents lethality of beta2 deficiency in mice. *J. Neurosci.* **1998**, *18*, 9192–9203. [CrossRef] [PubMed]

329. Heller-Stilb, B.; van Roeyen, C.; Rascher, K.; Hartwig, H.G.; Huth, A.; Seeliger, M.W.; Warskulat, U.; Haussinger, D. Disruption of the taurine transporter gene (taut) leads to retinal degeneration in mice. *FASEB J.* **2002**, *16*, 231–233. [CrossRef] [PubMed]

330. Bok, D.; Galbraith, G.; Lopez, I.; Woodruff, M.; Nusinowitz, S.; BeltrandelRio, H.; Huang, W.; Zhao, S.; Geske, R.; Montgomery, C.; et al. Blindness and auditory impairment caused by loss of the sodium bicarbonate cotransporter NBC3. *Nat. Genet.* **2003**, *34*, 313–319. [CrossRef]

331. Jin, Z.B.; Huang, X.F.; Lv, J.N.; Xiang, L.; Li, D.Q.; Chen, J.; Huang, C.; Wu, J.; Lu, F.; Qu, J. SLC7A14 linked to autosomal recessive retinitis pigmentosa. *Nat. Commun.* **2014**, *5*, 3517. [CrossRef]

332. Jadeja, S.; Barnard, A.R.; McKie, L.; Cross, S.H.; White, J.K.; Sanger Mouse Genetics, P.; Robertson, M.; Budd, P.S.; MacLaren, R.E.; Jackson, I.J. Mouse slc9a8 mutants exhibit retinal defects due to retinal pigmented epithelium dysfunction. *Investig. Ophthalmol. Vis. Sci.* **2015**, *56*, 3015–3026. [CrossRef]

333. Hori, K.; Katayama, N.; Kachi, S.; Kondo, M.; Kadomatsu, K.; Usukura, J.; Muramatsu, T.; Mori, S.; Miyake, Y. Retinal dysfunction in basigin deficiency. *Investig. Ophthalmol. Vis. Sci.* **2000**, *41*, 3128–3133.

334. Veleri, S.; Nellissery, J.; Mishra, B.; Manjunath, S.H.; Brooks, M.J.; Dong, L.; Nagashima, K.; Qian, H.; Gao, C.; Sergeev, Y.V.; et al. REEP6 mediates trafficking of a subset of Clathrin-coated vesicles and is critical for rod photoreceptor function and survival. *Hum. Mol. Genet.* **2017**, *26*, 2218–2230. [CrossRef]

335. Ettaiche, M.; Deval, E.; Pagnotta, S.; Lazdunski, M.; Lingueglia, E. Acid-sensing ion channel 3 in retinal function and survival. *Investig. Ophthalmol. Vis. Sci.* **2009**, *50*, 2417–2426. [CrossRef]

336. Li, L.; Jiao, X.; D'Atri, I.; Ono, F.; Nelson, R.; Chan, C.C.; Nakaya, N.; Ma, Z.; Ma, Y.; Cai, X.; et al. Mutation in the intracellular chloride channel CLCC1 associated with autosomal recessive retinitis pigmentosa. *PLoS Genet.* **2018**, *14*, e1007504. [CrossRef] [PubMed]

337. Wong, B.H.; Chan, J.P.; Cazenave-Gassiot, A.; Poh, R.W.; Foo, J.C.; Galam, D.L.; Ghosh, S.; Nguyen, L.N.; Barathi, V.A.; Yeo, S.W.; et al. Mfsd2a Is a Transporter for the Essential omega-3 Fatty Acid Docosahexaenoic Acid (DHA) in Eye and Is Important for Photoreceptor Cell Development. *J. Biol. Chem.* **2016**, *291*, 10501–10514. [CrossRef] [PubMed]

338. Mahimkar, R.M.; Visaya, O.; Pollock, A.S.; Lovett, D.H. The disintegrin domain of ADAM9: A ligand for multiple beta1 renal integrins. *Biochem. J.* **2005**, *385*, 461–468. [CrossRef] [PubMed]

339. Parry, D.A.; Toomes, C.; Bida, L.; Danciger, M.; Towns, K.V.; McKibbin, M.; Jacobson, S.G.; Logan, C.V.; Ali, M.; Bond, J.; et al. Loss of the metalloprotease ADAM9 leads to cone-rod dystrophy in humans and retinal degeneration in mice. *Am. J. Hum. Genet.* **2009**, *84*, 683–691. [CrossRef] [PubMed]

340. Vijayasarathy, C.; Ziccardi, L.; Sieving, P.A. Biology of retinoschisin. *Adv. Exp. Med. Biol.* **2012**, *723*, 513–518. [CrossRef]

341. Jablonski, M.M.; Dalke, C.; Wang, X.; Lu, L.; Manly, K.F.; Pretsch, W.; Favor, J.; Pardue, M.T.; Rinchik, E.M.; Williams, R.W.; et al. An ENU-induced mutation in Rs1h causes disruption of retinal structure and function. *Mol. Vis.* **2005**, *11*, 569–581.

342. Han, J.; Farmer, S.R.; Kirkland, J.L.; Corkey, B.E.; Yoon, R.; Pirtskhalava, T.; Ido, Y.; Guo, W. Octanoate attenuates adipogenesis in 3T3-L1 preadipocytes. *J. Nutr.* **2002**, *132*, 904–910. [CrossRef]

343. Zeng, Y.; Takada, Y.; Kjellstrom, S.; Hiriyanna, K.; Tanikawa, A.; Wawrousek, E.; Smaoui, N.; Caruso, R.; Bush, R.A.; Sieving, P.A. RS-1 Gene Delivery to an Adult Rs1h Knockout Mouse Model Restores ERG b-Wave with Reversal of the Electronegative Waveform of X-Linked Retinoschisis. *Investig. Ophthalmol. Vis. Sci.* **2004**, *45*, 3279–3285. [CrossRef]

344. Quinn, P.M.; Pellissier, L.P.; Wijnholds, J. The CRB1 Complex: Following the Trail of Crumbs to a Feasible Gene Therapy Strategy. *Front. Neurosci.* **2017**, *11*, 175. [CrossRef]

345. Mehalow, A.K.; Kameya, S.; Smith, R.S.; Hawes, N.L.; Denegre, J.M.; Young, J.A.; Bechtold, L.; Haider, N.B.; Tepass, U.; Heckenlively, J.R.; et al. CRB1 is essential for external limiting membrane integrity and photoreceptor morphogenesis in the mammalian retina. *Hum. Mol. Genet.* **2003**, *12*, 2179–2189. [CrossRef]

346. van de Pavert, S.A.; Kantardzhieva, A.; Malysheva, A.; Meuleman, J.; Versteeg, I.; Levelt, C.; Klooster, J.; Geiger, S.; Seeliger, M.W.; Rashbass, P.; et al. Crumbs homologue 1 is required for maintenance of photoreceptor cell polarization and adhesion during light exposure. *J. Cell Sci.* **2004**, *117*, 4169–4177. [CrossRef] [PubMed]

347. Quinn, P.M.J.; Wijnholds, J. Retinogenesis of the Human Fetal Retina: An Apical Polarity Perspective. *Genes* **2019**, *10*, 987. [CrossRef]

348. Moore, B.A.; Leonard, B.C.; Sebbag, L.; Edwards, S.G.; Cooper, A.; Imai, D.M.; Straiton, E.; Santos, L.; Reilly, C.; Griffey, S.M.; et al. Identification of genes required for eye development by high-throughput screening of mouse knockouts. *Commun. Biol.* **2018**, *1*, 236. [CrossRef] [PubMed]

349. Watson, J.R.; Owen, D.; Mott, H.R. Cdc42 in actin dynamics: An ordered pathway governed by complex equilibria and directional effector handover. *Small GTPases* **2017**, *8*, 237–244. [CrossRef]

350. Yokokura, S.; Wada, Y.; Nakai, S.; Sato, H.; Yao, R.; Yamanaka, H.; Ito, S.; Sagara, Y.; Takahashi, M.; Nakamura, Y.; et al. Targeted disruption of FSCN2 gene induces retinopathy in mice. *Investig. Ophthalmol. Vis. Sci.* **2005**, *46*, 2905–2915. [CrossRef] [PubMed]

351. Liu, X.; Zhao, M.; Xie, Y.; Li, P.; Wang, O.; Zhou, B.; Yang, L.; Nie, Y.; Cheng, L.; Song, X.; et al. Null Mutation of the Fascin2 Gene by TALEN Leading to Progressive Hearing Loss and Retinal Degeneration in C57BL/6J Mice. *G3* **2018**, *8*, 3221–3230. [CrossRef]

352. Saksens, N.T.; Krebs, M.P.; Schoenmaker-Koller, F.E.; Hicks, W.; Yu, M.; Shi, L.; Rowe, L.; Collin, G.B.; Charette, J.R.; Letteboer, S.J.; et al. Mutations in CTNNA1 cause butterfly-shaped pigment dystrophy and perturbed retinal pigment epithelium integrity. *Nat. Genet.* **2016**, *48*, 144–151. [CrossRef]

353. Maddox, D.M.; Collin, G.B.; Ikeda, A.; Pratt, C.H.; Ikeda, S.; Johnson, B.A.; Hurd, R.E.; Shopland, L.S.; Naggert, J.K.; Chang, B.; et al. A Mutation in Syne2 Causes Early Retinal Defects in Photoreceptors, Secondary Neurons, and Muller Glia. *Investig. Ophthalmol. Vis. Sci.* **2015**, *56*, 3776–3787. [CrossRef]

354. Yu, J.; Lei, K.; Zhou, M.; Craft, C.M.; Xu, G.; Xu, T.; Zhuang, Y.; Xu, R.; Han, M. KASH protein Syne-2/Nesprin-2 and SUN proteins SUN1/2 mediate nuclear migration during mammalian retinal development. *Hum. Mol. Genet.* **2011**, *20*, 1061–1073. [CrossRef]

355. Gordon, M.D.; Nusse, R. Wnt signaling: Multiple pathways, multiple receptors, and multiple transcription factors. *J. Biol. Chem.* **2006**, *281*, 22429–22433. [CrossRef]

356. Liu, C.; Nathans, J. An essential role for frizzled 5 in mammalian ocular development. *Development* **2008**, *135*, 3567–3576. [CrossRef] [PubMed]

357. Wang, Z.; Liu, C.H.; Sun, Y.; Gong, Y.; Favazza, T.L.; Morss, P.C.; Saba, N.J.; Fredrick, T.W.; He, X.; Akula, J.D.; et al. Pharmacologic Activation of Wnt Signaling by Lithium Normalizes Retinal Vasculature in a Murine Model of Familial Exudative Vitreoretinopathy. *Am. J. Pathol.* **2016**, *186*, 2588–2600. [CrossRef] [PubMed]

358. Berger, W.; van de Pol, D.; Bachner, D.; Oerlemans, F.; Winkens, H.; Hameister, H.; Wieringa, B.; Hendriks, W.; Ropers, H.H. An animal model for Norrie disease (ND): Gene targeting of the mouse ND gene. *Hum. Mol. Genet.* **1996**, *5*, 51–59. [CrossRef] [PubMed]

359. Junge, H.J.; Yang, S.; Burton, J.B.; Paes, K.; Shu, X.; French, D.M.; Costa, M.; Rice, D.S.; Ye, W. TSPAN12 regulates retinal vascular development by promoting Norrin- but not Wnt-induced FZD4/beta-catenin signaling. *Cell* **2009**, *139*, 299–311. [CrossRef] [PubMed]

360. Hackam, A.S. The Wnt signaling pathway in retinal degenerations. *IUBMB Life* **2005**, *57*, 381–388. [CrossRef]

361. Hawes, N.L.; Chang, B.; Hageman, G.S.; Nusinowitz, S.; Nishina, P.M.; Schneider, B.S.; Smith, R.S.; Roderick, T.H.; Davisson, M.T.; Heckenlively, J.R. Retinal degeneration 6 (rd6): A new mouse model for human retinitis punctata albescens. *Investig. Ophthalmol. Vis. Sci.* **2000**, *41*, 3149–3157.

362. Hawkes, W.G. Bibliography: Nurses and smoking. *J. N. Y. State Nurses Assoc.* **1990**, *21*, 14.

363. Chavali, V.R.; Khan, N.W.; Cukras, C.A.; Bartsch, D.U.; Jablonski, M.M.; Ayyagari, R. A CTRP5 gene S163R mutation knock-in mouse model for late-onset retinal degeneration. *Hum. Mol. Genet.* **2011**, *20*, 2000–2014. [CrossRef]

364. Cai, Z.; Simons, D.L.; Fu, X.Y.; Feng, G.S.; Wu, S.M.; Zhang, X. Loss of Shp2-mediated mitogen-activated protein kinase signaling in Muller glial cells results in retinal degeneration. *Mol. Cell Biol.* **2011**, *31*, 2973–2983. [CrossRef]

365. Chavez-Solano, M.; Ibarra-Sanchez, A.; Trevino, M.; Gonzalez-Espinosa, C.; Lamas, M. Fyn kinase genetic ablation causes structural abnormalities in mature retina and defective Muller cell function. *Mol. Cell Neurosci.* **2016**, *72*, 91–100. [CrossRef]

366. Ji, X.; Liu, Y.; Hurd, R.; Wang, J.; Fitzmaurice, B.; Nishina, P.M.; Chang, B. Retinal Pigment Epithelium Atrophy 1 (rpea1): A New Mouse Model With Retinal Detachment Caused by a Disruption of Protein Kinase C, theta. *Investig. Ophthalmol. Vis. Sci.* **2016**, *57*, 877–888. [CrossRef]

367. Ivanovic, I.; Anderson, R.E.; Le, Y.Z.; Fliesler, S.J.; Sherry, D.M.; Rajala, R.V. Deletion of the p85alpha regulatory subunit of phosphoinositide 3-kinase in cone photoreceptor cells results in cone photoreceptor degeneration. *Investig. Ophthalmol. Vis. Sci.* **2011**, *52*, 3775–3783. [CrossRef] [PubMed]

368. Rajala, R.V.; Ranjo-Bishop, M.; Wang, Y.; Rajala, A.; Anderson, R.E. The p110alpha isoform of phosphoinositide 3-kinase is essential for cone photoreceptor survival. *Biochimie* **2015**, *112*, 35–40. [CrossRef] [PubMed]

369. Yi, X.; Schubert, M.; Peachey, N.S.; Suzuma, K.; Burks, D.J.; Kushner, J.A.; Suzuma, I.; Cahill, C.; Flint, C.L.; Dow, M.A.; et al. Insulin receptor substrate 2 is essential for maturation and survival of photoreceptor cells. *J. Neurosci.* **2005**, *25*, 1240–1248. [CrossRef] [PubMed]

370. Kitahara, H.; Kajikawa, S.; Ishii, Y.; Yamamoto, S.; Hamashima, T.; Azuma, E.; Sato, H.; Matsushima, T.; Shibuya, M.; Shimada, Y.; et al. The Novel Pathogenesis of Retinopathy Mediated by Multiple RTK Signals is Uncovered in Newly Developed Mouse Model. *EBioMedicine* **2018**, *31*, 190–201. [CrossRef]

371. Mongan, M.; Wang, J.; Liu, H.; Fan, Y.; Jin, C.; Kao, W.Y.; Xia, Y. Loss of MAP3K1 enhances proliferation and apoptosis during retinal development. *Development* **2011**, *138*, 4001–4012. [CrossRef]

372. Toyofuku, T.; Nojima, S.; Ishikawa, T.; Takamatsu, H.; Tsujimura, T.; Uemura, A.; Matsuda, J.; Seki, T.; Kumanogoh, A. Endosomal sorting by Semaphorin 4A in retinal pigment epithelium supports photoreceptor survival. *Genes Dev.* **2012**, *26*, 816–829. [CrossRef]

373. Carter-Dawson, L.D.; LaVail, M.M. Rods and cones in the mouse retina. II. Autoradiographic analysis of cell generation using tritiated thymidine. *J. Comp. Neurol.* **1979**, *188*, 263–272. [CrossRef]

374. Swaroop, A.; Kim, D.; Forrest, D. Transcriptional regulation of photoreceptor development and homeostasis in the mammalian retina. *Nat. Rev. Neurosci.* **2010**, *11*, 563–576. [CrossRef]

375. Brzezinski, J.A.; Reh, T.A. Photoreceptor cell fate specification in vertebrates. *Development* **2015**, *142*, 3263–3273. [CrossRef]

376. Khidr, L.; Chen, P.L. RB, the conductor that orchestrates life, death and differentiation. *Oncogene* **2006**, *25*, 5210–5219. [CrossRef] [PubMed]

377. Roger, J.E.; Hiriyanna, A.; Gotoh, N.; Hao, H.; Cheng, D.F.; Ratnapriya, R.; Kautzmann, M.A.; Chang, B.; Swaroop, A. OTX2 loss causes rod differentiation defect in CRX-associated congenital blindness. *J. Clin. Investig.* **2014**, *124*, 631–643. [CrossRef] [PubMed]

378. Tran, N.M.; Zhang, A.; Zhang, X.; Huecker, J.B.; Hennig, A.K.; Chen, S. Mechanistically distinct mouse models for CRX-associated retinopathy. *PLoS Genet.* **2014**, *10*, e1004111. [CrossRef] [PubMed]

379. Omori, Y.; Kitamura, T.; Yoshida, S.; Kuwahara, R.; Chaya, T.; Irie, S.; Furukawa, T. Mef2d is essential for the maturation and integrity of retinal photoreceptor and bipolar cells. *Genes Cells* **2015**, *20*, 408–426. [CrossRef]

380. Kiyama, T.; Chen, C.K.; Wang, S.W.; Pan, P.; Ju, Z.; Wang, J.; Takada, S.; Klein, W.H.; Mao, C.A. Essential roles of mitochondrial biogenesis regulator Nrf1 in retinal development and homeostasis. *Mol. Neurodegener.* **2018**, *13*, 56. [CrossRef] [PubMed]

381. Wu, F.; Li, R.; Umino, Y.; Kaczynski, T.J.; Sapkota, D.; Li, S.; Xiang, M.; Fliesler, S.J.; Sherry, D.M.; Gannon, M.; et al. Onecut1 is essential for horizontal cell genesis and retinal integrity. *J. Neurosci.* **2013**, *33*, 13053–13065. [CrossRef]

382. Goding, C.R.; Arnheiter, H. MITF-the first 25 years. *Genes Dev.* **2019**, *33*, 983–1007. [CrossRef]

383. Zelinger, L.; Swaroop, A. RNA Biology in Retinal Development and Disease. *Trends Genet.* **2018**, *34*, 341–351. [CrossRef]

384. Barabino, A.; Plamondon, V.; Abdouh, M.; Chatoo, W.; Flamier, A.; Hanna, R.; Zhou, S.; Motoyama, N.; Hebert, M.; Lavoie, J.; et al. Loss of Bmi1 causes anomalies in retinal development and degeneration of cone photoreceptors. *Development* **2016**, *143*, 1571–1584. [CrossRef]

385. Susaki, K.; Kaneko, J.; Yamano, Y.; Nakamura, K.; Inami, W.; Yoshikawa, T.; Ozawa, Y.; Shibata, S.; Matsuzaki, O.; Okano, H.; et al. Musashi-1, an RNA-binding protein, is indispensable for survival of photoreceptors. *Exp. Eye Res.* **2009**, *88*, 347–355. [CrossRef]

386. McKinnon, P.J. Maintaining genome stability in the nervous system. *Nat. Neurosci.* **2013**, *16*, 1523–1529. [CrossRef] [PubMed]

387. Gregersen, L.H.; Svejstrup, J.Q. The Cellular Response to Transcription-Blocking DNA Damage. *Trends Biochem. Sci.* **2018**, *43*, 327–341. [CrossRef] [PubMed]

388. Lans, H.; Hoeijmakers, J.H.J.; Vermeulen, W.; Marteijn, J.A. The DNA damage response to transcription stress. *Nat. Rev. Mol. Cell Biol.* **2019**, *20*, 766–784. [CrossRef] [PubMed]

389. Sanchez, A.; De Vivo, A.; Uprety, N.; Kim, J.; Stevens, S.M., Jr.; Kee, Y. BMI1-UBR5 axis regulates transcriptional repression at damaged chromatin. *Proc. Natl. Acad. Sci. USA* **2016**, *113*, 11243–11248. [CrossRef] [PubMed]

390. Calses, P.C.; Dhillon, K.K.; Tucker, N.; Chi, Y.; Huang, J.W.; Kawasumi, M.; Nghiem, P.; Wang, Y.; Clurman, B.E.; Jacquemont, C.; et al. DGCR8 Mediates Repair of UV-Induced DNA Damage Independently of RNA Processing. *Cell Rep.* **2017**, *19*, 162–174. [CrossRef] [PubMed]

391. Burger, K.; Schlackow, M.; Potts, M.; Hester, S.; Mohammed, S.; Gullerova, M. Nuclear phosphorylated Dicer processes double-stranded RNA in response to DNA damage. *J. Cell Biol.* **2017**, *216*, 2373–2389. [CrossRef]

392. Montaldo, N.P.; Bordin, D.L.; Brambilla, A.; Rosinger, M.; Fordyce Martin, S.L.; Bjoras, K.O.; Bradamante, S.; Aas, P.A.; Furrer, A.; Olsen, L.C.; et al. Alkyladenine DNA glycosylase associates with transcription elongation to coordinate DNA repair with gene expression. *Nat. Commun.* **2019**, *10*, 5460. [CrossRef]

393. Faridounnia, M.; Folkers, G.E.; Boelens, R. Function and Interactions of ERCC1-XPF in DNA Damage Response. *Molecules* **2018**, *23*, 3205. [CrossRef]

394. de Araujo, P.R.; Gorthi, A.; da Silva, A.E.; Tonapi, S.S.; Vo, D.T.; Burns, S.C.; Qiao, M.; Uren, P.J.; Yuan, Z.M.; Bishop, A.J.; et al. Musashi1 Impacts Radio-Resistance in Glioblastoma by Controlling DNA-Protein Kinase Catalytic Subunit. *Am. J. Pathol.* **2016**, *186*, 2271–2278. [CrossRef]

395. Onn, L.; Portillo, M.; Ilic, S.; Cleitman, G.; Stein, D.; Kaluski, S.; Shirat, I.; Slobodnik, Z.; Einav, M.; Erdel, F.; et al. SIRT6 is a DNA double-strand break sensor. *Elife* **2020**, *9*. [CrossRef]

396. Calderwood, S.K. A critical role for topoisomerase IIb and DNA double strand breaks in transcription. *Transcription* **2016**, *7*, 75–83. [CrossRef] [PubMed]

397. Aleksandrov, R.; Dotchev, A.; Poser, I.; Krastev, D.; Georgiev, G.; Panova, G.; Babukov, Y.; Danovski, G.; Dyankova, T.; Hubatsch, L.; et al. Protein Dynamics in Complex DNA Lesions. *Mol. Cell* **2018**, *69*, 1046.e1045–1061.e1045. [CrossRef]

398. Nishi, R.; Wijnhoven, P.W.G.; Kimura, Y.; Matsui, M.; Konietzny, R.; Wu, Q.; Nakamura, K.; Blundell, T.L.; Kessler, B.M. The deubiquitylating enzyme UCHL3 regulates Ku80 retention at sites of DNA damage. *Sci. Rep.* **2018**, *8*, 17891. [CrossRef] [PubMed]

399. Xu, H.; Lin, Z.; Li, F.; Diao, W.; Dong, C.; Zhou, H.; Xie, X.; Wang, Z.; Shen, Y.; Long, J. Dimerization of elongator protein 1 is essential for Elongator complex assembly. *Proc. Natl. Acad. Sci. USA* **2015**, *112*, 10697–10702. [CrossRef] [PubMed]

400. Li, Y.; Hao, H.; Swerdel, M.R.; Cho, H.Y.; Lee, K.B.; Hart, R.P.; Lyu, Y.L.; Cai, L. Top2b is involved in the formation of outer segment and synapse during late-stage photoreceptor differentiation by controlling key genes of photoreceptor transcriptional regulatory network. *J. Neurosci. Res.* **2017**, *95*, 1951–1964. [CrossRef] [PubMed]

401. Valdes-Sanchez, L.; De la Cerda, B.; Diaz-Corrales, F.J.; Massalini, S.; Chakarova, C.F.; Wright, A.F.; Bhattacharya, S.S. ATR localizes to the photoreceptor connecting cilium and deficiency leads to severe photoreceptor degeneration in mice. *Hum. Mol. Genet.* **2013**, *22*, 1507–1515. [CrossRef]

402. Bian, C.; Zhang, C.; Luo, T.; Vyas, A.; Chen, S.H.; Liu, C.; Kassab, M.A.; Yang, Y.; Kong, M.; Yu, X. NADP(+) is an endogenous PARP inhibitor in DNA damage response and tumor suppression. *Nat. Commun.* **2019**, *10*, 693. [CrossRef]

403. Sundermeier, T.R.; Sakami, S.; Sahu, B.; Howell, S.J.; Gao, S.; Dong, Z.; Golczak, M.; Maeda, A.; Palczewski, K. MicroRNA-processing Enzymes Are Essential for Survival and Function of Mature Retinal Pigmented Epithelial Cells in Mice. *J. Biol. Chem.* **2017**, *292*, 3366–3378. [CrossRef]

404. Damiani, D.; Alexander, J.J.; O'Rourke, J.R.; McManus, M.; Jadhav, A.P.; Cepko, C.L.; Hauswirth, W.W.; Harfe, B.D.; Strettoi, E. Dicer inactivation leads to progressive functional and structural degeneration of the mouse retina. *J. Neurosci.* **2008**, *28*, 4878–4887. [CrossRef] [PubMed]

405. Ueki, Y.; Ramirez, G.; Salcedo, E.; Stabio, M.E.; Lefcort, F. Loss of Ikbkap Causes Slow, Progressive Retinal Degeneration in a Mouse Model of Familial Dysautonomia. *eNeuro* **2016**, *3*. [CrossRef] [PubMed]

406. Spoor, M.; Nagtegaal, A.P.; Ridwan, Y.; Borgesius, N.Z.; van Alphen, B.; van der Pluijm, I.; Hoeijmakers, J.H.; Frens, M.A.; Borst, J.G. Accelerated loss of hearing and vision in the DNA-repair deficient Ercc1(delta/-) mouse. *Mech. Ageing Dev.* **2012**, *133*, 59–67. [CrossRef] [PubMed]

407. Gorgels, T.G.; van der Pluijm, I.; Brandt, R.M.; Garinis, G.A.; van Steeg, H.; van den Aardweg, G.; Jansen, G.H.; Ruijter, J.M.; Bergen, A.A.; van Norren, D.; et al. Retinal degeneration and ionizing radiation hypersensitivity in a mouse model for Cockayne syndrome. *Mol. Cell Biol.* **2007**, *27*, 1433–1441. [CrossRef] [PubMed]

408. Eblimit, A.; Zaneveld, S.A.; Liu, W.; Thomas, K.; Wang, K.; Li, Y.; Mardon, G.; Chen, R. NMNAT1 E257K variant, associated with Leber Congenital Amaurosis (LCA9), causes a mild retinal degeneration phenotype. *Exp. Eye Res.* **2018**, *173*, 32–43. [CrossRef]

409. Peshti, V.; Obolensky, A.; Nahum, L.; Kanfi, Y.; Rathaus, M.; Avraham, M.; Tinman, S.; Alt, F.W.; Banin, E.; Cohen, H.Y. Characterization of physiological defects in adult SIRT6-/- mice. *PLoS ONE* **2017**, *12*, e0176371. [CrossRef] [PubMed]

410. Lim, D.; Park, C.W.; Ryu, K.Y.; Chung, H. Disruption of the polyubiquitin gene Ubb causes retinal degeneration in mice. *Biochem. Biophys. Res. Commun.* **2019**, *513*, 35–40. [CrossRef]

411. Semenova, E.; Wang, X.; Jablonski, M.M.; Levorse, J.; Tilghman, S.M. An engineered 800 kilobase deletion of Uchl3 and Lmo7 on mouse chromosome 14 causes defects in viability, postnatal growth and degeneration of muscle and retina. *Hum. Mol. Genet.* **2003**, *12*, 1301–1312. [CrossRef]

412. Pinelli, M.; Carissimo, A.; Cutillo, L.; Lai, C.H.; Mutarelli, M.; Moretti, M.N.; Singh, M.V.; Karali, M.; Carrella, D.; Pizzo, M.; et al. An atlas of gene expression and gene co-regulation in the human retina. *Nucleic Acids Res.* **2016**, *44*, 5773–5784. [CrossRef]

413. Hoshino, A.; Ratnapriya, R.; Brooks, M.J.; Chaitankar, V.; Wilken, M.S.; Zhang, C.; Starostik, M.R.; Gieser, L.; La Torre, A.; Nishio, M.; et al. Molecular Anatomy of the Developing Human Retina. *Dev. Cell* **2017**, *43*, 763.e764–779.e764. [CrossRef]

414. Graziotto, J.J.; Farkas, M.H.; Bujakowska, K.; Deramaudt, B.M.; Zhang, Q.; Nandrot, E.F.; Inglehearn, C.F.; Bhattacharya, S.S.; Pierce, E.A. Three gene-targeted mouse models of RNA splicing factor RP show late-onset RPE and retinal degeneration. *Investig. Ophthalmol. Vis. Sci.* **2011**, *52*, 190–198. [CrossRef]

415. Xu, M.; Xie, Y.A.; Abouzeid, H.; Gordon, C.T.; Fiorentino, A.; Sun, Z.; Lehman, A.; Osman, I.S.; Dharmat, R.; Riveiro-Alvarez, R.; et al. Mutations in the Spliceosome Component CWC27 Cause Retinal Degeneration with or without Additional Developmental Anomalies. *Am. J. Hum. Genet.* **2017**, *100*, 592–604. [CrossRef]

416. Chen, B.J.; Lam, T.C.; Liu, L.Q.; To, C.H. Post-translational modifications and their applications in eye research (Review). *Mol. Med. Rep.* **2017**, *15*, 3923–3935. [CrossRef] [PubMed]

417. Christiansen, J.R.; Kolandaivelu, S.; Bergo, M.O.; Ramamurthy, V. RAS-converting enzyme 1-mediated endoproteolysis is required for trafficking of rod phosphodiesterase 6 to photoreceptor outer segments. *Proc. Natl. Acad. Sci. USA* **2011**, *108*, 8862–8866. [CrossRef] [PubMed]

418. Christiansen, J.R.; Pendse, N.D.; Kolandaivelu, S.; Bergo, M.O.; Young, S.G.; Ramamurthy, V. Deficiency of Isoprenylcysteine Carboxyl Methyltransferase (ICMT) Leads to Progressive Loss of Photoreceptor Function. *J. Neurosci.* **2016**, *36*, 5107–5114. [CrossRef]

419. Bosch Grau, M.; Masson, C.; Gadadhar, S.; Rocha, C.; Tort, O.; Marques Sousa, P.; Vacher, S.; Bieche, I.; Janke, C. Alterations in the balance of tubulin glycylation and glutamylation in photoreceptors leads to retinal degeneration. *J. Cell Sci.* **2017**, *130*, 938–949. [CrossRef] [PubMed]

420. Sun, X.; Park, J.H.; Gumerson, J.; Wu, Z.; Swaroop, A.; Qian, H.; Roll-Mecak, A.; Li, T. Loss of RPGR glutamylation underlies the pathogenic mechanism of retinal dystrophy caused by TTLL5 mutations. *Proc. Natl. Acad. Sci. USA* **2016**, *113*, E2925–E2934. [CrossRef] [PubMed]

421. Blanks, J.C.; Spee, C. Retinal degeneration in the pcd/pcd mutant mouse: Accumulation of spherules in the interphotoreceptor space. *Exp. Eye Res.* **1992**, *54*, 637–644. [CrossRef]

422. Chen, J.; Qian, H.; Horai, R.; Chan, C.C.; Falick, Y.; Caspi, R.R. Comparative analysis of induced vs. spontaneous models of autoimmune uveitis targeting the interphotoreceptor retinoid binding protein. *PLoS ONE* **2013**, *8*, e72161. [CrossRef]

423. Yu, M.; Zou, W.; Peachey, N.S.; McIntyre, T.M.; Liu, J. A novel role of complement in retinal degeneration. *Investig. Ophthalmol. Vis. Sci.* **2012**, *53*, 7684–7692. [CrossRef]

424. Lyzogubov, V.V.; Bora, P.S.; Wu, X.; Horn, L.E.; de Roque, R.; Rudolf, X.V.; Atkinson, J.P.; Bora, N.S. The Complement Regulatory Protein CD46 Deficient Mouse Spontaneously Develops Dry-Type Age-Related Macular Degeneration-Like Phenotype. *Am. J. Pathol.* **2016**, *186*, 2088–2104. [CrossRef]

425. Jobling, A.I.; Waugh, M.; Vessey, K.A.; Phipps, J.A.; Trogrlic, L.; Greferath, U.; Mills, S.A.; Tan, Z.L.; Ward, M.M.; Fletcher, E.L. The Role of the Microglial Cx3cr1 Pathway in the Postnatal Maturation of Retinal Photoreceptors. *J. Neurosci.* **2018**, *38*, 4708–4723. [CrossRef]

426. Combadiere, C.; Feumi, C.; Raoul, W.; Keller, N.; Rodero, M.; Pezard, A.; Lavalette, S.; Houssier, M.; Jonet, L.; Picard, E.; et al. CX3CR1-dependent subretinal microglia cell accumulation is associated with cardinal features of age-related macular degeneration. *J. Clin. Investig.* **2007**, *117*, 2920–2928. [CrossRef]

427. Huang, H.; Liu, Y.; Wang, L.; Li, W. Age-related macular degeneration phenotypes are associated with increased tumor necrosis-alpha and subretinal immune cells in aged Cxcr5 knockout mice. *PLoS ONE* **2017**, *12*, e0173716. [CrossRef] [PubMed]

428. Zhang, X.; Zhu, J.; Chen, X.; Jie-Qiong, Z.; Li, X.; Luo, L.; Huang, H.; Liu, W.; Zhou, X.; Yan, J.; et al. Interferon Regulatory Factor 3 Deficiency Induces Age-Related Alterations of the Retina in Young and Old Mice. *Front. Cell Neurosci.* **2019**, *13*, 272. [CrossRef] [PubMed]

429. Zhang, Q.; Jiang, Y.; Miller, M.J.; Peng, B.; Liu, L.; Soderland, C.; Tang, J.; Kern, T.S.; Pintar, J.; Steinle, J.J. IGFBP-3 and TNF-alpha regulate retinal endothelial cell apoptosis. *Investig. Ophthalmol. Vis. Sci.* **2013**, *54*, 5376–5384. [CrossRef] [PubMed]

430. Ambati, J.; Anand, A.; Fernandez, S.; Sakurai, E.; Lynn, B.C.; Kuziel, W.A.; Rollins, B.J.; Ambati, B.K. An animal model of age-related macular degeneration in senescent Ccl-2- or Ccr-2-deficient mice. *Nat. Med.* **2003**, *9*, 1390–1397. [CrossRef] [PubMed]

431. Coffey, P.J.; Gias, C.; McDermott, C.J.; Lundh, P.; Pickering, M.C.; Sethi, C.; Bird, A.; Fitzke, F.W.; Maass, A.; Chen, L.L.; et al. Complement factor H deficiency in aged mice causes retinal abnormalities and visual dysfunction. *Proc. Natl. Acad. Sci. USA* **2007**, *104*, 16651–16656. [CrossRef]

432. Ueda, Y.; Mohammed, I.; Song, D.; Gullipalli, D.; Zhou, L.; Sato, S.; Wang, Y.; Gupta, S.; Cheng, Z.; Wang, H.; et al. Murine systemic thrombophilia and hemolytic uremic syndrome from a factor H point mutation. *Blood* **2017**, *129*, 1184–1196. [CrossRef]

433. Ma, W.; Silverman, S.M.; Zhao, L.; Villasmil, R.; Campos, M.M.; Amaral, J.; Wong, W.T. Absence of TGFbeta signaling in retinal microglia induces retinal degeneration and exacerbates choroidal neovascularization. *Elife* **2019**, *8*. [CrossRef]

434. Zhou, Y.; Li, S.; Huang, L.; Yang, Y.; Zhang, L.; Yang, M.; Liu, W.; Ramasamy, K.; Jiang, Z.; Sundaresan, P.; et al. A splicing mutation in aryl hydrocarbon receptor associated with retinitis pigmentosa. *Hum. Mol. Genet.* **2018**, *27*, 2563–2572. [CrossRef]

435. Swiderski, R.E.; Nakano, Y.; Mullins, R.F.; Seo, S.; Banfi, B. A mutation in the mouse ttc26 gene leads to impaired hedgehog signaling. *PLoS Genet.* **2014**, *10*, e1004689. [CrossRef]

436. Omori, Y.; Kubo, S.; Kon, T.; Furuhashi, M.; Narita, H.; Kominami, T.; Ueno, A.; Tsutsumi, R.; Chaya, T.; Yamamoto, H.; et al. Samd7 is a cell type-specific PRC1 component essential for establishing retinal rod photoreceptor identity. *Proc. Natl. Acad. Sci. USA* **2017**, *114*, E8264–E8273. [CrossRef] [PubMed]

437. Behnen, P.; Felline, A.; Comitato, A.; Di Salvo, M.T.; Raimondi, F.; Gulati, S.; Kahremany, S.; Palczewski, K.; Marigo, V.; Fanelli, F. A Small Chaperone Improves Folding and Routing of Rhodopsin Mutants Linked to Inherited Blindness. *iScience* **2018**, *4*, 1–19. [CrossRef] [PubMed]

438. Kroeger, H.; Chiang, W.C.; Felden, J.; Nguyen, A.; Lin, J.H. ER stress and unfolded protein response in ocular health and disease. *FEBS J.* **2019**, *286*, 399–412. [CrossRef] [PubMed]

439. Stuck, M.W.; Conley, S.M.; Naash, M.I. PRPH2/RDS and ROM-1: Historical context, current views and future considerations. *Prog. Retin. Eye Res.* **2016**, *52*, 47–63. [CrossRef]

440. Boon, C.J.; den Hollander, A.I.; Hoyng, C.B.; Cremers, F.P.; Klevering, B.J.; Keunen, J.E. The spectrum of retinal dystrophies caused by mutations in the peripherin/RDS gene. *Prog. Retin. Eye Res.* **2008**, *27*, 213–235. [CrossRef]

441. Liu, M.M.; Zack, D.J. Alternative splicing and retinal degeneration. *Clin. Genet.* **2013**, *84*, 142–149. [CrossRef]

442. Zhao, Y.; Hong, D.H.; Pawlyk, B.; Yue, G.; Adamian, M.; Grynberg, M.; Godzik, A.; Li, T. The retinitis pigmentosa GTPase regulator (RPGR)- interacting protein: Subserving RPGR function and participating in disk morphogenesis. *Proc. Natl. Acad. Sci. USA* **2003**, *100*, 3965–3970. [CrossRef]

443. Won, J.; Gifford, E.; Smith, R.S.; Yi, H.; Ferreira, P.A.; Hicks, W.L.; Li, T.; Naggert, J.K.; Nishina, P.M. RPGRIP1 is essential for normal rod photoreceptor outer segment elaboration and morphogenesis. *Hum. Mol. Genet.* **2009**, *18*, 4329–4339. [CrossRef]

444. Zhang, C.; Quan, R.; Wang, J. Development and application of CRISPR/Cas9 technologies in genomic editing. *Hum. Mol. Genet.* **2018**, *27*, R79–R88. [CrossRef]

445. Comitato, A.; Schiroli, D.; La Marca, C.; Marigo, V. Differential Contribution of Calcium-Activated Proteases and ER-Stress in Three Mouse Models of Retinitis Pigmentosa Expressing P23H Mutant RHO. *Adv. Exp. Med. Biol.* **2019**, *1185*, 311–316. [CrossRef]

446. Hahn, P.; Qian, Y.; Dentchev, T.; Chen, L.; Beard, J.; Harris, Z.L.; Dunaief, J.L. Disruption of ceruloplasmin and hephaestin in mice causes retinal iron overload and retinal degeneration with features of age-related macular degeneration. *Proc. Natl. Acad. Sci. USA* **2004**, *101*, 13850–13855. [CrossRef]

447. Kumar, M.V.; Nagineni, C.N.; Chin, M.S.; Hooks, J.J.; Detrick, B. Innate immunity in the retina: Toll-like receptor (TLR) signaling in human retinal pigment epithelial cells. *J. Neuroimmunol.* **2004**, *153*, 7–15. [CrossRef] [PubMed]

448. Shiose, S.; Chen, Y.; Okano, K.; Roy, S.; Kohno, H.; Tang, J.; Pearlman, E.; Maeda, T.; Palczewski, K.; Maeda, A. Toll-like receptor 3 is required for development of retinopathy caused by impaired all-trans-retinal clearance in mice. *J. Biol. Chem.* **2011**, *286*, 15543–15555. [CrossRef] [PubMed]

449. Vollrath, D.; Yasumura, D.; Benchorin, G.; Matthes, M.T.; Feng, W.; Nguyen, N.M.; Sedano, C.D.; Calton, M.A.; LaVail, M.M. Tyro3 Modulates Mertk-Associated Retinal Degeneration. *PLoS Genet.* **2015**, *11*, e1005723. [CrossRef] [PubMed]

450. Zhang, Y.; Seo, S.; Bhattarai, S.; Bugge, K.; Searby, C.C.; Zhang, Q.; Drack, A.V.; Stone, E.M.; Sheffield, V.C. BBS mutations modify phenotypic expression of CEP290-related ciliopathies. *Hum. Mol. Genet.* **2014**, *23*, 40–51. [CrossRef] [PubMed]

451. Rachel, R.A.; May-Simera, H.L.; Veleri, S.; Gotoh, N.; Choi, B.Y.; Murga-Zamalloa, C.; McIntyre, J.C.; Marek, J.; Lopez, I.; Hackett, A.N.; et al. Combining Cep290 and Mkks ciliopathy alleles in mice rescues sensory defects and restores ciliogenesis. *J. Clin. Investig.* **2012**, *122*, 1233–1245. [CrossRef] [PubMed]

452. Rao, K.N.; Zhang, W.; Li, L.; Ronquillo, C.; Baehr, W.; Khanna, H. Ciliopathy-associated protein CEP290 modifies the severity of retinal degeneration due to loss of RPGR. *Hum. Mol. Genet.* **2016**, *25*, 2005–2012. [CrossRef]

453. Schon, C.; Asteriti, S.; Koch, S.; Sothilingam, V.; Garcia Garrido, M.; Tanimoto, N.; Herms, J.; Seeliger, M.W.; Cangiano, L.; Biel, M.; et al. Loss of HCN1 enhances disease progression in mouse models of CNG channel-linked retinitis pigmentosa and achromatopsia. *Hum. Mol. Genet.* **2016**, *25*, 1165–1175. [CrossRef]

454. Quinn, P.M.; Mulder, A.A.; Henrique Alves, C.; Desrosiers, M.; de Vries, S.I.; Klooster, J.; Dalkara, D.; Koster, A.J.; Jost, C.R.; Wijnholds, J. Loss of CRB2 in Muller glial cells modifies a CRB1-associated retinitis pigmentosa phenotype into a Leber congenital amaurosis phenotype. *Hum. Mol. Genet.* **2019**, *28*, 105–123. [CrossRef]

455. Ng, L.; Liu, H.; St Germain, D.L.; Hernandez, A.; Forrest, D. Deletion of the Thyroid Hormone-Activating Type 2 Deiodinase Rescues Cone Photoreceptor Degeneration but Not Deafness in Mice Lacking Type 3 Deiodinase. *Endocrinology* **2017**, *158*, 1999–2010. [CrossRef]

456. van der Pluijm, I.; Garinis, G.A.; Brandt, R.M.; Gorgels, T.G.; Wijnhoven, S.W.; Diderich, K.E.; de Wit, J.; Mitchell, J.R.; van Oostrom, C.; Beems, R.; et al. Impaired genome maintenance suppresses the growth hormone–insulin-like growth factor 1 axis in mice with Cockayne syndrome. *PLoS Biol.* **2007**, *5*, e2. [CrossRef]

457. Chang, B.; Heckenlively, J.R.; Bayley, P.R.; Brecha, N.C.; Davisson, M.T.; Hawes, N.L.; Hirano, A.A.; Hurd, R.E.; Ikeda, A.; Johnson, B.A.; et al. The nob2 mouse, a null mutation in Cacna1f: Anatomical and functional abnormalities in the outer retina and their consequences on ganglion cell visual responses. *Vis. Neurosci.* **2006**, *23*, 11–24. [CrossRef] [PubMed]

458. Humphries, M.M.; Kiang, S.; McNally, N.; Donovan, M.A.; Sieving, P.A.; Bush, R.A.; Machida, S.; Cotter, T.; Hobson, A.; Farrar, J.; et al. Comparative structural and functional analysis of photoreceptor neurons of Rho-/- mice reveal increased survival on C57BL/6J in comparison to 129Sv genetic background. *Vis. Neurosci.* **2001**, *18*, 437–443. [CrossRef]

459. Liu, Q.; Saveliev, A.; Pierce, E.A. The severity of retinal degeneration in Rp1h gene-targeted mice is dependent on genetic background. *Investig. Ophthalmol. Vis. Sci.* **2009**, *50*, 1566–1574. [CrossRef] [PubMed]

460. Haider, N.B.; Zhang, W.; Hurd, R.; Ikeda, A.; Nystuen, A.M.; Naggert, J.K.; Nishina, P.M. Mapping of genetic modifiers of Nr2e3 rd7/rd7 that suppress retinal degeneration and restore blue cone cells to normal quantity. *Mamm. Genome* **2008**, *19*, 145–154. [CrossRef]

461. Threadgill, D.W.; Miller, D.R.; Churchill, G.A.; de Villena, F.P. The collaborative cross: A recombinant inbred mouse population for the systems genetic era. *ILAR J.* **2011**, *52*, 24–31. [CrossRef]

462. Churchill, G.A.; Gatti, D.M.; Munger, S.C.; Svenson, K.L. The Diversity Outbred mouse population. *Mamm. Genome* **2012**, *23*, 713–718. [CrossRef]

463. Cruz, N.M.; Yuan, Y.; Leehy, B.D.; Baid, R.; Kompella, U.; DeAngelis, M.M.; Escher, P.; Haider, N.B. Modifier genes as therapeutics: The nuclear hormone receptor Rev Erb alpha (Nr1d1) rescues Nr2e3 associated retinal disease. *PLoS ONE* **2014**, *9*, e87942. [CrossRef]

464. Danciger, M.; Ogando, D.; Yang, H.; Matthes, M.T.; Yu, N.; Ahern, K.; Yasumura, D.; Williams, R.W.; Lavail, M.M. Genetic modifiers of retinal degeneration in the rd3 mouse. *Investig. Ophthalmol. Vis. Sci.* **2008**, *49*, 2863–2869. [CrossRef]

465. van Wyk, M.; Schneider, S.; Kleinlogel, S. Variable phenotypic expressivity in inbred retinal degeneration mouse lines: A comparative study of C3H/HeOu and FVB/N rd1 mice. *Mol. Vis.* **2015**, *21*, 811–827.

466. Luhmann, U.F.; Carvalho, L.S.; Holthaus, S.M.; Cowing, J.A.; Greenaway, S.; Chu, C.J.; Herrmann, P.; Smith, A.J.; Munro, P.M.; Potter, P.; et al. The severity of retinal pathology in homozygous Crb1rd8/rd8 mice is dependent on additional genetic factors. *Hum. Mol. Genet.* **2015**, *24*, 128–141. [CrossRef] [PubMed]

467. Won, J.; Charette, J.R.; Philip, V.M.; Stearns, T.M.; Zhang, W.; Naggert, J.K.; Krebs, M.P.; Nishina, P.M. Genetic modifier loci of mouse Mfrp(rd6) identified by quantitative trait locus analysis. *Exp. Eye Res.* **2014**, *118*, 30–35. [CrossRef] [PubMed]

468. Maddox, D.M.; Ikeda, S.; Ikeda, A.; Zhang, W.; Krebs, M.P.; Nishina, P.M.; Naggert, J.K. An allele of microtubule-associated protein 1A (Mtap1a) reduces photoreceptor degeneration in Tulp1 and Tub Mutant Mice. *Investig. Ophthalmol. Vis. Sci.* **2012**, *53*, 1663–1669. [CrossRef]

469. Kong, Y.; Zhao, L.; Charette, J.R.; Hicks, W.L.; Stone, L.; Nishina, P.M.; Naggert, J.K. An FRMD4B variant suppresses dysplastic photoreceptor lesions in models of enhanced S-cone syndrome and of Nrl deficiency. *Hum. Mol. Genet.* **2018**, *27*, 3340–3352. [CrossRef] [PubMed]

470. Paskowitz, D.M.; LaVail, M.M.; Duncan, J.L. Light and inherited retinal degeneration. *Br. J. Ophthalmol.* **2006**, *90*, 1060–1066. [CrossRef] [PubMed]

471. Dellett, M.; Sasai, N.; Nishide, K.; Becker, S.; Papadaki, V.; Limb, G.A.; Moore, A.T.; Kondo, T.; Ohnuma, S. Genetic background and light-dependent progression of photoreceptor cell degeneration in Prominin-1 knockout mice. *Investig. Ophthalmol. Vis. Sci.* **2014**, *56*, 164–176. [CrossRef]

472. Naash, M.L.; Peachey, N.S.; Li, Z.Y.; Gryczan, C.C.; Goto, Y.; Blanks, J.; Milam, A.H.; Ripps, H. Light-induced acceleration of photoreceptor degeneration in transgenic mice expressing mutant rhodopsin. *Investig. Ophthalmol. Vis. Sci.* **1996**, *37*, 775–782.

473. Rascher, K.; Servos, G.; Berthold, G.; Hartwig, H.G.; Warskulat, U.; Heller-Stilb, B.; Haussinger, D. Light deprivation slows but does not prevent the loss of photoreceptors in taurine transporter knockout mice. *Vis. Res.* **2004**, *44*, 2091–2100. [CrossRef]

474. Smith, S.B.; Cope, B.K.; McCoy, J.R. Effects of dark-rearing on the retinal degeneration of the C57BL/6-mivit/mivit mouse. *Exp. Eye Res.* **1994**, *58*, 77–84. [CrossRef]

475. Maeda, A.; Maeda, T.; Imanishi, Y.; Sun, W.; Jastrzebska, B.; Hatala, D.A.; Winkens, H.J.; Hofmann, K.P.; Janssen, J.J.; Baehr, W.; et al. Retinol dehydrogenase (RDH12) protects photoreceptors from light-induced degeneration in mice. *J. Biol. Chem.* **2006**, *281*, 37697–37704. [CrossRef]

476. Ettaiche, M.; Guy, N.; Hofman, P.; Lazdunski, M.; Waldmann, R. Acid-sensing ion channel 2 is important for retinal function and protects against light-induced retinal degeneration. *J. Neurosci.* **2004**, *24*, 1005–1012. [CrossRef] [PubMed]

477. Peng, Y.W.; Zallocchi, M.; Wang, W.M.; Delimont, D.; Cosgrove, D. Moderate light-induced degeneration of rod photoreceptors with delayed transducin translocation in shaker1 mice. *Investig. Ophthalmol. Vis. Sci.* **2011**, *52*, 6421–6427. [CrossRef] [PubMed]

478. Tian, M.; Wang, W.; Delimont, D.; Cheung, L.; Zallocchi, M.; Cosgrove, D.; Peng, Y.W. Photoreceptors in whirler mice show defective transducin translocation and are susceptible to short-term light/dark changes-induced degeneration. *Exp. Eye Res.* **2014**, *118*, 145–153. [CrossRef] [PubMed]

479. Li, G.; Anderson, R.E.; Tomita, H.; Adler, R.; Liu, X.; Zack, D.J.; Rajala, R.V. Nonredundant role of Akt2 for neuroprotection of rod photoreceptor cells from light-induced cell death. *J. Neurosci.* **2007**, *27*, 203–211. [CrossRef]

480. Datta, S.; Cano, M.; Ebrahimi, K.; Wang, L.; Handa, J.T. The impact of oxidative stress and inflammation on RPE degeneration in non-neovascular AMD. *Prog. Retin. Eye Res.* **2017**, *60*, 201–218. [CrossRef]

481. Khan, J.C.; Thurlby, D.A.; Shahid, H.; Clayton, D.G.; Yates, J.R.; Bradley, M.; Moore, A.T.; Bird, A.C.; Genetic Factors in AMD Study. Smoking and age related macular degeneration: The number of pack years of cigarette smoking is a major determinant of risk for both geographic atrophy and choroidal neovascularisation. *Br. J. Ophthalmol.* **2006**, *90*, 75–80. [CrossRef]

482. Cano, M.; Thimmalappula, R.; Fujihara, M.; Nagai, N.; Sporn, M.; Wang, A.L.; Neufeld, A.H.; Biswal, S.; Handa, J.T. Cigarette smoking, oxidative stress, the anti-oxidant response through Nrf2 signaling, and Age-related Macular Degeneration. *Vis. Res.* **2010**, *50*, 652–664. [CrossRef]

483. Fujihara, M.; Nagai, N.; Sussan, T.E.; Biswal, S.; Handa, J.T. Chronic cigarette smoke causes oxidative damage and apoptosis to retinal pigmented epithelial cells in mice. *PLoS ONE* **2008**, *3*, e3119. [CrossRef]

484. Ebrahimi, K.B.; Cano, M.; Rhee, J.; Datta, S.; Wang, L.; Handa, J.T. Oxidative Stress Induces an Interactive Decline in Wnt and Nrf2 Signaling in Degenerating Retinal Pigment Epithelium. *Antioxid. Redox Signal.* **2018**, *29*, 389–407. [CrossRef]

485. Farese, R.V., Jr.; Veniant, M.M.; Cham, C.M.; Flynn, L.M.; Pierotti, V.; Loring, J.F.; Traber, M.; Ruland, S.; Stokowski, R.S.; Huszar, D.; et al. Phenotypic analysis of mice expressing exclusively apolipoprotein B48 or apolipoprotein B100. *Proc. Natl. Acad. Sci. USA* **1996**, *93*, 6393–6398. [CrossRef]

486. Schmidt-Erfurth, U.; Rudolf, M.; Funk, M.; Hofmann-Rummelt, C.; Franz-Haas, N.S.; Aherrahrou, Z.; Schlotzer-Schrehardt, U. Ultrastructural changes in a murine model of graded Bruch membrane lipoidal degeneration and corresponding VEGF164 detection. *Investig. Ophthalmol. Vis. Sci.* **2008**, *49*, 390–398. [CrossRef] [PubMed]

487. Malek, G.; Johnson, L.V.; Mace, B.E.; Saloupis, P.; Schmechel, D.E.; Rickman, D.W.; Toth, C.A.; Sullivan, P.M.; Bowes Rickman, C. Apolipoprotein E allele-dependent pathogenesis: A model for age-related retinal degeneration. *Proc. Natl. Acad. Sci. USA* **2005**, *102*, 11900–11905. [CrossRef] [PubMed]

488. Perusek, L.; Maeda, T. Vitamin A derivatives as treatment options for retinal degenerative diseases. *Nutrients* **2013**, *5*, 2646–2666. [CrossRef] [PubMed]

489. Perusek, L.; Maeda, A.; Maeda, T. Supplementation with vitamin a derivatives to rescue vision in animal models of degenerative retinal diseases. *Methods Mol. Biol.* **2015**, *1271*, 345–362. [CrossRef]

490. Guadagni, V.; Novelli, E.; Piano, I.; Gargini, C.; Strettoi, E. Pharmacological approaches to retinitis pigmentosa: A laboratory perspective. *Prog. Retin. Eye Res.* **2015**, *48*, 62–81. [CrossRef] [PubMed]

491. Cai, X.; McGinnis, J.F. Oxidative stress: The achilles' heel of neurodegenerative diseases of the retina. *Front. Biosci. Landmark. Ed.* **2012**, *17*, 1976–1995. [CrossRef]

492. Komeima, K.; Rogers, B.S.; Campochiaro, P.A. Antioxidants slow photoreceptor cell death in mouse models of retinitis pigmentosa. *J. Cell Physiol.* **2007**, *213*, 809–815. [CrossRef]

493. Ebert, S.; Weigelt, K.; Walczak, Y.; Drobnik, W.; Mauerer, R.; Hume, D.A.; Weber, B.H.; Langmann, T. Docosahexaenoic acid attenuates microglial activation and delays early retinal degeneration. *J. Neurochem.* **2009**, *110*, 1863–1875. [CrossRef]

494. Yu, M.; Yan, W.; Beight, C. Lutein and Zeaxanthin Isomers Reduce Photoreceptor Degeneration in the Pde6b (rd10) Mouse Model of Retinitis Pigmentosa. *Biomed. Res. Int.* **2018**, *2018*, 4374087. [CrossRef]

495. Komeima, K.; Rogers, B.S.; Lu, L.; Campochiaro, P.A. Antioxidants reduce cone cell death in a model of retinitis pigmentosa. *Proc. Natl. Acad. Sci. USA* **2006**, *103*, 11300–11305. [CrossRef]

496. Barone, I.; Novelli, E.; Piano, I.; Gargini, C.; Strettoi, E. Environmental enrichment extends photoreceptor survival and visual function in a mouse model of retinitis pigmentosa. *PLoS ONE* **2012**, *7*, e50726. [CrossRef]

497. Sundin, O.H.; Leppert, G.S.; Silva, E.D.; Yang, J.M.; Dharmaraj, S.; Maumenee, I.H.; Santos, L.C.; Parsa, C.F.; Traboulsi, E.I.; Broman, K.W.; et al. Extreme hyperopia is the result of null mutations in MFRP, which encodes a Frizzled-related protein. *Proc. Natl. Acad. Sci. USA* **2005**, *102*, 9553–9558. [CrossRef] [PubMed]

498. Sundin, O.H. The mouse's eye and Mfrp: Not quite human. *Ophthalmic Genet.* **2005**, *26*, 153–155. [CrossRef] [PubMed]

499. Kameya, S.; Hawes, N.L.; Chang, B.; Heckenlively, J.R.; Naggert, J.K.; Nishina, P.M. Mfrp, a gene encoding a frizzled related protein, is mutated in the mouse retinal degeneration 6. *Hum. Mol. Genet.* **2002**, *11*, 1879–1886. [CrossRef] [PubMed]

500.	Almoallem, B.; Arno, G.; De Zaeytijd, J.; Verdin, H.; Balikova, I.; Casteels, I.; de Ravel, T.; Hull, S.; Suzani, M.; Destree, A.; et al. The majority of autosomal recessive nanophthalmos and posterior microphthalmia can be attributed to biallelic sequence and structural variants in MFRP and PRSS56. *Sci. Rep.* **2020**, *10*, 1289. [CrossRef] [PubMed]

501.	Chekuri, A.; Sahu, B.; Chavali, V.R.M.; Voronchikhina, M.; Soto-Hermida, A.; Suk, J.J.; Alapati, A.N.; Bartsch, D.U.; Ayala-Ramirez, R.; Zenteno, J.C.; et al. Long-Term Effects of Gene Therapy in a Novel Mouse Model of Human MFRP-Associated Retinopathy. *Hum. Gene Ther.* **2019**, *30*, 632–650. [CrossRef] [PubMed]

502.	Gibson, F.; Walsh, J.; Mburu, P.; Varela, A.; Brown, K.A.; Antonio, M.; Beisel, K.W.; Steel, K.P.; Brown, S.D. A type VII myosin encoded by the mouse deafness gene shaker-1. *Nature* **1995**, *374*, 62–64. [CrossRef]

503.	Lentz, J.J.; Gordon, W.C.; Farris, H.E.; MacDonald, G.H.; Cunningham, D.E.; Robbins, C.A.; Tempel, B.L.; Bazan, N.G.; Rubel, E.W.; Oesterle, E.C.; et al. Deafness and retinal degeneration in a novel USH1C knock-in mouse model. *Dev. Neurobiol.* **2010**, *70*, 253–267. [CrossRef]

504.	Karan, G.; Lillo, C.; Yang, Z.; Cameron, D.J.; Locke, K.G.; Zhao, Y.; Thirumalaichary, S.; Li, C.; Birch, D.G.; Vollmer-Snarr, H.R.; et al. Lipofuscin accumulation, abnormal electrophysiology, and photoreceptor degeneration in mutant ELOVL4 transgenic mice: A model for macular degeneration. *Proc. Natl. Acad. Sci. USA* **2005**, *102*, 4164–4169. [CrossRef]

505.	Grishchuk, Y.; Stember, K.G.; Matsunaga, A.; Olivares, A.M.; Cruz, N.M.; King, V.E.; Humphrey, D.M.; Wang, S.L.; Muzikansky, A.; Betensky, R.A.; et al. Retinal Dystrophy and Optic Nerve Pathology in the Mouse Model of Mucolipidosis IV. *Am. J. Pathol.* **2016**, *186*, 199–209. [CrossRef]

506.	Amir, N.; Zlotogora, J.; Bach, G. Mucolipidosis type IV: Clinical spectrum and natural history. *Pediatrics* **1987**, *79*, 953–959. [PubMed]

507.	Park, H.; Qazi, Y.; Tan, C.; Jabbar, S.B.; Cao, Y.; Schmid, G.; Pardue, M.T. Assessment of axial length measurements in mouse eyes. *Optom. Vis. Sci.* **2012**, *89*, 296–303. [CrossRef]

508.	Ruppersburg, C.C.; Hartzell, H.C. The Ca2+-activated Cl- channel ANO1/TMEM16A regulates primary ciliogenesis. *Mol. Biol. Cell* **2014**, *25*, 1793–1807. [CrossRef] [PubMed]

509.	He, M.; Ye, W.; Wang, W.J.; Sison, E.S.; Jan, Y.N.; Jan, L.Y. Cytoplasmic Cl(-) couples membrane remodeling to epithelial morphogenesis. *Proc. Natl. Acad. Sci. USA* **2017**, *114*, E11161–E11169. [CrossRef] [PubMed]

510.	Gupta, A.; Fabian, L.; Brill, J.A. Phosphatidylinositol 4,5-bisphosphate regulates cilium transition zone maturation in Drosophila melanogaster. *J. Cell Sci.* **2018**, *131*. [CrossRef]

511.	Bhatia, V.; Valdes-Sanchez, L.; Rodriguez-Martinez, D.; Bhattacharya, S.S. Formation of 53BP1 foci and ATM activation under oxidative stress is facilitated by RNA:DNA hybrids and loss of ATM-53BP1 expression promotes photoreceptor cell survival in mice. *F1000Res* **2018**, *7*, 1233. [CrossRef]

512.	Muller, B.; Ellinwood, N.M.; Lorenz, B.; Stieger, K. Detection of DNA Double Strand Breaks by gammaH2AX Does Not Result in 53bp1 Recruitment in Mouse Retinal Tissues. *Front. Neurosci.* **2018**, *12*, 286. [CrossRef]

9

Antisense Oligonucleotide Screening to Optimize the Rescue of the Splicing Defect Caused by the Recurrent Deep-Intronic *ABCA4* Variant c.4539+2001G>A in Stargardt Disease

Alejandro Garanto [1],*, Lonneke Duijkers [2], Tomasz Z. Tomkiewicz [1] and Rob W. J. Collin [1],*

[1]   Department of Human Genetics and Donders Institute for Brain, Cognition and Behaviour, Radboud University Medical Center, 6525GA Nijmegen, The Netherlands; tomasz.tomkiewicz@radboudumc.nl

[2]   Department of Human Genetics, Radboud University Medical Center, 6525GA Nijmegen, The Netherlands; lonneke.duijkers@radboudumc.nl

*   Correspondence: alex.garanto@radboudumc.nl (A.G.); rob.collin@radboudumc.nl (R.W.J.C.);

Abstract: Deep-sequencing of the *ABCA4* locus has revealed that ~10% of autosomal recessive Stargardt disease (STGD1) cases are caused by deep-intronic mutations. One of the most recurrent deep-intronic variants in the Belgian and Dutch STGD1 population is the c.4539+2001G>A mutation. This variant introduces a 345-nt pseudoexon to the *ABCA4* mRNA transcript in a retina-specific manner. Antisense oligonucleotides (AONs) are short sequences of RNA that can modulate splicing. In this work, we designed 26 different AONs to perform a thorough screening to identify the most effective AONs to correct splicing defects associated with c.4539+2001G>A. All AONs were tested in patient-derived induced pluripotent stem cells (iPSCs) that were differentiated to photoreceptor precursor cells (PPCs). AON efficacy was assessed through RNA analysis and was based on correction efficacy, and AONs were grouped and their properties assessed. We (a) identified nine AONs with significant correction efficacies (>50%), (b) confirmed that a single nucleotide mismatch was sufficient to significantly decrease AON efficacy, and (c) found potential correlations between efficacy and some of the parameters analyzed. Overall, our results show that AON-based splicing modulation holds great potential for treating Stargardt disease caused by splicing defects in *ABCA4*.

Keywords: antisense oligonucleotides; Stargardt disease; inherited retinal diseases; splicing modulation; RNA therapy; ABCA4; iPSC-derived photoreceptor precursor cells

1. Introduction

Stargardt disease (STGD1; MIM:248200) is an autosomal recessive condition affecting the retina, and was first described in 1909 by the German ophthalmologist Karl Stargardt [1]. The clinical hallmark of STGD1 is progressive bilateral impairment of central vision. Impairment in visual acuity and progressive bilateral atrophy of photoreceptors and the retinal pigment epithelium (RPE) are accompanied by the accumulation of toxic fluorescent deposits of lipofuscin in the macula [2,3]. The underlying genetic causes of the disease are mutations in the *ABCA4* gene that encodes the ATP-binding cassette transporter type 4 subfamily A (ABCA4). The *ABCA4* protein belongs to the superfamily of membrane-bound ATP-binding cassette transporters [4]. It translocates the visual cycle metabolites, all-*trans*-retinal and *N*-retinylidene-phosphatidyl ethanolamine (*N*-retinylidene-PE), from the lumen to the cytoplasmic side of photoreceptor disc membranes [5]. The decrease in *ABCA4* activity causes an accumulation of toxic retinal derivatives, which eventually results in RPE and photoreceptor cell death [6,7]. Over 900 disease-associated variants in *ABCA4* have been described [8,9], causing a wide range of phenotypes ranging from STGD1 to cone–rod dystrophy, depending on the severity of the mutation [10,11].

STGD1 cases can be explained by biallelic mutations in either the coding sequence or in the intronic regions of *ABCA4* [12]. Around 10% of cases carry intronic variants that result in the insertion of pseudoexons (PEs) into the final *ABCA4* mRNA transcript [4,9,13–20]. Such mutations are an ideal target for antisense oligonucleotide (AON) therapy. AONs are short synthetic RNA molecules that can interfere with the processing of pre-mRNA [21] and thereby modulate splicing. Modified AONs employed to correct splicing defects have been extensively studied in the field of inherited retinal diseases (IRDs) for genes such as *CEP290* [22–27], *USH2A* [28], *CHM* [29], *OPN1* [30], or *ABCA4* [18,20,31]. The first splicing modulation strategy described for a retinal disease was targeting a recurring deep-intronic variant (c.2991+1655A>G) in the *CEP290* gene, underlying recessive Leber congenital amaurosis (LCA; MIM:611755). This mutation results in the generation of a cryptic splice donor site leading to a 128-nt pseudoexon with a premature stop codon between exons 26 and 27. AONs used to block the pseudoexon showed successful restoration of the original mRNA both in vivo and in vitro [22,24–27] and have recently shown promising results in the first clinical trial with AONs for IRDs [32].

Another mutation that causes a pre-mRNA splicing defect and is amenable to AON therapy is the c.4539+2001G>A variant in *ABCA4* [13–15], which is recurrently found in the Belgian and Dutch STGD1 population. Recently, our group described the molecular mechanism by which c.4539+2001G>A and the adjacent c.4539+2028C>T mutations in *ABCA4* lead to insertion of a retina-specific 345-nt pseudoexon that is predicted to result in premature termination of protein synthesis (p.Arg1514Leufs*36). The c.4539+2001G>A variant enhances a predicted exonic splice enhancer and creates a new SRp55 motif. This was the first reported insertion of a pseudoexon into a retinal gene due to the creation of new exonic splicing enhancer (ESE) motifs rather than the generation of new cryptic splice sites, although other examples have been described previously [33,34]. By using AON technology, we were able to restore correct splicing with two of the four AONs (AON1–4) that were used (AON1 and AON4) [18].

In this study, we performed an in-depth screening of a large set of AONs targeting the entire pseudoexon region to identify the most effective AON(s) against the splicing defect caused by the c.4539+2001G>A mutation. In total, 26 AONs were screened in retinal precursor cells differentiated from patient-derived induced pluripotent stem cell (iPSC), and their efficacy in correcting splicing defects was assessed. Subsequently, properties of the most effective AONs were compared in order to identify potential parameters for a better design of AONs in the future.

2. Materials and Methods

2.1. Study Design

The objectives of this study were to (1) perform an in-depth screening of AONs targeting the pseudoexon introduced by the recurrent c.4539+2001G>A deep-intronic variant in *ABCA4*, (2) identify the best AON(s) to correct the pre-mRNA splicing defect caused by this mutation using patient-derived photoreceptor precursor cells (PPCs), and (3) identify potential correlations between AON characteristics and their efficacy that can provide new insights into a better AON design. Twenty-two new AONs targeting the pseudoexon were designed and tested together with four previously described AONs [18]. Fibroblast cells obtained from a skin biopsy of a Stargardt individual carrying the deep-intronic variant were cultured, reprogrammed into iPSCs, and subsequently differentiated to PPCs. All 26 AONs and two sense oligonucleotides (SONs) were designed along the pseudoexon. Upon AON delivery, subsequent RNA analysis by RT-PCR was performed to assess the efficacy of the splicing redirection for each AON. After semiquantification of the rescue, AONs were classified into different groups, and the properties of the AONs were compared to identify parameters that could improve the AON design. Two separate differentiation experiments were performed. RNA analysis was performed in triplicate to reduce technical variability.

2.2. AON Design

Previously, four AONs were designed targeting the top SC35 motifs and the mutation itself [18]. For the detailed screening that was the subject of this study, the entire pseudoexon plus the flanking regions were analyzed for their RNA structure to identify the open and closed regions. Subsequently, AONs were designed according to previously described guidelines independently of the potential motifs that they were targeting [35,36]. All AON sequences and properties are provided in Table 1. After AON design, targeted regions were analyzed to predict potential exonic splicing enhancer (ESE) motifs using either an ESE finder (http://krainer01.cshl.edu/cgi-bin/tools/ESE3/esefinder.cgi?process=home), which allows for the detection of SRSF1, SRSF2, SRSF5, and SRSF6, or using RBPmap (http://rbpmap.technion.ac.il/index.html), which allows for the identification of 94 potential binding sites for RNA binding proteins. All AONs were 2'OMe-PS (2'O-methyl phosphorothioate) and were purchased from Eurogentec (Liege, Belgium). Sequences and general parameters of the 26 AONs and 2 SONs are depicted in Table 1.

2.3. Subjects

A skin biopsy was collected from a Dutch individual with STGD1 carrying the *ABCA4* variants c.4539+2001G>A (p.Arg1514Leufs*36) and c.4892T>C (p.Leu1631Pro) to establish a fibroblast cell line, as described previously [18]. Our research was conducted according to the tenets of the Declaration of Helsinki and after gathering written informed consent from the STGD1 individual. The procedures for obtaining human skin biopsies to establish primary fibroblast cell lines were approved by the local ethical committee (2015-1543).

2.4. iPSC Differentiation into Photoreceptor Precursor Cells (PPCs)

Fibroblast cells were reprogrammed into iPSCs, as previously described [18]. PPCs were obtained after following a 2D differentiation protocol [37]. Briefly, iPSCs were dissociated with ReLeSR (Stemcell Technologies) and plated in 12-well plates coated with matrigel (Corning, Tewksbury, MA, USA) to form a monolayer. Essential-Flex E8 medium was changed to differentiation medium (CI) when reaching confluence. The CI medium consisted of DMEM/F12 supplemented with nonessential amino acids (NEAA, Sigma Aldrich, Saint Louis, CA, USA), B27 supplements (Thermo Fisher Scientific, Waltham, MA, USA), N2 supplements (Thermo Fisher Scientific), 100 ng/μL of insulin growth factor-1 (IGF-1, Sigma Aldrich), 10 ng/μL of recombinant fibroblast growth factor basic (bFGF, Sigma Aldrich), 10 μg/μL of Heparin (Sigma Aldrich), 200 μg/mL of recombinant human COCO (R&D Systems, Minneapolis, MN, USA), and 100 μg/mL of Primocin (Invivogen, Toulouse, France). Half of the medium was replaced every day for 30 days. On day 28, PPCs were treated with 1 μM of AON. AONs were first mixed with the medium without any transfection reagent and were subsequently added to the cells. Twenty-four hours later, cycloheximide (CHX) was added to the medium (final concentration 100 μg/mL), and on day 30 (48 h post-AON delivery and 24 h post-CHX treatment), cells were collected.

2.5. RNA Analysis

RNA was isolated from patient-derived PPCs using the Nucleospin RNA kit (Machery Nagel, Düren, Germany) following the manufacturer's instructions. One microgram of total RNA was used for cDNA synthesis using SuperScript VILO Master Mix (Thermo Fisher Scientific) and was subsequently diluted with H_2O to a final concentration of 20 ng/μL. Reverse transcription-PCR (RT-PCR) was performed with 10 μM of each primer, 2 μM of dNTPs, 2.5 mM of $MgCl_2$, 1 U of Taq polymerase (Roche, Basel, Switzerland), and 80 ng of cDNA in a total reaction of 25 μL using the following PCR conditions: 2 min at 94 °C, followed by 35 cycles of 30 s at 94 °C, 30 s at 58 °C, and 70 s at 72 °C, with a final extension of 2 min at 72 °C. Actin was amplified to serve as a loading control. All PCR products were resolved on 2% agarose gels and were confirmed by Sanger. Fiji software was used to perform a semiquantitative analysis of the bands in which the values were normalized against the housekeeping gene *ACTB* [38]. For that, the band representing the 345-nt pseudoexon, plus half of the value of the heteroduplexes, and the partial pseudoexon skipping band were counted as aberrant. The other half of the heteroduplexes together with the correct band were considered to be correct transcripts. We observed a nonspecific band that was not considered for the analysis. The list of primers is provided in the Supplementary Materials, Table S1.

2.6. qPCR

The cDNA samples were obtained as described above from iPSCs at day 0, and the nontreated PPCs at day 30 (both replicates) were used for quantitative real-time PCR (qPCR) to assess the differentiation process: qPCR was performed using GoTaq qPCR master mix (Promega, Madison, WI, USA). Three technical replicates were done for each of the two biological replicates. The list of primers is provided in the Supplementary Materials, Table S1.

2.7. AON Classification and Common Properties

Once the rescue was assessed, AONs were classified into 5 groups: Highly effective (>75% correction), effective (between 75% and 50%), moderately effective (between 50% and 25%), poorly effective (between 25% and 0%), and noneffective (no correction detected). For the study of the properties of each group, the groups poorly effective and noneffective were combined into one single group, as well as the highly effective and effective groups, generating three new groups: Effective, moderately effective, and poorly effective. Using this information, several potential correlations between AON properties, target motifs, and their efficacy were assessed, with the aim of establishing possible improvements in the AON design. Statistical analyses were performed using GraphPad Prism. Given the low numbers for some of the groups, normality could not be assessed, and therefore nonparametric tests were used.

Table 1. Antisense oligonucleotide (AON) sequences and general parameters.

AON#	Sequence (5' to 3')	L	Tm	GC	FE-A	FE-D	BE	Remarks
AON1	ACAGGAGUCCUCAGCAUUG	19	51.1	53	−0.1	−12.4	16.2	Specific for c.4539+2001G>A-pseudoexon
AON2	UUUUGUCCAGGACCAAGG	19	51.1	53	−1.6	−15.6	23.1	Previously reported in Reference [18]
AON3	CUGUUACAUUUGUCCAGG	19	46.8	42	−0.9	−7.3	20.7	Previously reported in Reference [18]
AON4	GGGCACAGAGGACUGAGA	19	55.4	63	−0.8	−5.9	30.6	Previously reported in Reference [18]
AON5	GAGAGAAAAUAUUGCUUGAGAA	22	47.4	32	1.7	−5.0	27.5	Previously reported in Reference [18]
AON6	GCAGAUGAGCUGUGAUUCAA	20	49.7	45	−2.5	−8.8	24.0	
AON7	UAUGAUGCAGCAGAUGAGCUG	21	52.4	48	−3.9	−12.2	24.1	
AON8	UGGGAUCCUAUGAUGCAGC	20	53.8	55	−1.1	−17.4	19.4	
AON9	AGAGGACUGAGACAAGUUCC	20	51.8	50	−4.2	−10.0	23.1	
AON10	GCUCCUCUUGGGCACAGA	20	55.9	60	−5.1	−12.0	28.4	
AON11	CCUCAGCAUUGACAGCAA	18	48	50	−0.6	−3.2	16.1	
AON12	ACAGGAGCCCUCAGCAUUG	19	53.2	58	−0.4	−9.3	11.1	One mismatch in c.4539+2001G>A-pseudoexon
AON13	UGGAGGCAGCCACAGGAG	18	54.9	67	−1.3	−11.8	31.4	One mismatch in c.4539+2028C>T-pseudoexon
AON14	GAUGCUGGAGGGUUUUGAGUG	21	54.4	52	−1.7	−12.6	27.1	Perfect match in c.4539+2001G>A-pseudoexon
AON15	GAUGCUGGAGAGUUUUGAGUG	21	52.4	48	−1.7	−14.2	20.2	Specific for c.4539+2028C>T-pseudoexon
AON16	GCCUUGACGUCCUGAUGCU	19	53.2	58	1.4	−10.3	20.4	One mismatch in c.4539+2001G>A-pseudoexon
AON17	GCCAAGAGCUCAGGGUACAG	20	55.9	60	−0.9	−19.9	31.8	
AON18	CUUGGCCUCCCCUCCUC	18	57.2	72	1.4	−8.3	29.4	
AON19	AACACCAUGUAGGUAGGC	18	48	50	−1.6	−6.8	21.2	
AON20	GUUUAGGAAAUGAAACACCAUG	22	49.2	36	−0.7	−4.5	23.0	
AON21	GACCGCGUGGAAGUAAGG	18	52.6	61	−0.3	−14.9	22.1	
AON22	AUAAGUUUCUAAGCUGGACAG	21	48.5	38	−0.4	−8.1	27.2	
AON23	GGACCAAGGACCAACACUAC	20	53.8	55	−0.6	−9.7	27.9	
AON24	GGCUGUUACAUUUUGUCCAGG	21	52.4	48	−1.0	−7.5	28.5	
AON25	GGCAGGAACUGGCUUGCCUU	20	55.9	60	−8.6	−20.2	27.2	
AON26	AGAAGUGAAAGAAAAUGGCAGG	22	51.1	41	1.9	−3.0	23.3	
SON1	CAAUGCUGAGGACUCCUGU	19	51.1	53	−0.7	−11	6.0	Sense sequence of AON1 / Previously reported in Reference [18]
SON2	UCUCAGUCCUCUGUGCCCC	19	55.4	63	−0.9	−5.6	3.4	Sense sequence of AON4

The nucleotides underlined represent the possible mismatch in relation to the mutation present in the pseudoexon (c.4539+2001G>A or c.4539+2028C>T). L: Length in nt; Tm: Melting temperature in °C; GC: GC content in %; FE-A: Free energy AON molecule; FE-D: Free energy AON dimer; BE: Binding energy to the target region. All energy values are in arbitrary units obtained using RNAstructure software (https://rna.urmc.rochester.edu/RNAstructureWeb/Servers/bifold/bifold.html).

3. Results

Previously, we showed that the variants c.4539+2001G>A and c.4539+2028C>T cause the insertion of a 345-nt pseudoexon in a retina-specific manner. Four AONs (AON1 to AON4) targeting this region were designed according to previously described guidelines [35,36,39] and were assessed in PPCs. Our results showed that two AONs (AON1 and AON4) were able to restore correct *ABCA4* splicing by skipping the pseudoexon in a mutation-dependent manner. AON1 was specific for the c.4539+2001G>A variant and was not able to correct the splicing defect caused by the c.4539+2028C>T mutation, suggesting that one nucleotide mismatch can already impair rescue efficacy. Here, we screened the entire pseudoexon region in order to identify potential new targets that can promote splicing redirection with a higher efficacy by designing 22 new AONs.

3.1. Screening and Selection of AONs

The entire pseudoexon (345 nt) together with its flanking regions were subjected to AON design. A total of 22 new AONs were designed throughout the entire region (Figure 1A). The AON design parameters, such as melting temperature (Tm), GC content, and free energy were assessed in order to have optimal sequences when possible (e.g., Tm > 48 °C, GC content between 40% and 60%). Subsequently, to further assess what AONs were targeting, we predicted the RNA structure of the region using mfold software [40]. We also checked the ESE motifs that were present in the region using an ESE finder (http://rulai.cshl.edu/) or the potential RNA binding protein sites using RBPmap (http://rbpmap.technion.ac.il/). Overall, all AONs were covering the pseudoexon or its splice sites and were targeting all types of regions (predicted to be more closed or open) and motifs.

Patient-derived iPSCs heterozygously carrying the c.4539+2001G>A mutation in conjunction with another *ABCA4* mutation on the other allele were differentiated into PPCs. Differentiation of the cells was assessed by qPCR. The results showed a differentiation toward retinal lineage with a clear increase in *ABCA4* expression (Supplementary Materials, Figure S1). As we already described, the 345-nt pseudoexon was only visible upon inhibition of nonsense-mediated decay (NMD) (Figure 1B). Therefore, PPCs were first treated with the corresponding AON and after 24 h were subjected to cycloheximide (CHX) treatment to inhibit NMD. RNA analysis was performed by RT-PCR (Figure 1B). We then semiquantified the amount of aberrant transcript (Figure 1C). Remarkably, three AONs were able to almost completely rescue the splicing defect (AON4, AON17, and AON18). Interestingly, we also observed that four AONs (AON7, AON13, AON14, and AON16) caused the appearance of additional bands. Some of them represented partial pseudoexon skipping, while others turned out to be potential artifacts due to mis-splicing, although we could not exactly determine the splicing sites. Sequencing results determined that the partial-exon skipping observed in AON14 and AON16-treated samples was a partial skipping of exon 30 (previously described in Reference [18]) together with partial skipping of the first 142 nt of the pseudoexon (splice acceptor site in c.4539+2035). In the case of AON13, we identified partial pseudoexon exclusion, but we could not determine the splice acceptor site. In the case of AON7, we could not determine both splice sites (acceptor and donor), and it was probably an aberrant mRNA caused by the AON treatment. Using the average of the cells not treated with AONs but subjected to CHX treatment and the ones treated with the sense oligonucleotide (SON), we established the basal levels (~29%) of the *ABCA4* aberrant transcript (Figure 1C). These values were used to establish the percentage of correction for each AON (Figure 2A). Five groups were determined: Highly effective (correction >75%, n = 3), effective (75%–50%, n = 6), moderately effective (50%–25%, n = 8), poorly effective (25%–0%, n = 9), and noneffective (0% or even increasing the amount of pseudoexon). These groups are depicted in Figure 2A according to different colors in the graph.

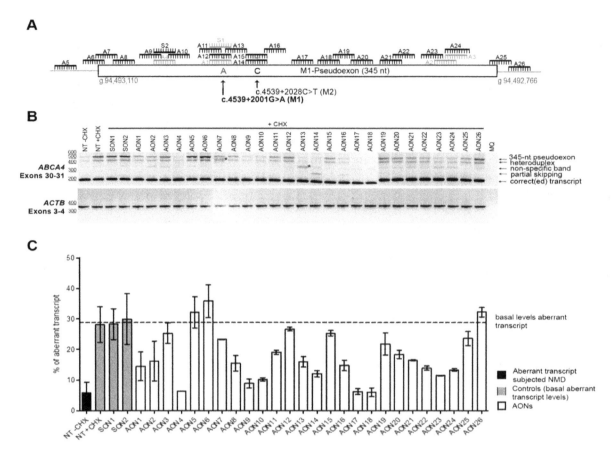

Figure 1. AON-based pseudoexon skipping efficacy. (**A**) Schematic representation of the 345-nt pseudoexon insertion caused by the c.4539+2001G>A mutation and the location of the 26 AONs and the 2 sense oligonucleotides (SONs). Blue oligonucleotides refer to previously studied molecules [18]. Red asterisks represent mismatches with the pseudoexon sequence created only by the c.4539+2001G>A mutation (namely an A at position c.4539+2001 and a C at position c.4539+2028). (**B**) Representative image of an RT-PCR performed on patient-derived photoreceptor precursor cells (PPCs) upon AON treatment. *ACTB* was used to normalize samples. An heteroduplex band was observed in all samples, containing the correct and the pseudoexon-included transcripts. AON-derived partial skipping was observed in samples AON14 and AON16. Double bands highlighted with an * (lanes AON7 and AON13) indicate artifacts derived from the AON treatment, and splice sites could not be identified upon Sanger sequencing. In most of the lanes, we identified a PCR artifact (nonspecific band). (**C**) Percentage of aberrant transcript after semiquantification. NT: Nontreated; CHX: Cycloheximide. Error bars indicate average ± SD.

3.2. Analysis of the Properties of the AONs

Once the efficacy of all AONs was estimated, we subdivided them into three larger groups: Effective (*n* = 9 comprising all AONs with an efficacy > 50%), moderately effective (*n* = 8 with efficacies between 25% and 50%), and poorly effective (*n* = 7, the rest). AONs containing a mismatch (AON12 and AON15) were not used in these analyses, as the decrease in the efficacy was due to the mismatch. This was shown by the fact that both AON1 and AON14 (perfectly matching the c.4539+2001G>A allele, but containing a mismatch for the PE induced by the c.4539+2028C>T mutation) correct the splice defect associated with c.4539+2001G>A.

We first analyzed the basic parameters: Melting temperature (Tm), GC content, and length (Figure 2B). We found a statistically significant correlation (two-tailed Spearman test) for the Tm and GC content parameters ($p = 0.0012$ and $p = 0.0041$, respectively). In both cases, the higher the value was, the more efficient the AON was (Supplementary Materials, Figure S2). The Tm average of the three groups ranged from 54.21 °C (effective) to 50.19 °C (poorly effective). The differences in Tm between groups was statistically different ($p = 0.0292$, nonparametric one-way ANOVA), while the GC content was nearly significant ($p = 0.0611$). When comparing all different groups separately, statistically significant differences were observed between the groups of effective AONs and poorly effective AONs for Tm ($p = 0.0256$, Mann–Whitney test) and GC content ($p = 0.0127$). No differences were observed for the length of the AONs.

Other important parameters when designing AONs are the free energy of the AON molecule itself, the dimer, and the binding energy to the target. The free energy of the AON molecule and its dimer did not show any correlation nor difference between groups. Interestingly, the binding energy showed a significant correlation ($p = 0.0391$) with efficacy. We analyzed the groups separately, and although no statistically significant differences were found, the effective group showed a trend toward significance when compared to the moderately effective ($p = 0.0673$, Mann–Whitney test) and the poorly effective ($p = 0.0712$, Mann–Whitney test) groups. Consistently, the highest binding energies corresponded to the three most effective AONs (AON4, AON17, and AON18). Interestingly, when these three values were separated, the tendency of the effective group disappeared. In contrast, these three AONs only showed a statistically significant higher binding energy compared to the other three groups (Figure 2C).

Next, we checked the common serine and arginine-rich splicing factors (SRSFs): SF2 (SRSF1), SC35 (SRSF2), SRp40 (SRSF4), and SRp55 (SRSF5)) using an ESE finder (Supplementary Materials, Figure S3). All motifs that were partially or completely covered by an AON were counted and assigned to the particular AON. We did not find any correlation between the percentage of correction and the presence of these motifs. However, we noticed that the strength of some of the motifs was different between groups. For that, we categorized all the motifs found by assigning them a number according to the strength of the predicted score (lowest = 1, second lowest = 2, etc.). After that, the average for each AON was calculated. Interestingly, a statistically significant correlation ($p = 0.0066$, two-tailed Spearman test) was observed for the categorized SRp40 motifs. In this case, the strongest motifs were correlating with the poorly or moderately effective AONs, and the lowest with the effective ones (Figure 2D). However, when pooling all groups together, differences were not statistically significant. No other differences were detected for any of the other three SRSF motifs, except for SC35, where significant differences were observed when comparing effective versus moderately effective AONs ($p = 0.0316$, Mann–Whitney test; Supplementary Materials, Figure S3).

Finally, we used RBPmap to predict potential RNA protein-binding motifs. Again, each motif detected in the region was assigned to each AON when partial or complete overlap occurred. First, manual filtering of the motifs was done by checking which motifs were common to all AONs in each group. Unfortunately, none of the motifs were shared between all effective AONs. AON18 was the one behaving differently than the rest, almost not sharing any motif with the others. When AON18 was left out of the filtering, SRSF3 appeared as a common motif not only in the effective group, but also in the poorly and moderately effective groups. When assessed in more detail (Figure 2D), a statistically significant negative correlation was observed ($p = 0.0188$, two-tailed Spearman test). The analysis per group revealed a significant difference between the effective and poorly effective groups ($p = 0.0431$) and close to significance between the moderately and poorly effective groups ($p = 0.0622$). Categorized SRSF3 did not show significant differences. The second most recurrent motif in the poorly effective group was MBNL1. Given the fact that all but one poorly acting AON contained this predicted motif, we performed statistical analyses to determine whether the presence of MBNL1 motifs correlated with the lower performance of some AONs. Indeed, a significant correlation was observed ($p = 0.0025$), implying an association between the presence of these motifs and a low AON performance (Figure 2D). When differences between groups were assessed, only the effective group showed a statistically significant lower number of MBNL1 when compared to the poorly effective group ($p = 0.0309$). The total amount of motifs detected by RBPmap showed a nearly significant negative correlation with efficiency ($p = 0.0522$). However, when groups were analyzed separately, this trend completely disappeared (Supplementary Materials, Figure S4).

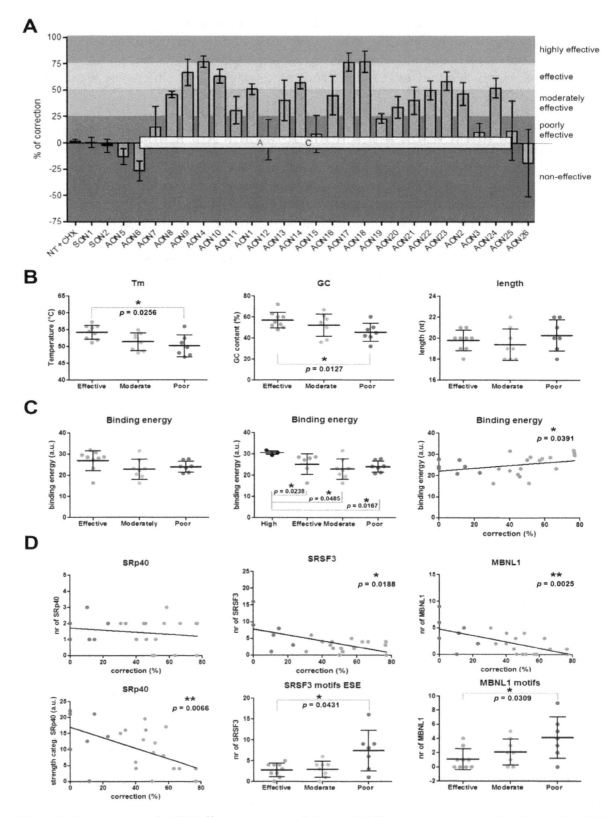

Figure 2. Assessment of AON efficacy and correlations. (**A**) Percentage of correction for each AON. AONs are located according to their position in the c.4539+2001G>A-specific pseudoexon. Colors indicate the efficacy classification that was established. (**B–C**) Representation of the statistical analyses for general parameters taken into account for AON design. (**D**) Analysis of the influence of certain motifs in AON efficacy. Error bars in all graphs indicate average ± SD.

4. Discussion

The fact that the eye is an isolated, immunoprivileged, and easily accessible organ makes it a very attractive model for molecular therapies. In addition, IRDs are progressive diseases that offer a window of opportunity for treatment. However, the high genetic heterogeneity in IRDs hampers the development of new therapies. AONs have been shown to be an auspicious approach to treat splicing defects causing IRDs. They have been shown to be safe and easy to deliver to the retina without the necessity of any vector. Furthermore, recent results from a phase 1/2 clinical trial to correct the splicing defect introduced by a deep-intronic mutation in *CEP290* showed the great potential that these molecules hold. In this study, we screened 26 AONs targeting a pseudoexon product of a recurrent deep-intronic mutation (c.4539+2001G>A) in the *ABCA4* gene with the intention of identifying the most promising AON molecules to eventually treat STGD1.

We designed and tested 26 different AONs located across the 345-nt pseudoexon. In total, three highly effective AONs were identified: AON4, AON17, and AON18. All of them showed similar efficacies (76.42%–76.97%). Another six AONs (AON1, AON9, AON10, AON14, AON23, and AON24) corrected the pre-mRNA splicing defect with an efficacy of more than 50%. Previously, we showed that AON1 was only effective when the change c.4539+2001G>A was present, as the pseudoexon containing the change c.4539+2028C>T was not removed. This highlighted the fact that for 2'OMe/PS chemically modified AONs, one mismatch could dramatically affect the splicing redirection efficacy. Here, we demonstrated again that one mismatch was enough to prevent AON-based splicing modulation. For that, we generated the same AON1 but with a wild-type nucleotide (AON12). Furthermore, we also designed an AON specific for the c.4539+2028C>T variant (AON15) and a corresponding AON with a wild-type change (AON14). As expected, the mutation-specific AON (AON15) did not redirect splicing in this cell line, while the one perfectly matching the target did (AON14). Interestingly, AON14, although its correction efficacy was around 50%, is not considered a very promising AON for future studies since it was one of the four AONs (together with AON7, AON13, and AON16) that showed novel aberrant bands in RT-PCR. In this particular case, both AON14 and AON16 caused an unexpected (AONs binding on top of the novel splice acceptor site at position c.4539+2035) partial pseudoexon exclusion together with an already described partial exon 30 skipping [18]. However, this was clearly induced by these two AONs, which bind in the same region. However, for AON7 and AON13, we were not able to determine how the aberrant band was generated due to the lack of predicted splicing sites, and therefore we considered them artifacts. We previously observed a similar effect for another variant, and we concluded that this was either a PCR artifact or, due to the fact that AONs can interfere with RNA structure and the splicing machinery, some aberrant mis-spliced transcripts that may have appeared [20].

After classifying the AONs into three groups, we tried to identify common properties that could eventually lead to a better AON design. When analyzing the groups, we found correlations with the Tm and the GC content. Previously published guidelines [35,36,39] have indicated that Tm should be above 48 °C and the GC content between 40% and 60%. Based on our analyses, it seems that if the temperature is higher than 51 °C and the GC content close to 60%, the chances of designing an AON with a good efficacy are higher. According to previous guidelines, the binding energy should stay between 21 and 28. However, our best AON molecules had binding energies to the target of more than 30. Moreover, based on correlations that we were able to identify, AONs targeting predicted SRSF3 or MBNL1, as well as strong predicted SRp40 motifs, might show poorer efficacies. Although some of these parameters have been shown before to be relevant to AON design, it is important to mention that the efficacy of an AON molecule also can depend on the type of cell, tissue, or organ. In that sense, the parameters established above might be valid only for AONs delivered to retinal cells, and further confirmation in cells of other origins needs to be addressed. Unfortunately, this comparison was not possible in our case due to the fact that although *ABCA4* is lowly expressed in fibroblast cells, the splicing defects observed for some mutations, including c.4539+2001G>A, are not recapitulated in those cells. Most probably this is because the splicing retinal machinery may have different efficacies or recognition sites [41,42].

In our previous studies, AON1 showed an efficacy of ~75% [18]. However, in this study, only ~51% correction was detected, although the PPCs were derived from the same patient iPSC line. One explanation could be that in our previous study, we only detected around 25% of pseudoexon insertion, while in this study we were able to detect more pseudoexon-including transcripts (~30%). This could therefore have modified the correction ratio. In addition, the inhibition of NMD by CHX is not always complete, and therefore variability in the detection of the pseudoexon transcript (subjected to NMD) might have been variable between experiments and samples. Another possible explanation could be differences between the AON batches. All of these factors, either alone or in combination, could have influenced the differences observed between the two studies.

Finally, as discussed above, AON4, AON17, and AON18 showed the highest efficacies. However, AON18 did not show that much similarity to the other two AONs other than a high binding energy. AON18 did not share obvious targeted predicted motifs with either of the two highly effective AONs (Supplementary Materials, Figure S5). We also checked the secondary structure of the RNA and all three AON target partially closed regions. Therefore, the slightly higher efficacy might have been related to the binding to the target itself and the disruption of the secondary structure rather than the motifs that were blocked by the molecule. In addition, when comparing the sequences to see which one could be a potential candidate for further development, we observed that all three AONs contained stretches of Gs and Cs (which are recommended to be avoided). AON4 and AON17 contained a G stretch of four and three Gs, respectively, while AON18 contained two stretches of three and four Cs. Nevertheless, given their efficacy, all three molecules might be potential good candidates for further therapeutic studies.

5. Conclusions

In conclusion, we designed 26 AONs targeting a 345-nt pseudoexon caused by the recurrent c.4539+2001G>A deep-intronic mutation in *ABCA4*. In total, nine AONs showed promising efficacies (correction above 50%). We identified three AONs promoting a correction superior to 75%. For AON design, we suggest increasing the minimum Tm to 50 or 51 °C, the GC content close to 60%, and the binding energy to around 30 to target retinal pseudoexons, although this needs to be tested and confirmed using other targets. Overall, we demonstrated that AON-based splicing modulation holds great potential for treating Stargardt disease caused by splicing defects in *ABCA4*.

6. Patents

A.G. and R.W.J.C. are inventors on a filed patent (PCT/EP2017/1082627) that is related to the contents of this manuscript.

Author Contributions: Conceptualization: A.G. and R.W.J.C.; methodology and experimental work: A.G. and L.D.; results analysis: A.G., L.D., and R.W.J.C.; writing and reviewing the manuscript: all authors; funding acquisition: A.G. and R.W.J.C.

Acknowledgments: The authors would like to thank the Stem Cell Technology Center of the Radboudumc for providing iPSCs.

References

1. Stargardt, K. Über familiäre, progressive Degeneration in der Maculagegend des Auges. *Albrecht von Graefes Archiv für Ophthalmologie* **1909**, *71*, 534–550. [CrossRef]

2. Birnbach, C.D.; Jarvelainen, M.; Possin, D.E.; Milam, A.H. Histopathology and immunocytochemistry of the neurosensory retina in fundus flavimaculatus. *Ophthalmology* **1994**, *101*, 1211–1219. [CrossRef]

3. Sahel, J.A.; Marazova, K.; Audo, I. Clinical characteristics and current therapies for inherited retinal degenerations. *Cold Spring Harb. Perspect. Med.* **2014**, *5*, a017111. [CrossRef] [PubMed]

4. Zernant, J.; Xie, Y.A.; Ayuso, C.; Riveiro-Alvarez, R.; Lopez-Martinez, M.A.; Simonelli, F.; Testa, F.; Gorin, M.B.; Strom, S.P.; Bertelsen, M.; et al. Analysis of the *ABCA4* genomic locus in Stargardt disease. *Hum. Mol. Genet.* **2014**, *23*, 6797–6806. [CrossRef] [PubMed]

5. Vasiliou, V.; Vasiliou, K.; Nebert, D.W. Human ATP-binding cassette (ABC) transporter family. *Hum. Genom.* **2009**, *3*, 281–290. [CrossRef]

6. Molday, R.S. Insights into the Molecular Properties of *ABCA4* and Its Role in the Visual Cycle and Stargardt Disease. *Prog. Mol. Biol. Transl. Sci.* **2015**, *134*, 415–431. [PubMed]

7. Molday, R.S.; Zhong, M.; Quazi, F. The role of the photoreceptor ABC transporter *ABCA4* in lipid transport and Stargardt macular degeneration. *Biochim. Biophys. Acta* **2009**, *1791*, 573–583. [CrossRef]

8. Quazi, F.; Lenevich, S.; Molday, R.S. *ABCA4* is an N-retinylidene-phosphatidylethanolamine and phosphatidylethanolamine importer. *Nat. Commun.* **2012**, *3*, 925. [CrossRef]

9. Cornelis, S.S.; Bax, N.M.; Zernant, J.; Allikmets, R.; Fritsche, L.G.; den Dunnen, J.T.; Ajmal, M.; Hoyng, C.B.; Cremers, F.P. In Silico Functional Meta-Analysis of 5,962 *ABCA4* Variants in 3,928 Retinal Dystrophy Cases. *Hum. Mutat.* **2017**, *38*, 400–408. [CrossRef]

10. Maugeri, A.; van Driel, M.A.; van de Pol, D.J.; Klevering, B.J.; van Haren, F.J.; Tijmes, N.; Bergen, A.A.; Rohrschneider, K.; Blankenagel, A.; Pinckers, A.J.; et al. The 2588G→C mutation in the ABCR gene is a mild frequent founder mutation in the Western European population and allows the classification of ABCR mutations in patients with Stargardt disease. *Am. J. Hum. Genet.* **1999**, *64*, 1024–1035. [CrossRef]

11. Sheffield, V.C.; Stone, E.M. Genomics and the eye. *N. Engl. J. Med.* **2011**, *364*, 1932–1942. [CrossRef] [PubMed]

12. Zernant, J.; Collison, F.T.; Lee, W.; Fishman, G.A.; Noupuu, K.; Yuan, B.; Cai, C.; Lupski, J.R.; Yannuzzi, L.A.; Tsang, S.H.; et al. Genetic and clinical analysis of *ABCA4*-associated disease in African American patients. *Hum. Mutat.* **2014**, *35*, 1187–1194. [CrossRef] [PubMed]

13. Braun, T.A.; Mullins, R.F.; Wagner, A.H.; Andorf, J.L.; Johnston, R.M.; Bakall, B.B.; Deluca, A.P.; Fishman, G.A.; Lam, B.L.; Weleber, R.G.; et al. Non-exomic and synonymous variants in *ABCA4* are an important cause of Stargardt disease. *Hum. Mol. Genet.* **2013**, *22*, 5136–5145. [CrossRef] [PubMed]

14. Bauwens, M.; De Zaeytijd, J.; Weisschuh, N.; Kohl, S.; Meire, F.; Dahan, K.; Depasse, F.; De Jaegere, S.; De Ravel, T.; De Rademaeker, M.; et al. An augmented *ABCA4* screen targeting noncoding regions reveals a deep intronic founder variant in Belgian Stargardt patients. *Hum. Mutat.* **2015**, *36*, 39–42. [CrossRef] [PubMed]

15. Bax, N.M.; Sangermano, R.; Roosing, S.; Thiadens, A.A.; Hoefsloot, L.H.; van den Born, L.I.; Phan, M.; Klevering, B.J.; Westeneng-van Haaften, C.; Braun, T.A.; et al. Heterozygous deep-intronic variants and deletions in *ABCA4* in persons with retinal dystrophies and one exonic *ABCA4* variant. *Hum. Mutat.* **2015**, *36*, 43–47. [CrossRef] [PubMed]

16. Sangermano, R.; Bax, N.M.; Bauwens, M.; van den Born, L.I.; De Baere, E.; Garanto, A.; Collin, R.W.; Goercharn-Ramlal, A.S.; den Engelsman-van Dijk, A.H.; Rohrschneider, K.; et al. Photoreceptor Progenitor mRNA Analysis Reveals Exon Skipping Resulting from the *ABCA4* c.5461-10T→C Mutation in Stargardt Disease. *Ophthalmology* **2016**, *123*, 1375–1385. [CrossRef] [PubMed]

17. Zernant, J.; Lee, W.; Nagasaki, T.; Collison, F.T.; Fishman, G.A.; Bertelsen, M.; Rosenberg, T.; Gouras, P.; Tsang, S.H.; Allikmets, R. Extremely hypomorphic and severe deep intronic variants in the *ABCA4* locus result in varying Stargardt disease phenotypes. *Mol. Case Stud.* **2018**, *4*, a002733. [CrossRef]

18. Albert, S.; Garanto, A.; Sangermano, R.; Khan, M.; Bax, N.M.; Hoyng, C.B.; Zernant, J.; Lee, W.; Allikmets, R.; Collin, R.W.J.; et al. Identification and Rescue of Splice Defects Caused by Two Neighboring Deep-Intronic *ABCA4* Mutations Underlying Stargardt Disease. *Am. J. Hum. Genet.* **2018**, *102*, 517–527. [CrossRef]

19. Sangermano, R.; Khan, M.; Cornelis, S.S.; Richelle, V.; Albert, S.; Garanto, A.; Elmelik, D.; Qamar, R.; Lugtenberg, D.; van den Born, L.I.; et al. *ABCA4* midigenes reveal the full splice spectrum of all reported noncanonical splice site variants in Stargardt disease. *Genome Res.* **2018**, *28*, 100–110. [CrossRef]

20. Sangermano, R.; Garanto, A.; Khan, M.; Runhart, E.H.; Bauwens, M.; Bax, N.M.; van den Born, L.I.; Khan, M.I.; Cornelis, S.S.; Verheij, J.B.G.M.; et al. Deep-intronic *ABCA4* variants explain missing heritability in Stargardt disease and allow correction of splice defects by antisense oligonucleotides. *Genet. Med.* **2019**. [CrossRef]

21. Shen, X.; Corey, D.R. Chemistry, mechanism and clinical status of antisense oligonucleotides and duplex RNAs. *Nucleic Acids Res.* **2018**, *46*, 1584–1600. [CrossRef] [PubMed]

22. Collin, R.W.; den Hollander, A.I.; van der Velde-Visser, S.D.; Bennicelli, J.; Bennett, J.; Cremers, F.P. Antisense Oligonucleotide (AON)-based Therapy for Leber Congenital Amaurosis Caused by a Frequent Mutation in CEP290. *Mol. Ther. Nucleic Acids* **2012**, *1*, e14. [CrossRef] [PubMed]

23. Gerard, X.; Perrault, I.; Hanein, S.; Silva, E.; Bigot, K.; Defoort-Delhemmes, S.; Rio, M.; Munnich, A.; Scherman, D.; Kaplan, J.; et al. AON-mediated Exon Skipping Restores Ciliation in Fibroblasts Harboring the Common Leber Congenital Amaurosis CEP290 Mutation. *Mol. Ther. Nucleic Acids* **2012**, *1*, e29. [CrossRef] [PubMed]

24. Garanto, A.; Chung, D.C.; Duijkers, L.; Corral-Serrano, J.C.; Messchaert, M.; Xiao, R.; Bennett, J.; Vandenberghe, L.H.; Collin, R.W. In vitro and in vivo rescue of aberrant splicing in CEP290-associated LCA by antisense oligonucleotide delivery. *Hum. Mol. Genet.* **2016**, *25*, 2552–2563. [PubMed]

25. Parfitt, D.A.; Lane, A.; Ramsden, C.M.; Carr, A.J.; Munro, P.M.; Jovanovic, K.; Schwarz, N.; Kanuga, N.; Muthiah, M.N.; Hull, S.; et al. Identification and Correction of Mechanisms Underlying Inherited Blindness in Human iPSC-Derived Optic Cups. *Cell Stem Cell* **2016**, *18*, 769–781. [CrossRef] [PubMed]

26. Duijkers, L.; van den Born, L.I.; Neidhardt, J.; Bax, N.M.; Pierrache, L.H.M.; Klevering, B.J.; Collin, R.W.J.; Garanto, A. Antisense Oligonucleotide-Based Splicing Correction in Individuals with Leber Congenital Amaurosis due to Compound Heterozygosity for the c.2991+1655A>G Mutation in CEP290. *Int. J. Mol. Sci.* **2018**, *19*, 753. [CrossRef] [PubMed]

27. Dulla, K.; Aguila, M.; Lane, A.; Jovanovic, K.; Parfitt, D.A.; Schulkens, I.; Chan, H.L.; Schmidt, I.; Beumer, W.; Vorthoren, L.; et al. Splice-Modulating Oligonucleotide QR-110 Restores CEP290 mRNA and Function in Human c.2991+1655A>G LCA10 Models. *Mol. Ther. Nucleic Acids* **2018**, *12*, 730–740. [CrossRef] [PubMed]

28. Slijkerman, R.W.; Vache, C.; Dona, M.; Garcia-Garcia, G.; Claustres, M.; Hetterschijt, L.; Peters, T.A.; Hartel, B.P.; Pennings, R.J.; Millan, J.M.; et al. Antisense Oligonucleotide-based Splice Correction for USH2A-associated Retinal Degeneration Caused by a Frequent Deep-intronic Mutation. *Mol. Ther. Nucleic Acids* **2016**, *5*, e381. [CrossRef]

29. Garanto, A.; van der Velde-Visser, S.D.; Cremers, F.P.M.; Collin, R.W.J. Antisense Oligonucleotide-Based Splice Correction of a Deep-Intronic Mutation in CHM Underlying Choroideremia. *Adv. Exp. Med. Biol.* **2018**, *1074*, 83–89.

30. Bonifert, T.; Gonzalez Menendez, I.; Battke, F.; Theurer, Y.; Synofzik, M.; Schols, L.; Wissinger, B. Antisense Oligonucleotide Mediated Splice Correction of a Deep Intronic Mutation in OPA1. *Mol. Ther. Nucleic Acids* **2016**, *5*, e390. [CrossRef]

31. Bauwens, M.; Garanto, A.; Sangermano, R.; Naessens, S.; Weisschuh, N.; De Zaeytijd, J.; Khan, M.; Sadler, F.; Balikova, I.; Van Cauwenbergh, C.; et al. *ABCA4*-associated disease as a model for missing heritability in autosomal recessive disorders: Novel noncoding splice, cis-regulatory, structural, and recurrent hypomorphic variants. *Genet. Med. Off. J. Am. Coll. Med. Genet.* **2019**. [CrossRef] [PubMed]

32. Cideciyan, A.V.; Jacobson, S.G.; Drack, A.V.; Ho, A.C.; Charng, J.; Garafalo, A.V.; Roman, A.J.; Sumaroka, A.; Han, I.C.; Hochstedler, M.D.; et al. Effect of an intravitreal antisense oligonucleotide on vision in Leber congenital amaurosis due to a photoreceptor cilium defect. *Nat. Med.* **2019**, *25*, 225–228. [CrossRef] [PubMed]

33. Homolova, K.; Zavadakova, P.; Doktor, T.K.; Schroeder, L.D.; Kozich, V.; Andresen, B.S. The deep intronic c.903+469T>C mutation in the MTRR gene creates an SF2/ASF binding exonic splicing enhancer, which leads to pseudoexon activation and causes the cblE type of homocystinuria. *Hum. Mutat.* **2010**, *31*, 437–444. [CrossRef] [PubMed]

34. Rincon, A.; Aguado, C.; Desviat, L.R.; Sanchez-Alcudia, R.; Ugarte, M.; Perez, B. Propionic and methylmalonic acidemia: Antisense therapeutics for intronic variations causing aberrantly spliced messenger RNA. *Am. J. Hum. Genet.* **2007**, *81*, 1262–1270. [CrossRef] [PubMed]
35. Aartsma-Rus, A. Overview on AON design. *Methods Mol. Biol.* **2012**, *867*, 117–129. [PubMed]
36. Collin, R.W.; Garanto, A. Applications of antisense oligonucleotides for the treatment of inherited retinal diseases. *Curr. Opin. Ophthalmol.* **2017**, *28*, 260–266. [CrossRef] [PubMed]
37. Flamier, A.; Barabino, A.; Gilbert, B. Differentiation of Human Embryonic Stem Cells into Cone Photoreceptors. *Bio-Protoc.* **2016**, *6*, e1870. [CrossRef]
38. Schindelin, J.; Arganda-Carreras, I.; Frise, E.; Kaynig, V.; Longair, M.; Pietzsch, T.; Preibisch, S.; Rueden, C.; Saalfeld, S.; Schmid, B.; et al. Fiji: An open-source platform for biological-image analysis. *Nat. Methods* **2012**, *9*, 676–682. [CrossRef] [PubMed]
39. Slijkerman, R.; Kremer, H.; van Wijk, E. Antisense Oligonucleotide Design and Evaluation of Splice-Modulating Properties Using Cell-Based Assays. *Methods Mol. Biol.* **2018**, *1828*, 519–530.
40. Zuker, M. Mfold web server for nucleic acid folding and hybridization prediction. *Nucleic Acid Res.* **2013**, *31*, 3406–3415. [CrossRef]
41. Garanto, A.; Riera, M.; Pomares, E.; Permanyer, J.; de Castro-Miro, M.; Sava, F.; Abril, J.F.; Marfany, G.; Gonzalez-Duarte, R. High transcriptional complexity of the retinitis pigmentosa CERKL gene in human and mouse. *Investig. Ophthalmol. Vis. Sci.* **2011**, *52*, 5202–5214. [CrossRef] [PubMed]
42. Murphy, D.; Cieply, B.; Carstens, R.; Ramamurthy, V.; Stoilov, P. The Musashi 1 Controls the Splicing of Photoreceptor-Specific Exons in the Vertebrate Retina. *PLoS Genet.* **2016**, *12*, e1006256. [CrossRef] [PubMed]

10

Molecular Strategies for *RPGR* Gene Therapy

Jasmina Cehajic Kapetanovic [1,2,*], **Michelle E McClements** [1],
Cristina Martinez-Fernandez de la Camara [1,2] **and Robert E MacLaren** [1,2]

[1]   Nuffield Laboratory of Ophthalmology, University of Oxford, Oxford OX3 9DU, UK
[2]   Oxford Eye Hospital, Oxford University Hospitals NHS Foundation Trust, Oxford OX3 9DU, UK
*   Correspondence: FRCOphthenquiries@eye.ox.ac.uk

Abstract: Mutations affecting the *Retinitis Pigmentosa GTPase Regulator* (*RPGR*) gene are the commonest cause of X-linked and recessive retinitis pigmentosa (RP), accounting for 10%–20% of all cases of RP. The phenotype is one of the most severe amongst all causes of RP, characteristic for its early onset and rapid progression to blindness in young people. At present there is no cure for *RPGR*-related retinal disease. Recently, however, there have been important advances in *RPGR* research from bench to bedside that increased our understanding of *RPGR* function and led to the development of potential therapies, including the progress of adeno-associated viral (AAV)-mediated gene replacement therapy into clinical trials. This manuscript discusses the advances in molecular research, which have connected the RPGR protein with an important post-translational modification, known as glutamylation, that is essential for its optimal function as a key regulator of photoreceptor ciliary transport. In addition, we review key pre-clinical research that addressed challenges encountered during development of therapeutic vectors caused by high infidelity of the *RPGR* genomic sequence. Finally, we discuss the structure of three current phase I/II clinical trials based on three AAV vectors and *RPGR* sequences and link the rationale behind the use of the different vectors back to the bench research that led to their development.

Keywords: *Retinitis Pigmentosa GTPase Regulator*; gene therapy; adeno-associated viral; Retinitis Pigmentosa (RP)

1. Introduction

Inherited retinal diseases, most of which are retinitis pigmentosa (RP), affect 1 in 4000 people worldwide. The hallmark of this heterogeneous group of disorders is premature degeneration of rod and cone photoreceptors that leads to early vision loss. RP can be inherited as an autosomal recessive, dominant, X-linked, oligogenic, or mitochondrial trait. X-linked RP is one of the most severe forms of retinal degeneration and it accounts for 10%–20% of all RP cases [1–3]. To date, only 3 genes have been identified to be associated with X-linked pattern of inheritance. Mutations in the *Retinitis pigmentosa GTPase regulator* (*RPGR*) gene accounts for over 70% of X-linked RP cases whereas less common forms of the disease are caused by retinitis pigmentosa 2 (*RP2*) and 23 (*RP23* or *OFD1*) genes [4,5].

RPGR-related X-linked RP is characterised by severe disease in males with early onset and rapidly progressing sight loss that leads to legal blindness commonly by the fourth decade of life [2]. The classic rod-cone phenotype with peripheral pigmentary retinopathy, waxy optic disc pallor and vascular attenuation makes it often indistinguishable from other forms of RP. Less commonly, a cone-rod phenotype manifests with early central cone degeneration and accompanying loss of visual acuity. Female carriers of the *RPGR* disease are typically asymptomatic with a characteristic phenotype that manifests as a radial streak pattern originating from the fovea [6,7]. Rarely, however, skewed X-inactivation leads to more severe male-like phenotype with associated visual impairment [8].

At present, there is no approved treatment for retinitis pigmentosa caused by mutations in *RPGR*. Several treatment options have been under investigation and with the emergence of novel gene-based therapies for inherited retinal disease, this seems the most logical strategy to develop for the *RPGR* disease. Due to its severe phenotype, relatively high incidence and the fact that more commonly mutated genes such as *ABCA4* or *USH2A* are too large to be packaged into AAV vectors, the *RPGR* disease has drawn significant interest amongst scientific and clinical research communities over the last years. However, due to the inherent instability in the retina-specific RPGR^{ORF15} isoform sequence [9–12] the production of the therapeutic AAV-mediated *RPGR* vector has been very challenging. In attempts to improve the sequence stability and fidelity several approaches have been explored including codon optimisation [13–15], which has allowed generation of vectors for use in human trials. In this review we discuss recent advances in the understanding of *RPGR* gene structure and its evolutionary conservation that has led to an improved understanding of protein's molecular function and mechanisms implicated in the pathogenesis of RPRG-related retinal dystrophy. The pre-clinical development of gene therapy vectors that has resulted in their progression into three phase I/II clinical trials is covered in detail, including discussion on three different *RPGR* cDNA sequences used in the trials.

2. Structure and Function of *Retinitis Pigmentosa GTPase Regulator (RPGR)*

The human *RPGR* gene is located on the short arm of the X-chromosome (Xp21.1). The gene exhibits a complex expression pattern with 10 alternatively spliced isoforms, five of which are protein coding [16]. The first transcript to be identified in association with X-linked retinitis pigmentosa, was the constitutive RPGR^{Ex1-19} isoform. In humans, the RPGR^{Ex1-19} isoform contains 19 exons and expresses a full-length messenger RNA transcript of 2448 bp, which generates an 815 amino acid sequence that forms ~90 kDa protein in a variety of tissues [17]. Since this initial characterisation, multiple alternative transcripts have been identified, including the retina-specific RPGR^{ORF15} variant [10,16,18]. This variant contains exons 1–14 of constitutive RPGR with the exon ORF15 derived from alternatively spliced exon 15 and intron 15 (Figure 1A). The RPGR^{ORF15} isoform is 3459 bp, encoding a 1152 amino acid sequence which forms a ~200 kDa protein. As with the widely expressed variant, amino acids 54–367 (exons 3–10) form a regulator of chromosome condensation 1 (RCC1)-like domain. The alternative ORF15 exon consists of a highly repetitive purine-rich sequence coding for multiple acidic glutamate-glycine repeats. This is followed by a C-terminal tail region rich in basic amino acid residues, called the basic domain.

The reason for this complex expression pattern of the RPGR protein remains largely unknown, but may be related to the functional role of its splice isoforms in various cell types. The RPGR protein is widely expressed in vertebrate tissue including eye, brain, lung, testis and kidney. In the eye, the two major isoforms, RPGR^{Ex1-19} and RPGR^{ORF15} are predominantly localised to the photoreceptor connecting cilia [19] and less consistently, to the nuclei and photoreceptor outer segments of some species [20]. The connecting cilium is a critical junction between the inner and outer photoreceptor segments, controlling the bidirectional transport of opsin and other proteins involved in the phototransduction cascade and the overall health and viability of the photoreceptors. Attempts are ongoing to elucidate further the expression patterns of RPGR through evolutionary characterisation of RPGR domains across species and via molecular interactions of RPGR with other proteins in order to shed light on the exact role of the RPGR protein.

The RCC1-like domain, present in both major splice forms, adopts a seven-bladed β-propeller structure and it is strongly conserved across evolution, in vertebrates and invertebrates [9]. This domain has been implicated in a regulatory role of small GTPases. It is thought to enable RPGR to act as a Ran guanine nucleotide exchange factor and RPGR has been shown to upregulate the guanine nucleotide exchange factor RAB8A, associating with the GDP-bound form of RAB8A to stimulate GDP/GTP nucleotide exchange [21]. The RCC1-like region also interacts with: RPGR interaction protein 1 (RPGRIP1), which links it to the connecting cilium of photoreceptor cells [19]; the lipid trafficking protein phosphodiesterase 6D (PDE6D) [22]; two chromosome-associated proteins important for the structural maintenance of chromosomes, SMC1 and SMC3 [23] and two ciliary disease-associated proteins nephrocystin-5 (NPHP5) [24] and centrosomal protein 290 (CEP290) [25].

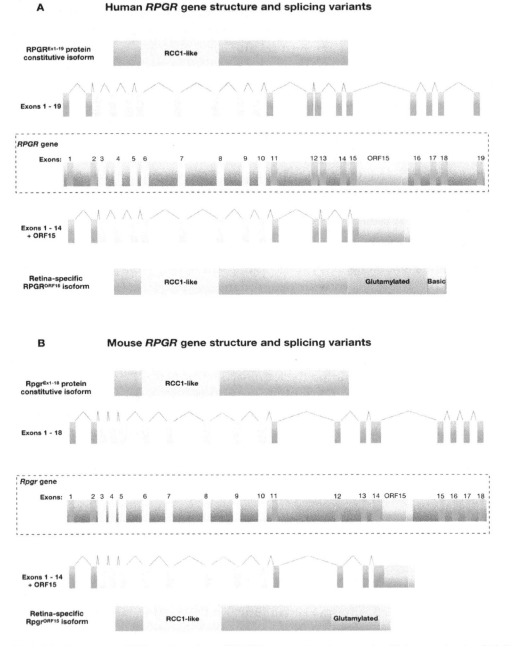

Figure 1. *Retinitis Pigmentosa GTPase Regulator (RPGR) gene structure and splicing variants.* (**A**) Human *RPGR* gene exon-intron structure showing the combination of exons 1 to 19 to create the constitutive protein isoform, and alternative splicing of exon 15/intron 15 that creates the RPGR^{ORF15} variant. (**B**) Mouse RPGR gene exon-intron structure showing the combination of exons 1 to 18 to create the constitutive protein isoform and alternative splicing of intron 14 creates the RPGR^{OFR15} variant.

The retina-specific ORF15 domain is also highly evolutionarily conserved across varied species, indicating a functional importance (Table 1). However, in contrast to the RCC1-like domain, the ORF15 domain is unique to vertebrates, suggesting a role that is unique to the ciliary-derived photoreceptors of "simple" vertebrate eyes, compared to the rhabdomeric photoreceptors of "compound" invertebrate eyes. Hence, the ciliary-based transport of cargoes such as rhodopsin, which is at least 10 times more abundant in vertebrates than invertebrates, fits with this hypothesis. ORF15 homology and a region of high AG content of >80% is identifiable in a range of species although the length varies—the mouse

ORF15 is shorter than the human ORF15, Figure 1A). This purine-rich region of ORF15 (97.5% purines within 1kb in humans) encodes the glutamine-glycine rich domain that ends in a basic C-terminal domain, which is also highly conserved, suggesting that it constitutes another functional region. This basic domain, which is unique to RPGR^{ORF15}, interacts with at least two proteins, a chaperone protein nucleophosmin and a scaffold protein whirlin [26]. Neither protein is unique to vertebrate photoreceptors, but nucleophosmin is present in metaphase centrosomes during cell division, while whirlin helps to maintain ciliary structures within the eye and ear.

Table 1. Evolutionary conservation of DNA and amino acid sequences of RPGR^{ORF15} variants across selected species. All data were extracted from NCBI database files with comparisons performed in Geneious Prime 2017.10.2. For *Homo sapiens*, details were extracted from gene files NG_009553.1 and 6103 combined with mRNA file NM_001034853.2. * The conserved basic domain of the human *RPGR^{ORF15}* coding sequence was used for predictions of ORF15 locations in all other species sequences by homology alignment. For *Mus musculus* data, gene files NC_000086.7 and 19893 were aligned with the basic domain of human *RPGR^{ORF15}* and the partial sequence file AF286473.1 to identify the predicted ORF15 variant. For *Canis lupus familiaris* data, gene files 403726 and AF148801.1 were aligned with the basic domain of human *RPGR^{ORF15}* and the partial sequence file AF385629.1. For *Pan troglodytes* data, files 4465569 and XM_024352988 were used. For *Gorilla gorilla gorilla*, files 101149059, the basic domain of human *RPGR^{ORF15}* and the partial sequence AY855163.1 were combined. For *Macaca mulatta*, files 714316, the basic domain of human *RPGR^{ORF15}* and the partial sequence file AY855162.1 were combined. Finally, *Xenopus tropicalis* sequence predictions were achieved from files 733454 and XM_018091818.1.

Species	DNA Sequence				Amino Acid Sequence	
	Coding Sequence Prior to ORF15	Percentage of Purine Bases	Region with Homology to Human ORF15 *	Percentage of Purine Bases	ORF15 Amino Acid Length (Percentage Glu-Gly) *	Glutamylation Region (Percentage Glu-Gly) *
Homo sapiens	1 to 14 1.7 kb	54%	ORF15 1.7 kb	89%	567 (67%)	351 (88%)
Mus musculus	1 to 14 2.5 kb	57%	Intron 14 1.5 kb	86%	488 (60%)	273 (84%)
Canis lupus familiaris	1 to 13 2.5 kb	58%	Exon 14/ Intron 14 1.5 kb	88%	522 (66%)	331 (72%)
Pan troglodytes	1 to 14 1.7 kb	54%	Exon 15/ Intron 15 1.7 kb	89%	560 (66%)	330 (88%)
Gorilla gorilla gorilla	1 to 14 1.7 kb	54%	Exon 15/ Intron 15 1.7 kb	89%	549 (66%)	321 (88%)
Macaca mulatta	1 to 14 1.7 kb	53%	Exon 15/ Intron 15 1.7 kb	89%	549 (65%)	323 (86%)
Xenopus tropicalis	1 to 13 1.6 kb	57%	Exon 14/ Intron 14/ Exon 15 2.0 kb	77%	679 (45%)	232 (82%)

The function of the repetitive glutamine-glycine-rich domain itself has been difficult to establish due to its variable length and relatively poor conservation at the individual amino acid level, although the overall charge and repeat structure length remain conserved in vertebrates. However, recent evidence shows that this intrinsically disordered region is heavily glutamylated [27], a post-translational protein modification that adds glutamates to target proteins to affect their stabilisation and folding. This process is known to be essential for the function of tubulins in intracellular trafficking [28]. Furthermore, this glutamylation has been shown to be achieved by tubulin tyrosine ligase like-5

(TTLL5) enzyme, which interacts directly with the basic domain of the OFR15 to bring it into the proximity of glutamylation sites along the glutamine-glycine-rich repetitive region [29]. The role of the ORF15 region is of course critically important to photoreceptor function, because otherwise ORF15 mutations would not be pathogenic since the RPGR^{EX1-19} variant is still expressed in these cells. Hence in-frame deletions in the ORF15 region lead to progressive loss of function as the deletion length increases [13].

3. Molecular Mechanisms and Pathogenesis of RPGR-Related X-Linked Retinitis Pigmentosa (RP)

Molecular mechanisms and pathogenesis of RPGR-related X-linked RP have been under investigation for several decades. The drive to better understand the disease process comes from the high incidence with mutations in the gene encoding RPGR accounting at least 70% of X-linked RP and up to 20% of all RP cases [2–4]. Moreover, the disease is associated with one of the most severe phenotypes among inherited retinal diseases with central visual loss occurring early in adult life [2]. This coupled with the developments in genetic therapies has given impetus to a large number of studies aimed to uncover the pathogenic mechanisms.

Despite ubiquitous expression of the constitutive RPGR variant in ciliated cells throughout the body, the RPGR^{Ex1-19} has yet to show a firm association with any human disease. The RPGR-related phenotype seems to be confined to the retina and several studies have established an essential role for RPGR^{ORF15} in photoreceptor function and survival [10,11]. Genetic studies have shown that mutations in the RPGR^{ORF15} result in abnormal protein transport across the connecting cilium, which can lead to photoreceptor cell death [12,30,31]. However, there are reports in the literature that describe RPGR-related X-linked retinitis pigmentosa syndrome comprising of retinitis pigmentosa, recurrent respiratory tract infections and hearing loss [32,33]. These findings point to the abnormalities in respiratory and auditory cilia in addition to the photoreceptors. In addition, as photoreceptors develop from ciliated progenitors, it has been postulated that the axoneme may play a role in their early development. Sperm axonemes were thus studies in patients with X-linked retinitis pigmentosa and a significant increase in abnormal sperm tails was observed [34]. Similar findings have been reported in another syndromic ciliopathy, the Usher syndrome [35].

Mutations in *RPGR* account for ~70% of cases of X-linked RP and have been identified across exons 1–15, yet up to 60% of mutations occur in the ORF15 region [10,30]. The repetitive nature of the glutamate-glycine region in ORF15 is prone to adopt unusual double helix DNA conformations or triplexes that are thought to promote polymerase arrest and block replication and transcription. These imperfections are likely to contribute to genome instability and account for the high frequency of mutations in this region, known as the mutation 'hot spot' of the *RPGR*. Surprisingly, no disease-causing mutations have been reported in exons 16–19 [36].

The most common mutations are small deletions that lead to frameshifts followed by nonsense mutations [30]. Within ORF15, the most common mutations are microdeletions 1–2, or 4–5 bp [10], that cause frameshifts leading to truncated forms of the protein and in particular, loss of the C-terminus. Small in-frame deletions or insertions (and missense changes) that can alter the length of ORF15 region by a few base-pairs (e.g., up to 36, equivalent to 9 amino acids in this population based study [37], are seemingly well tolerated [38]. Thus, despite being a coding region, this domain has a surprisingly high rate of tolerable indels within primate lineages, suggesting a rapidly evolving region [9]. However, recent evidence shows that larger deletions in the ORF15 region significantly affect the degree of RPGR glutamylation, which may subsequently influence its function and ability to associate with the cilium and other interacting factors [29]. Thus, frame shift mutations that lead to loss of the C-terminal basic domain are invariably disease causing [12]. In addition, mutations that lead to the loss of TTLL5 enzyme, the basic domain-binding partner that mediates RPGR glutamylation, abort glutamylation process and cause RPGR-like phenotype in humans [39]. This further supports the critical role of glutamylation in normal RPGR^{ORF15} function. It remains intriguing that despite its ubiquitous expression, the RPGR^{Ex1-19} is unable to compensate for the loss of function of RPGR^{ORF15} in the retina to rescue the phenotype. It is possible that the alternative splicing in the retina could favour the RPGR^{ORF15} variant, so the majority of transcripts will be the RPGR^{ORF15} isoform, with few constitutive variants available to compensate. One study failed to identify the constitutive transcript in the retina [18], which supports the finding that the constitutive isoform is expressed early in development in a mouse before its levels decline and the RPGR^{ORF15} becomes the predominant isoform [26]. Notably, the constitutive variant lacks the glutamate-glycine repetitive region and given the importance of this domain for the normal function of RPGR^{ORF15} in the photoreceptors, perhaps it is not so surprising that the constitutive variant cannot offer the same functional benefit as the RPGR^{ORF15} variant.

4. Clinical and Genetic Diagnosis of RPGR-Related X-Linked RP

The diagnosis of RPGR-related retinal dystrophy is made on the basis of presenting symptoms and retinal signs seen on clinical examination and various imaging modalities. In addition, study of family history showing X-linked inheritance (no male to male transmission) and genetic testing identifying the pathogenic mutation are important in confirming the diagnosis. In cases of uncertain diagnosis and unequivocal genetic test results we have adopted several important steps, which are discussed below, in order to minimise the risk of establishing an incorrect diagnosis, and administering the patient with an incorrect gene if recruited into a gene therapy clinical trial.

RPGR-related retinal dystrophy is associated with a very heterogeneous phenotype that ranges from pan-retinal rod-cone to predominant cone dystrophy (Figure 2). The phenotype is generally more severe with faster progression compared to other forms of RP and median age of legal blindness of approximately 45 years old, which is much younger than in other RP genotypes [40]. Most patients lose their peripheral vision first, followed by the loss of central vision. Recent evidence suggests that the rod-cone phenotype is found in 70% of patients, the cone-rod in 23% and the cone phenotype in 7% of patients with X-linked RPGR related retinal dystrophy [2]. The study shows that the onset of symptoms was in early childhood in rod-cone dystrophy (median age 5 years) and in third decade in cone-rod and cone dystrophy, although the age range was very wide (between 0 and 60 years). However, cone-rod and cone dystrophies were associated with a more severe phenotype and the probability of being blind at the age of 40, with visual acuity of less than 0.05 LogMAR (3/60 or 20/400) observed in 55% of patients with cone-rod and cone dystrophy compared to only 20% in rod-cone dystrophy.

The RPGR phenotype (Figure 2) has been associated with anatomical changes including central retinal thinning of the outer nuclear layer as seen on retinal cross-sections taken by optical coherence tomography [40,41]. The junction between the inner and outer photoreceptor segments, better known as the ellipsoid zone, can be used as an important predictor of central retinal function and for monitoring of disease progression. [42]. Thus, the disruption of the ellipsoid zone can be detected with corresponding early reduction in visual acuity and retinal sensitivity as measured by microperimetry. In addition, autofluorescence can be used to assess the health of the retinal pigment epithelium with early signs of hyper-autofluorescence indicating accumulation of lipofuscin and related metabolites as a by-product of photoreceptor outer segment degradation. Later in the disease process, areas of hypo-autofluorescence become evident indicating outer retinal atrophy with loss of retinal pigment epithelium cells. The RPGR phenotype is often associated with para-foveal hyper-autofluorescent rings, which decline exponentially with disease progression [43]. Constriction areas are correlated highly with baseline area and age, where younger subjects had greatest rate of progression. No correlation with genotype was observed in this study. In the cone-rod phenotype, however, the area of hypo-autofluorescence associated with a surrounding hyper-autofluorescent ring tends to increase in size with disease progression and is inversely related to electroretinogram amplitude [44]. Ongoing natural history studies are promising to shed more light on the natural progression of the RPGR disease phenotypes and provide better understanding and interpretation of clinical trial endpoints used in current interventional gene therapy trials (Table 2).

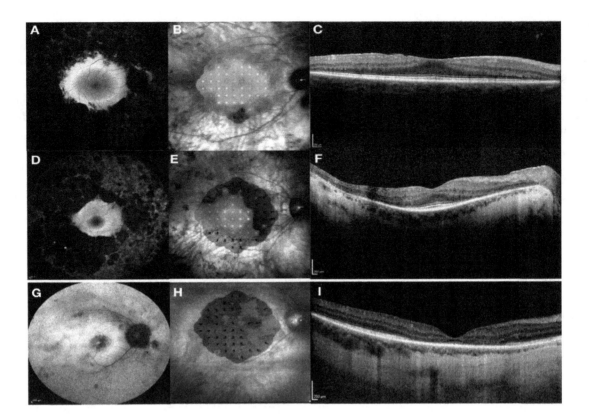

Figure 2. Clinical phenotypes associated with *RPGR* retinal degeneration—rod-cone phenotype (early stage (**A–C**) and a more advanced stage (**D–F**)) and cone-rod phenotype (**G–I**). The phenotypes are captured by Heidelberg fundus autofluorescence, (left column), MAIA microperimetry measuring central retinal sensitivity (central column; sensitivity is represented by a heat map: green/yellow—normal/mildly reduced; red/purple—reduced; black—not measurable) and Heidelberg optical coherence tomography showing retinal structures in cross-section (right column). In rod-cone phenotype there is extensive peripheral retinal atrophy with relative preservation of central retina as seen on autofluorescence associated with para-foveal hyper-autofluorescent ring (**A**). This is confirmed by near normal central retinal sensitivity (**B**) and preservation of ellipsoid zone (**C**). In more advanced stages of the disease there is reduction in size of the para-foveal hyper-autofluorescent ring (**D**) with corresponding reduction in retinal sensitivity (**E**) and length of ellipsoid zone (**F**). In contrast, in cone-rod phenotype there is early loss of para-foveal photoreceptors with associated hypo-fluorescent ring and marked reduction of retinal sensitivity with corresponding loss of the ellipsoid zone.

Female carriers of *RPGR* mutations also show high phenotypic variability [7] (Figure 3). The carrier phenotype includes asymptomatic females with near-normal clinical appearance, macular pattern reflex with different degrees of pigmentary retinopathy and severely affected females with clinical phenotype that results from skewed X chromosome inactivation and is indistinguishable from the male pattern. Female carriers with male pattern dystrophy should be considered for *RPGR* gene therapy as discussed below.

The molecular diagnosis using next-generation sequencing (NGS) is usually a robust approach in determining pathogenic variants in RP. However, the ORF15 region of RPGR is not normally sequenced with NGS methods and is currently only performed upon specific request. Moreover, sequencing of the ORF15 region in *RPGR* is notoriously difficult and error-prone. Overlapping reading frames and polymorphic deletions/insertions add further complexity to the detection of true mutations. Additional precautions must, therefore, be taken with interpreting the sequencing data so that small deletions are not confused with artefacts that would lead to spurious results. In cases of uncertainty, testing should be repeated. In addition, the full RP panel should be performed to exclude other pathogenic variants including the sequencing of *RP2* and *OFD1* X-linked genes. This comprehensive molecular genetic analysis together with the *RPGR* phenotype and a clear family history of X-linked inheritance, including evidence of a carrier phenotype, forms the basis of inclusion criteria into gene therapy clinical trials. In addition, a recent study describes an in vitro assay for determining the pathogenicity of *RPGR* missense variations [45]. The strategy is based on the RPGR protein interaction network, which is disrupted by missense variations in RCC1-like domain in RPGR, and could help to differentiate between causative missense mutations and non-disease-causing polymorphisms.

Table 2. Summary of clinical trials for RPGR-related X-linked retinitis pigmentosa (RP).

Clinical Trial (clinicaltrials.gov)	Intervention/ Observation	Clinical Centre/s	Sponsor
Phase I/II/III NCT03116113 multicenter, open-label Part 1: non-randomised, dose-selection study 18 participants Part 2: dose expansion study (randomised to low dose, high dose, control) 63 participants Start date: March 2017	Subretinal delivery of AAV8-hRK-coRPGR^{ORF15}	Oxford, UK Manchester, UK Southampton, UK Florida, USA Oregon, USA Pennsylvania, USA	Nightstar Therapeutics (now Biogen Inc), UK
Phase I/II NCT03252847 Non-randomised, open-label, dose-escalation trial 36 participants Start date: July 2017	Subretinal delivery of AAV2/5-hRK-RPGR^{ORF15}	London, UK	MeiraGTx, UK
Phase I/II NCT03316560 Non-randomised, open-label, multicenter, dose-escalation trial 30 participants with RPGR ORF15 mutations Start date: April 2018	Subretinal delivery of rAAV2tYF-GRK1-coRPGR^{ORF15}	Colorado, USA Massachusetts, USA New York, USA North Carolina, USA Ohio, USA Oregon, USA Pennsylvania, USA Texas, USA	Applied Genetic Technologies Corporation (AGTC), USA
Prospective natural history study of XLRP with genetically confirmed mutation in RPGR 150 participants Start date: December 2017	Observational study	Multiple centres in UK, Germany, Holland, France, USA	Nightstar Therapeutics (now Biogen Inc), UK
Prospective natural history study of XLRP NCT03349242 Start date: December 2017	Observational study	Massachusetts, USA Michigan, USA	MeiraGTx, UK
Prospective natural history study of XLRP caused by RPGR-ORF15 mutations 45 participants NCT03314207 Start date: December 2017	Observational study	New York, USA North Carolina, USA Ohio, USA Oregon, USA Texas, USA	Applied Genetic Technologies Corporation (AGTC), USA

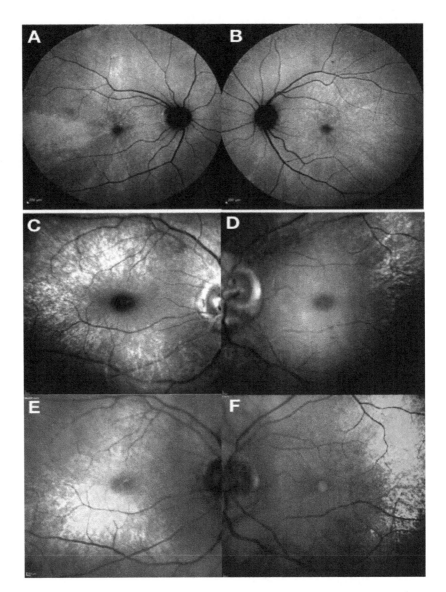

Figure 3. Clinical phenotype of *RPGR* female carriers. Fundus autofluorescence (Heidelberg) showing a typical macular radial pattern or 'tapetal' reflex in a female carrier of an *RPGR* mutation (**A,B**). Random X-chromosome inactivation generates clones of normal or affected photoreceptors giving rise to this mosaic pattern. Blue reflectance (**C,D**) and multicoloured (**E,F**) modes using Heidelberg scanning laser ophthalmoscope can be very helpful in showing the macular reflex.

5. Treatment Options for RPGR-Related X-Linked RP

Several non-gene based treatment approaches have been investigated for the preservation of vision in X-linked RP including a nutritional supplement, docosahexaenoic acid [46] and a ciliary neurotrophic factor [47] both of which were unable to prevent photoreceptor degeneration and visual loss. For patients with advanced disease, electronic retinal devices have demonstrated proof-of-concept in their ability to restore crude vision [48,49]. However, the unpredictability of benefit for individual patients and the high price of these devices make it economically difficult to maintain their availability for the treatment of patients with RP. Another potential strategy, optogenetics, is under investigation and has shown promising results for vision restoration in advanced retinal degeneration [50,51].

Emerging gene-based therapy using the AAV vector is currently the most promising therapeutic strategy for RPGR X-linked RP. The size of the coding sequence of RPGR^{ORF15} (3.5 kb) is within the AAV carrying capacity and the relatively high prevalence and disease severity have justified development of this therapy. However, the repetitive sequence of ORF15 not only makes it a hotspot for mutations but also creates challenges for therapeutic vector production. Attempts to generate AAV vectors for RPGR gene-supplementation strategies have been thwarted by the poor sequence stability of the ORF15 region and transgene production has struggled to control spontaneous mutations and maintain the complete sequence [13,52–55]. AAV gene therapy in two RPGR X-linked RP canine models that carry different ORF15 mutations [55] provided proof of concept for treating RPGR mutations within the ORF15 region. AAV2/5-mediated sub retinal gene delivery of a full-length human RPGR-ORF15 cDNA [10], driven by either the human interphotoreceptor retinoid-binding protein (hIRBP) promoter or the human G-protein-coupled receptor kinase 1 (hGRK1) promoter, prevented photoreceptor degeneration and preserved retinal function in both canine models. However, the AAV2/5.RPGR vector was found to have multiple mutations within the purine-rich exon 15 region that led to toxic effects in mice at higher doses [52] thus posing safety questions for human applications. In an attempt to improve the sequence stability, a step-wise cloning approach was used to generate the correct full-length RPGR^{ORF15} coding sequence (the purine-rich region was generated first and then ligated to the rest of the DNA sequence) [53], which was packaged into the AAV8.GRK1.RPGR^{ORF15} vector and evaluated in the *Rpgr*-KO mouse. However, despite improved stability, some vector preparations were still ridden with micro-deletions that led to expression of alternatively spliced truncated forms of the RPGR protein that was mislocalised to photoreceptor inner segments and only a partial rescue of the phenotype in treated mice. The truncated forms of the protein were further investigated for their ability to rescue the RPGR phenotype in the *Rpgr*-KO mouse [13]. The short (314 out of 348 ORF15 codons deleted) and the long (126 out of 348 codons deleted) forms of the *RPGR*^{ORF15} were tested. The long form demonstrated significant improvement in the disease phenotype, whilst the short form failed to localise correctly in the photoreceptors and showed no functional rescue of the phenotype. Importantly, as discussed above, large deletions in the ORF15 region can affect the glutamylation of the protein and lead to impaired function. Indeed, a follow-up study by the same group tested these truncated vectors [29] for their glutamylation capacity. Unsurprisingly, the long form demonstrated significantly impaired glutamylation (only 30% of the full length protein), whereas the short form showed no detectable glutamylation of the RPGR protein.

To circumvent these issues, the research team of Fischer and colleagues (2017) generated a full-length, human, codon-optimised version of RGPR^{ORF15} to stabilise the sequence, remove cryptic splice sites and increase expression levels from the therapeutic transgene [14]. This enabled reliable cloning and vector production. The resulting AAV8.coRPGR^{ORF15} vector was shown to offer therapeutic rescue in two mouse models of X-linked RP (*Rpgr*$^{-/y}$ and *Rd9*). This vector is now being used in a Phase I/II/III gene therapy clinical trial in humans (NCT03116113). In addition, the codon optimised form of the RPGR vector used in the canine studies [15] and the truncated form of the RPGR with near-total OFR15 deletion [13] are also being tested in ongoing clinical trials (NCT03316560 and NCT03252847 respectively) as will be discussed further in the next section. A very recent study used a bioinformatics approach as an alternative method to develop a molecularly stable *RPGR* gene therapy vector [56]. The strategy identified regions of genomic instability within ORF15 and made synonymous substitutions to reduce the repetitive sequence and thus increase the molecular stability of *RPGR*. The codon optimized construct was validated in vitro in pull-down experiments and in a murine model, demonstrating production of functional RPGR protein.

6. Gene Therapy Clinical Trials for RPGR-Related X-Linked RP

The results of the pre-clinical studies described above support the use of AAV-based gene therapy for RPGR-related X-linked RP in humans, in the early to mid-stage of the disease. Ideally, patients with moderately reduced visual acuity and constricted visual fields, but a preserved central ellipsoid zone, should be recruited into gene therapy trials for best expected therapeutic benefits. Interestingly, development of RPGR therapy from bench to bedside has resulted in setting-up of three multi-centre dose-escalation gene-therapy clinical trials (see Table 2 for details). Each trial is using a different combination of AAV vector variant and *RPGR* coding sequence (Figure 4). Specifically, the Nightstar

Therapeutics (now Biogen Inc) sponsored trial (NCT03116113) is using the wild-type AAV8 vector with a human rhodopsin kinase promoter and a human codon optimised full-length RPGR^{ORF15} cDNA sequence (AAV2/8.hRK.$coRPGR^{ORF15}$). The second trial sponsored by Meira GTx (NCT03252847) is using a wild-type AAV2/5 capsid with a truncated, non-codon optimised *RPGR* sequence under control of the human rhodopsin kinase promoter (AAV2/5.hRK.$RPGR^{ORF15}$). The third trial conducted by Applied Genetic Technologies Corporation (NCT03316560) is using mutated AAV2 capsids (capsids with single tyrosine to phenylalanine (YF) mutations) packaged with full-length, codon optimised human *RPGR^{ORF15}* sequence also driven by the rhodopsin kinase promoter (AAV2tYF.GRK1.$coRPGR^{ORF15}$).

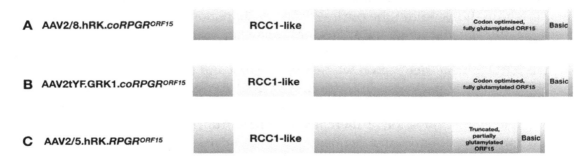

Figure 4. AAV vector constructs used in current gene therapy trials: (**A**) the Nightstar Therapeutics (now Biogen Inc) trial, NCT03116113; (**B**) the Applied Genetic Technologies Corporation trial, NCT03316560; (**C**) the MeiraGTx trial, NCT03252847.

The pre-clinical studies that led to the development of vectors used in human trials were described in detail in the previous section. However, the rationale for using the three different vectors deserves further discussion. The coding sequence used in the Meira GTx trial is an abbreviated form of human *RPGR^{ORF15}* sequence. The rationale provided for using the truncated form, which arose through a spontaneous mutation resulting in deletion of one third of the ORF15 region, was because the deletion led it to become more stable, thereby reducing the rate of further recombination errors and potential mutations. Interestingly, the authors also showed that further shortening of this critical ORF15 region significantly affects the protein function, leading to mislocalisation of the protein in photoreceptors and no functional or morphological rescue in a mouse model, confirming the importance of the ORF15 region for photoreceptor function. Importantly, a further study demonstrated that the post-translational glutamylation is reduced by over 70% in this abbreviated form of the RPGR^{ORF15}, significantly affecting trafficking of molecules critical for photoreceptor function [29]. However, since RPGR is not expressed highly in photoreceptors, it is possible that over-expression of RPGR with gene therapy can compensate for the reduced trafficking ability. The truncated construct was shown to rescue the photoreceptor function in a murine model of X-linked RP [13]. However, the mouse *RPGR^{ORF15}* is naturally shorter than the human *RPGR^{ORF15}* with an abbreviated ORF15 region (see Figure 2 and Table 1) much like the engineered abbreviated human construct used in the human trial. Thus, it may not be so surprising that the abbreviated human construct led to the rescue in a murine model, as the two sequences are very similar and the murine model has a milder phenotype compared to humans. The efficacy of this shortened version of *RPGR^{ORF15}* has not been evaluated in canine models of X-linked RP and the results from human trials are awaited in anticipation.

The constructs used in the AGTC and the Nightstar Therapeutics (now Biogen Inc.) trials are very similar and encode the full-length human wild-type RPGR^{ORF15} protein. Both constructs applied codon optimisation that was shown by Fischer et al. to confer greater sequence stability with higher expression levels than wild-type RPGR sequence, whilst not affecting the glutamylation pattern in the RPGR protein. The codon-optimised RPGR rescued the disease phenotype in two mouse models of X-linked RP [14] and was recently also validated in the RPGR canine model [15] showing transduction of both rods and cones and preserving the outer nuclear layer structure in the treated retina. The results of the phase I/II trials are expected in the near future.

7. Summary

X-linked RPGR-related RP is a heterogenous group of disorders with no clear genotype–phenotype correlation. Both rod-cone and cone-rod retinal dystrophies are seen with relatively early onset and rapid progression to blindness that is related to mutations that cause loss of function of this key photoreceptor protein. The complex expression pattern of the *RPGR* gene through cryptic splice sites that create multiple isoforms poses challenges in elucidating its function. However, mounting evidence suggests that retina-specific RPGR^{ORF15} is unique to vertebrates and plays a crucial role in regulating protein trafficking between inner and outer segments as well as in microtubular organisation. Importantly, RPGR^{ORF15} contains a characteristic repetitive purine-rich region that is highly glutamylated and only the glutamylated RPGR^{ORF15} is fully functional. Thus, any mutations that reduce the glutamylation process adversely affect RPGR protein function. In addition, the ORF15 region created challenges for the researches interested in developing *RPGR* gene-based therapies as the repetitive region made it unstable and prone to mutations. The current approach in developing a codon-optimised version of the RGPR^{ORF15} to stabilise the sequence, remove cryptic splice sites and increase expression levels from the therapeutic transgene is now being used in humans, following proof-of-concept studies in murine and canine models of X-linked RP. This approach has allowed the rapid progression towards the first in-human gene therapy trial (NCT03116113) for X-linked RP, which began in March 2017. In parallel, two additional independent research consortia have been developing gene therapies for the RPGR disease. With recent approval of gene replacement therapy Luxturna, for the treatment of *RPE65*-related retinal disease, the precedence for approval of future gene-based therapies has been set and results of the RPGR early phase clinical trials are awaited with great expectation.

References

1. Tee, J.J.; Smith, A.J.; Hardcastle, A.J.; Michaelides, M. *RPGR*-associated retinopathy: Clinical features, molecular genetics, animal models and therapeutic options. *Br. J. Ophthalmol.* **2016**, *100*, 1022–1027. [CrossRef]

2. Talib, M.; van Schooneveld, M.J.; Thiadens, A.A.; Fiocco, M.; Wijnholds, J.; Florijn, R.J.; Schalij-Delfos, N.E.; van Genderen, M.M.; Putter, H.; Cremers, F.P.M.; et al. Clinical and genetic characteristics of male patients with *RPGR*-associated retinal dystrophies: A long-term follow-up study. *Retina* **2019**, *39*, 1186–1199. [CrossRef]

3. Pelletier, V.; Jambou, M.; Delphin, N.; Zinovieva, E.; Stum, M.; Gigarel, N.; Dollfus, H.; Hamel, C.; Toutain, A.; Dufier, J.L.; et al. Comprehensive survey of mutations in RP2 and RPGR in patients affected with distinct retinal dystrophies: Genotype-phenotype correlations and impact on genetic counseling. *Hum. Mutat.* **2007**, *28*, 81–91. [CrossRef]

4. Branham, K.; Othman, M.; Brumm, M.; Karoukis, A.J.; Atmaca-Sonmez, P.; Yashar, B.M.; Schwartz, S.B.; Stover, N.B.; Trzupek, K.; Wheaton, D.; et al. Mutations in *RPGR* and RP2 account for 15% of males with simplex retinal degenerative disease. *Investig. Ophthalmol. Vis. Sci.* **2012**, *53*, 8232–8237. [CrossRef]

5. Webb, T.R.; Parfitt, D.A.; Gardner, J.C.; Martinez, A.; Bevilacqua, D.; Davidson, A.E.; Zito, I.; Thiselton, D.L.; Ressa, J.H.; Apergi, M.; et al. Deep intronic mutation in *OFD1*, identified by targeted genomic next-generation sequencing, causes a severe form of X-linked retinitis pigmentosa (RP23). *Hum. Mol. Genet.* **2012**, *21*, 3647–3654. [CrossRef]

6. Comander, J.; Weigel-DiFranco, C.; Sandberg, M.A.; Berson, E.L. Visual function in carriers of X-linked retinitis pigmentosa. *Ophthalmology* **2015**, *122*, 1899–1906. [CrossRef]

7. Nanda, A.; Salvetti, A.P.; Clouston, P.; Downes, S.M.; MacLaren, R.E. Exploring the Variable Phenotypes of *RPGR* Carrier Females in Assessing their Potential for Retinal Gene Therapy. *Genes* **2018**, *9*, 643. [CrossRef]

8. Wu, H.; Luo, J.; Yu, H.; Rattner, A.; Mo, A.; Wang, Y.; Smallwood, P.M.; Erlanger, B.; Wheelan, S.J.; Nathans, J. Cellular resolution maps of X chromosome inactivation: Implications for neural development, function, and disease. *Neuron* **2014**, *81*, 103–119. [CrossRef]

9.   Raghupathy, R.K.; Gautier, P.; Soares, D.C.; Wright, A.F.; Shu, X. Evolutionary characterization of the retinitis pigmentosa GTPase regulator gene. *Investig. Ophthalmol. Vis. Sci.* **2015**, *56*, 6255–6264. [CrossRef]

10. Vervoort, R.; Lennon, A.; Bird, A.C.; Tulloch, B.; Axton, R.; Miano, M.G.; Meindl, A.; Meitinger, T.; Ciccodicola, A.; Wright, A.F. Mutational hot spot within a new *RPGR* exon in X-linked retinitis pigmentosa. *Nat. Genet.* **2000**, *25*, 462–466. [CrossRef]

11. Vervoort, R.; Wright, A.F. Mutations of *RPGR* in X-linked retinitis pigmentosa (RP3). *Hum. Mutat.* **2002**, *19*, 486–500. [CrossRef]

12. Megaw, R.D.; Soares, D.C.; Wright, A.F. RPGR: Its role in photoreceptor physiology, human disease, and future therapies. *Exp. Eye Res.* **2015**, *138*, 32–41. [CrossRef]

13. Pawlyk, B.S.; Bulgakov, O.V.; Sun, X.; Adamian, M.; Shu, X.; Smith, A.J.; Berson, E.L.; Ali, R.R.; Khani, S.; Wright, A.F.; et al. Photoreceptor rescue by an abbreviated human *RPGR* gene in a murine model of X-linked retinitis pigmentosa. *Gene. Ther.* **2015**, *23*, 196–204. [CrossRef]

14. Fischer, M.D.; McClements, M.E.; Martinez-Fernandez De La Camara, C.; Bellingrath, J.S.; Dauletbekov, D.; Ramsden, S.C.; Hickey, D.G.; Barnard, A.R.; MacLaren, R.E. Codon-optimized RPGR improves stability and efficacy of AAV8 gene therapy in two mouse models of X-linked retinitis pigmentosa. *Mol. Ther.* **2017**, *25*, 1854–1865. [CrossRef]

15. Beltran, W.A.; Cideciyan, A.V.; Boye, S.E.; Ye, G.J.; Iwabe, S.; Dufour, V.L.; Marinho, L.F.; Swider, M.; Kosyk, M.S.; Sha, J.; et al. Optimization of retinal gene therapy for X-linked retinitis pigmentosa due to *RPGR* mutations. *Mol. Ther.* **2017**, *25*, 1866–1880. [CrossRef]

16. Hong, D.H.; Li, T. Complex expression pattern of RPGR reveals a role for purine-rich exonic splicing enhancers. *Investig. Ophthalmol. Vis. Sci.* **2002**, *43*, 3373–3382.

17. Meindl, A.; Dry, K.; Herrmann, K.; Manson, E.; Ciccodicola, A.; Edgar, A.; Carvalho, M.R.; Achatz, H.; Hellebrand, H.; Lennon, A.; et al. A gene (RPGR) with homology to the RCC1 guanine nucleotide exchange factor is mutated in X–linked retinitis pigmentosa (RP3). *Nat. Genet.* **1996**, *13*, 35–42. [CrossRef]

18. Kirschner, R.; Erturk, D.; Zeitz, C.; Sahin, S.; Ramser, J.; Cremers, F.P.; Ropers, H.H.; Berger, W. DNA sequence comparison of human and mouse retinitis pigmentosa GTPase regulator (*RPGR*) identifies tissue-specific exons and putative regulatory elements. *Hum. Genet.* **2001**, *109*, 271–278. [CrossRef]

19. Hong, D.H.; Pawlyk, B.; Sokolov, M.; Strissel, K.J.; Yang, J.; Tulloch, B.; Wright, A.F.; Arshavsky, V.Y.; Li, T. RPGR isoforms in photoreceptor connecting cilia and the transitional zone of motile cilia. *Investig. Ophthalmol. Vis. Sci.* **2003**, *44*, 2413–2421. [CrossRef]

20. Mavlyutov, T.A.; Zhao, H.; Ferreira, P.A. Species-specific subcellular localization of RPGR and RPGRIP isoforms: Implications for the phenotypic variability of congenital retinopathies among species. *Hum. Mol. Genet.* **2002**, *11*, 1899–1907. [CrossRef]

21. Murga-Zamalloa, C.A.; Atkins, S.J.; Peranen, J.; Swaroop, A.; Khanna, H. Interaction of retinitis pigmentosa GTPase regulator (RPGR) with RAB8A GTPase: Implications for cilia dysfunction and photoreceptor degeneration. *Hum. Mol. Genet.* **2010**, *19*, 3591–3598. [CrossRef]

22. Zhang, H.; Liu, X.-H.; Zhang, K.; Chen, C.-K.; Frederick, J.M.; Prestwich, G.D.; Baehr, W. Photoreceptor cGMP phosphodiesterase delta subunit (PDEδ) functions as a prenyl-binding protein. *J. Biol. Chem.* **2004**, *279*, 407–413. [CrossRef]

23. Khanna, H.; Hurd, T.W.; Lillo, C.; Shu, X.; Parapuram, S.K.; He, S.; Akimoto, M.; Wright, A.F.; Margolis, B.; Williams, D.S.; et al. RPGR-ORF15, which is mutated in retinitis pigmentosa, associates with SMC1, SMC3, and microtubule transport proteins. *J. Biol. Chem.* **2005**, *280*, 33580–33587. [CrossRef]

24. Otto, E.A.; Loeys, B.; Khanna, H.; Hellemans, J.; Sudbrak, R.; Fan, S.; Muerb, U.; O'Toole, J.F.; Helou, J.; Attanasio, M.; et al. Nephrocystin-5, a ciliary IQ domain protein, is mutated in Senior-Loken syndrome and interacts with RPGR and calmodulin. *Nat. Genet.* **2005**, *37*, 282–288. [CrossRef]

25. Chang, B.; Khanna, H.; Hawes, N.; molecular, D.J.H. In-frame deletion in a novel centrosomal/ciliary protein CEP290/NPHP6 perturbs its interaction with RPGR and results in early-onset retinal degeneration in the rd16 mouse. *Hum. Mol. Genet.* **2006**, *15*, 1847–1857. [CrossRef]

26. Wright, R.N.; Hong, D.-H.; Perkins, B. RpgrORF15 Connects to the usher protein network through direct interactions with multiple whirlin isoforms. *Investig. Opthalmol. Vis. Sci.* **2012**, *53*, 1519. [CrossRef]

27. Rao, K.N.; Anand, M.; Khanna, H. The carboxyl terminal mutational hotspot of the ciliary disease protein RPGRORF15 (retinitis pigmentosa GTPase regulator) is glutamylated in vivo. *Biol. Open* **2016**, *5*, 424–428. [CrossRef]

28. Natarajan, K.; Gadadhar, S.; Souphron, J.; Magiera, M.M.; Janke, C. Molecular interactions between tubulin tails and glutamylases reveal determinants of glutamylation patterns. *EMBO Rep.* **2017**, *18*, 1013–1026. [CrossRef]

29. Sun, X.; Park, J.H.; Gumerson, J.; Wu, Z.; Swaroop, A.; Qian, H.; Roll-Mecak, A.; Li, T. Loss of RPGR glutamylation underlies the pathogenic mechanism of retinal dystrophy caused by TTLL5 mutations. *Proc. Natl. Acad. Sci. USA* **2016**, *113*, E2925–E2934. [CrossRef]

30. Shu, X.; McDowall, E.; Brown, A.F.; Wright, A.F. The human retinitis pigmentosa GTPase regulator gene variant database. *Hum. Mutat.* **2008**, *29*, 605–608. [CrossRef]

31. Hosch, J.; Lorenz, B.; Stieger, K. RPGR: Role in the photoreceptor cilium, human retinal disease, and gene therapy. *Ophthalmic Genet.* **2011**, *32*, 1–11. [CrossRef]

32. Iannaccone, A.; Breuer, D.K.; Wang, X.F.; Kuo, S.F.; Normando, E.M.; Filippova, E.; Baldi, A.; Hiriyanna, S.; MacDonald, C.B.; Baldi, F.; et al. Clinical and immunohistochemical evidence for an X linked retinitis pigmentosa syndrome with recurrent infections and hearing loss in association with an RPGR mutation. *J. Med. Genet.* **2003**, *40*, e118. [CrossRef]

33. Zito, I.; Downes, S.M.; Patel, R.J.; Cheetham, M.E.; Ebenezer, N.D.; Jenkins, S.A.; Bhattacharya, S.S.; Webster, A.R.; Holder, G.E.; Bird, A.C.; et al. RPGR mutation associated with retinitis pigmentosa, impaired hearing, and sinorespiratory infections. *J. Med. Genet.* **2003**, *40*, 609–615. [CrossRef]

34. Hunter, D.G.; Fishman, G.A.; Kretzer, F.L. Abnormal axonemes in X-linked retinitis pigmentosa. *Arch. Ophthal.* **1988**, *106*, 362–368. [CrossRef]

35. Hunter, D.G.; Fishman, G.A.; Mehta, R.S.; Kretzer, F.L. Abnormal sperm and photoreceptor axonemes in Usher's syndrome. *Arch. Ophthalmol.* **1986**, *104*, 385–389. [CrossRef]

36. He, S.; Parapuram, S.K.; Hurd, T.W.; Behnam, B.; Margolis, B.; Swaroop, A.; Khanna, H. Retinitis pigmentosa GTPase regulator (RPGR) protein isoforms in mammalian retina: Insights into X-linked retinitis pigmentosa and associated ciliopathies. *Vision Res.* **2008**, *48*, 366–376. [CrossRef]

37. Jacobi, F.K.; Karra, D.; Broghammer, M.; Blin, N.; Pusch, C.M. Mutational risk in highly repetitive exon ORF15 of the RPGR multidisease gene is not associated with haplotype background. *Int. J. Mol. Med.* **2005**, *16*, 1175–1178. [CrossRef]

38. Karra, D.; Jacobi, F.K.; Broghammer, M.; Blin, N.; Pusch, C.M. Population haplotypes of exon ORF15 of the retinitis pigmentosa GTPase regulator gene in Germany: Implications for screening for inherited retinal disorders. *Mol. Diagn. Ther.* **2006**, *10*, 115–123. [CrossRef]

39. Sergouniotis, P.I.; Chakarova, C.; Murphy, C.; Becker, M.; Lenassi, E.; Arno, G.; Lek, M.; MacArthur, D.G.; Bhattacharya, S.S.; Moore, A.T.; et al. UCL-Exomes Consortium Biallelic variants in TTLL5, encoding a tubulin glutamylase, cause retinal dystrophy. *Am. J. Hum. Genet.* **2014**, *94*, 760–769. [CrossRef]

40. Sandberg, M.A.; Rosner, B.; Weigel-DiFranco, C.; Dryja, T.P.; Berson, E.L. Disease course of patients with X-linked retinitis pigmentosa due to RPGR gene mutations. *Investig. Ophthalmol. Vis. Sci.* **2007**, *48*, 1298–1304. [CrossRef]

41. Huang, W.C.; Wright, A.F.; Roman, A.J.; Cideciyan, A.V.; Manson, F.D.; Gewaily, D.Y.; Schwartz, S.B.; Sadigh, S.; Limberis, M.P.; Bell, P.; et al. RPGR-associated retinal degeneration in human X-linked RP and a murine model. *Investig. Ophthalmol. Vis. Sci.* **2012**, *53*, 5594–5608. [CrossRef]

42. Mitamura, Y.; Mitamura-Aizawa, S.; Nagasawa, T.; Katome, T.; Eguchi, H.; Naito, T. Diagnostic imaging in patients with retinitis pigmentosa. *J. Med. Investig.* **2012**, *59*, 1–11. [CrossRef]

43. Tee, J.J.L.; Kalitzeos, A.; Webster, A.R.; Peto, T.; Michaelides, M. Quantitative analysis of hyperautofluorescent rings to characterize the natural history and progression in RPGR-associated retinopathy. *Retina* **2018**, *38*, 2401–2414. [CrossRef]

44. Robson, A.G.; Michaelides, M.; Luong, V.A.; Holder, G.E.; Bird, A.C.; Webster, A.R.; Moore, A.T.; Fitzke, F.W. Functional correlates of fundus autofluorescence abnormalities in patients with RPGR or RIMS1 mutations causing cone or cone rod dystrophy. *Br. J. Ophthalmol.* **2008**, *92*, 95–102. [CrossRef]

45. Zhang, Q.; Giacalone, J.C.; Searby, C.; Stone, E.M.; Tucker, B.A.; Sheffield, V.C. Disruption of RPGR protein interaction network is the common feature of RPGR missense variations that cause XLRP. *Proc. Natl. Acad. Sci. USA* **2019**, *116*, 1353–1360. [CrossRef]

46. Hoffman, D.R.; Hughbanks-Wheaton, D.K.; Pearson, N.S.; Fish, G.E.; Spencer, R.; Takacs, A.; Klein, M.; Locke, K.G.; Birch, D.G. Four-year placebo-controlled trial of docosahexaenoic acid in X-linked retinitis pigmentosa (DHAX trial): A randomized clinical trial. *JAMA Ophthalmol.* **2014**, *132*, 866–873. [CrossRef]

47. Beltran, W.A.; Wen, R.; Acland, G.M.; Aguirre, G.D. Intravitreal injection of ciliary neurotrophic factor (CNTF) causes peripheral remodeling and does not prevent photoreceptor loss in canine RPGR mutant retina. *Exp. Eye Res.* **2007**, *84*, 753–771. [CrossRef]

48. Ho, A.C.; Humayun, M.S.; Dorn, J.D.; da Cruz, L.; Dagnelie, G.; Handa, J.; Barale, P.O.; Sahel, J.A.; Stanga, P.E.; Hafezi, F.; et al. Long-term results from an epiretinal prosthesis to restore sight to the blind. *Ophthalmology* **2015**, *122*, 1547–1554. [CrossRef]

49. Edwards, T.L.; Cottriall, C.L.; Xue, K.; Simunovic, M.P.; Ramsden, J.D.; Zrenner, E.; MacLaren, R.E. Assessment of the Electronic Retinal Implant α AMS in Restoring Vision to Blind Patients with End-Stage Retinitis Pigmentosa. *Ophthalmology* **2018**, *125*, 432–443. [CrossRef]

50. Cehajic-Kapetanovic, J.; Eleftheriou, C.; Allen, A.E.; Milosavljevic, N.; Pienaar, A.; Bedford, R.; Davis, K.E.; Bishop, P.N.; Lucas, R.J. Restoration of Vision with Ectopic Expression of Human Rod Opsin. *Curr. Biol.* **2015**, *25*, 2111–2122. [CrossRef]

51. Eleftheriou, C.G.; Cehajic-Kapetanovic, J.; Martial, F.P.; Milosavljevic, N.; Bedford, R.A.; Lucas, R.J. Meclofenamic acid improves the signal to noise ratio for visual responses produced by ectopic expression of human rod opsin. *Mol. Vis.* **2017**, *23*, 334–345.

52. Hong, D.H.; Pawlyk, B.S.; Adamian, M.; Sandberg, M.A.; Li, T. A single, abbreviated RPGR-ORF15 variant reconstitutes RPGR function in vivo. *Investig. Ophthalmol. Vis. Sci.* **2005**, *46*, 435–441. [CrossRef]

53. Deng, W.T.; Dyka, F.M.; Dinculescu, A.; Li, J.; Zhu, P.; Chiodo, V.A.; Boye, S.L.; Conlon, T.J.; Erger, K.; Cossette, T.; et al. Stability and Safety of an AAV Vector for Treating RPGR-ORF15 X-Linked Retinitis Pigmentosa. *Hum. Gene. Ther.* **2015**, *26*, 593–602. [CrossRef]

54. Wu, Z.; Hiriyanna, S.; Qian, H.; Mookherjee, S.; Campos, M.M.; Gao, C.; Fariss, R.; Sieving, P.A.; Li, T.; Colosi, P.; et al. A long-term efficacy study of gene replacement therapy for RPGR-associated retinal degeneration. *Hum. Mol. Genet.* **2015**, *24*, 3956–3970. [CrossRef]

55. Beltran, W.A.; Cideciyan, A.V.; Lewin, A.S.; Iwabe, S.; Khanna, H.; Sumaroka, A.; Chiodo, V.A.; Fajardo, D.S.; Román, A.J.; Deng, W.T.; et al. Gene therapy rescues photoreceptor blindness in dogs and paves the way for treating human X-linked retinitis pigmentosa. *Proc. Natl. Acad. Sci. USA* **2012**, *109*, 2132–2137. [CrossRef]

56. Giacalone, J.C.; Andorf, J.L.; Zhang, Q.; Burnight, E.R.; Ochoa, D.; Reutzel, A.J.; Collins, M.M.; Sheffield, V.C.; Mullins, R.F.; Han, I.C.; et al. Development of a Molecularly Stable Gene Therapy Vector for the Treatment of RPGR-Associated X-Linked Retinitis Pigmentosa. *Hum. Gene. Ther.* **2019**, *30*, 967–974. [CrossRef]

Permissions

List of Contributors

Raquel Boia and Inês Dinis Aires
Coimbra Institute for Clinical and Biomedical Research (iCBR), Faculty of Medicine, University of Coimbra, 3000-548 Coimbra, Portugal
Center for Innovative Biomedicine and Biotechnology (CIBB), University of Coimbra, 3000-548 Coimbra, Portugal

Xandra Pereiro, Noelia Ruzafa and Elena Vecino
Department of Cell Biology and Histology, University of the Basque Country UPV/EHU, 48940 Leioa, Vizcaya, Spain

António Francisco Ambrósio and Ana Raquel Santiago
Coimbra Institute for Clinical and Biomedical Research (iCBR), Faculty of Medicine, University of Coimbra, 3000-548 Coimbra, Portugal
Center for Innovative Biomedicine and Biotechnology (CIBB), University of Coimbra, 3000-548 Coimbra, Portugal
Association for Innovation and Biomedical Research on Light and Image (AIBILI), 3000-548 Coimbra, Portugal

Emilie Picard, Jenny Youale and Yves Courtois
Centre de Recherche des Cordeliers, INSERM, Sorbonne Université, USPC, Université Paris Descartes, Team 17, F-75006 Paris, France

Alejandra Daruich
Centre de Recherche des Cordeliers, INSERM, Sorbonne Université, USPC, Université Paris Descartes, Team 17, F-75006 Paris, France
Ophthalmology Department, Necker-Enfants Malades University Hospital, APHP, 75015 Paris, France

Francine Behar-Cohen
Centre de Recherche des Cordeliers, INSERM, Sorbonne Université, USPC, Université Paris Descartes, Team 17, F-75006 Paris, France
Ophtalmopole, Cochin Hospital, AP-HP, Assistance Publique Hôpitaux de Paris, 24 rue du Faubourg Saint-Jacques, 75014 Paris, France

Ben Shaberman and Todd Durham
Foundation Fighting Blindness, 7168 Columbia Gateway Drive, Suite 100, Columbia, MD 21046, USA

Bright Asare-Bediako, Yvonne Adu-Agyeiwaah and Mariana Dupont
Vision Science Graduate Program, School of Optometry, University of Alabama at Birmingham, Birmingham, AL 35233, USA

Sunil K. Noothi, Sergio Li Calzi, Cristiano P. Vieira, Dibyendu Chakraborty and Maria B. Grant
Department of Ophthalmology and Visual Sciences, School of Medicine, The University of Alabama at Birmingham, Birmingham, AL 35294, USA

Baskaran Athmanathan and Prabhakara R. Nagareddy
Division of Cardiac Surgery, Department of Surgery, Ohio State University Wexner Medical Center, Columbus, OH 43210, USA

Bryce A. Jones
Department of Pharmacology and Physiology, Georgetown University, Washington, DC 20057, USA

Xiaoxin X. Wang and Moshe Levi
Department of Biochemistry and Molecular & Cellular Biology, Georgetown University, Washington, DC 20057, USA

Ivana Trapani
Telethon Institute of Genetics and Medicine (TIGEM), 80078 Pozzuoli, Italy
Medical Genetics, Department of Translational Medicine, Federico II University, 80131 Naples, Italy

Sriganesh Ramachandra Rao and Steven J. Fliesler
Research Service, VA Western NY Healthcare System, Buffalo, NY 14215, USA
Departments of Ophthalmology and Biochemistry and Neuroscience Graduate Program, The State University of New York- University at Buffalo, Buffalo, NY 14209, USA

Pravallika Kotla, Mai N. Nguyen and Steven J. Pittler
Department of Optometry and Vision Science, Vision Science Research Center, University of Alabama at Birmingham, School of Optometry, Birmingham, AL 35294, USA

Jasmina Cehajic Kapetanovic, Alun R. Barnard and Robert E. MacLaren
Nuffield Laboratory of Ophthalmology, University of Oxford, Oxford OX3 9DU, UK
Oxford Eye Hospital, Oxford University Hospitals NHS Foundation Trust, Oxford OX3 9DU, UK

Gayle B. Collin, Navdeep Gogna, Bo Chang, Jai Pinkney, Lillian F. Hyde, Lisa Stone, Jürgen K. Naggert, Patsy M. Nishina and Mark P. Krebs
The Jackson Laboratory, Bar Harbor, Maine, ME 04609, USA

Nattaya Damkham
The Jackson Laboratory, Bar Harbor, Maine, ME 04609, USA
Department of Immunology, Faculty of Medicine Siriraj Hospital, Mahidol University, Bangkok 10700, Thailand
Siriraj Center of Excellence for Stem Cell Research, Faculty of Medicine Siriraj Hospital, Mahidol University, Bangkok 10700, Thailand

Alejandro Garanto, Tomasz Z. Tomkiewicz and Rob W. J. Collin
Department of Human Genetics and Donders Institute for Brain, Cognition and Behaviour, Radboud University Medical Center, 6525GA Nijmegen, The Netherlands

Lonneke Duijkers
Department of Human Genetics, Radboud University Medical Center, 6525GA Nijmegen, The Netherlands

Michelle E McClements
Nuffield Laboratory of Ophthalmology, University of Oxford, Oxford OX3 9DU, UK

Cristina Martinez-Fernandez de la Camara
Nuffield Laboratory of Ophthalmology, University of Oxford, Oxford OX3 9DU, UK
Oxford Eye Hospital, Oxford University Hospitals NHS Foundation Trust, Oxford OX3 9DU, UK

Index